Alternative Medicine Guide

The Enzyme Cure

How Plant Enzymes Can Help You Relieve 36 Health Problems

by **LITA LEE, Ph.D.,** *with*

LISA TURNER *and* **BURTON GOLDBERG**

 FUTURE MEDICINE PUBLISHING
TIBURON, CALIFORNIA

Future Medicine Publishing, Inc.
1640 Tiburon Blvd., Suite 2
Tiburon, CA 94920

Editor: Richard Leviton
Senior Editor: Stephanie Marohn
Assistant Editor: Christine Schultz-Touge
Associate Editor: John Anderson

Art Director: Janine White
Production Assistant: Gail Gongoll

Manufactured in the United States of America.

10 9 8 7 6 5 4 3 2 1

Library of Congress Cataloging-in-Publication Data
Lee, Lita.
    The enzyme cure : how plant enzymes can help you relieve 36 health problems / by Lita Lee with Lisa Turner and Burton Goldberg.
          p.   cm.
    Includes bibliographical references and index.
    ISBN 1-887299-22-X (paperback)
    1. Plant enzymes—Therapeutic use. I. Turner, Lisa. II. Goldberg, Burton, 1926-   . III. Title. IV. Title: Alternative medicine guide
RM666.E55L44   1998
615'.35--dc21   98-38395
                                                           CIP

Contents

PART ONE—
What You Need to Know About Enzymes

PART TWO—
An A-Z of Health Conditions
With Enzyme Therapy Success Stories

PART THREE—
Appendices

About the Author

Lita Lee, Ph.D., has been in practice as an enzyme therapist since 1987. Originally trained as a chemist, Dr. Lee received a doctorate in chemistry in 1967 from the University of Colorado at Boulder, and has over 30 years of experience in chemical and medical research. Dr. Lee spent the early years of her career as a research chemist at SRI International in Menlo Park, California, and several other chemical corporations. An abiding interest in health and healing led her from the chemistry laboratory to the medical laboratory and finally to clinical practice in 1981.

Since 1980, Dr. Lee has been training in clinical nutrition with individual doctors. Unlike in conventional medical schools, the nutritional model of these doctors clearly draws the link between nutritional deficiencies and the development of health disorders. Dr. Lee's strong scientific background informs her work as an enzyme therapist, particularly her specialty of developing nutritional protocols for balancing body chemistry, with a focus on enzyme therapy, hormonal balancing, and protection from environmental toxins.

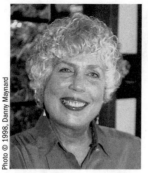

Photo © 1998, Danny Maynard

To contact **Lita Lee, Ph.D.**: P.O. Box 516, Lowell, OR 97452; tel.: 541-937-1123; fax: 541-937-1132.

With a chemist's understanding of the negative health effects of our increasingly polluted environment, Dr. Lee has undertaken the mission of informing the public on the dangers of toxins and radiation and providing guidance for reducing or eliminating exposure. With this in mind, she authored the *Radiation Protection Manual* (self-published, 3rd Edition, 1990) and, from 1991 to 1994, published *Earthletter*, a quarterly newsletter supplying information on the latest developments in the field of environmental health and radiation protection, including political issues involving nutrition, medicine, and the environment. Dr. Lee continues to cover these subjects as well as enzyme therapy in her current quarterly newsletter *To Your Health*.

Acknowledgments

I am very grateful to the following people whose help has made this book possible:

Howard Loomis, D.C., the enzyme pioneer who developed the formulas which I have used since 1987 along with objective tests to determine enzyme deficiencies. Loomis' enzymes have changed my life and made it possible for me to help hundreds of people with severe digestive disturbances and other problems caused by enzyme deficiencies.

Raymond Peat, Ph.D., a pioneer in hormonal balancing who has also revealed the importance of the anti-aging steroids. My writings and therapies would not have been possible without his prolific research, and dozens of articles and books, and the many interviews I've had with him over the last five years.

Lisa Turner, author and journalist, for her help in weaving my 11 years of writings into a book format.

My editors Richard Leviton and Stephanie Marohn, the staff at Future Medicine Publishing, and Burton Goldberg, all of whom have made natural healing therapies available to the general public.

My family—my husband, John, and twins, Sean and Veronica—and my staff, whose love, support, and encouragement never wavered these last 11 years.

Important Information

Burton Goldberg and the editors of *Alternative Medicine* are proud of the public and professional praise accorded Future Medicine Publishing's series of books. This latest book in the series continues the groundbreaking tradition of its predecessors.

The health of you and your loved ones is important. Treat this book as an educational tool which will enable you to better understand, assess, and choose the best course of treatment when a health problem arises, and how to prevent health problems from developing in the first place. It could save your life.

Remember that this book on enzyme therapy is different. It is not yet another catalog of mainstream medicine's conventional treatments and drugs used to treat health problems. This book is about alternative approaches to health—approaches generally not understood and, at this time, not endorsed by the medical establishment. We urge you to discuss the treatments described in this book with your doctor. If your doctor is open-minded, you may actually educate him or her. We have been gratified to learn that many of our readers have found their physicians open to the new ideas presented to them.

Use this book wisely. As many of the treatments described in this book are, by definition, alternative, they have not been investigated, approved, or endorsed by any government or regulatory agency. National, state, and local laws may vary regarding the use and application of many of the treatments discussed. Accordingly, this book should not be substituted for the advice and care of a physician or other licensed health-care professional. Pregnant women, in particular, are urged to consult a physician before commencing any therapy. Ultimately, you the reader must take responsibility for your health. The authors and publisher disclaim any responsibility for how you use the information in this book.

All of the factual information in this book has been drawn from the scientific literature. To protect privacy, all patient names have been changed. Branded products and services discussed in the book are evaluated solely on Lita Lee's independent and direct experience with them. Reference to them does not imply an endorsement nor a superiority over other branded products and services which may provide similar or superior results.

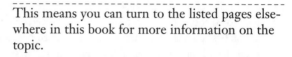

User's Guide

One of the features of this book is that it is interactive, thanks to the following 12 icons:

This means you can turn to the listed pages elsewhere in this book for more information on the topic.

This tells you where to contact a physician, group, or publication, or how to obtain substances mentioned in the text. This is an editorial service to our readers. Most importantly, the use of this icon empowers you right now, by giving you a source to acquire something vital to your health, quickly and easily. Whenever possible, we give you complete contact information for all substances mentioned in the text. All items are based on recommendations from the clinical practice of physicians in this book. The publisher has no financial interest in any clinic, physician, or product discussed in this book.

QUICK DEFINITION

Many times the text mentions a medical term that requires explanation. We don't want to interrupt the text, so instead we put the explanation in the margins under this icon. This gives you the option of proceeding with the text or taking a moment to learn more about an important term.

CAUTION

This sign tells you there may be some risks, uncertainties, side effects, or special contraindications regarding a procedure or substance.

EDITOR'S NOTE

This icon indicates a message to the reader from Future Medicine Publishing's editor.

Here we refer you to our book, *Alternative Medicine Definitive Guide to Cancer*, for more information on a particular topic.

Here we refer you to our book, *Alternative Medicine Definitive Guide to Headaches*, for more information on a particular topic.

Here we refer you to our book, *Alternative Medicine Guide to Heart Disease*, for more information on a particular topic.

Here we refer you to our book, *Alternative Medicine Guide to Chronic Fatigue, Fibromyalgia, and Environmental Illness*, for more information on a particular topic.

Here we refer you to our book, *Alternative Medicine Guide to Women's Health 1*, for more information on a particular topic. The first book in the Women's Health Series covers infertility, endometriosis, vaginitis, menstrual problems, ovarian cysts, PMS, fibroids, and urinary tract infections.

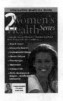

Here we refer you to our book, *Alternative Medicine Guide to Women's Health 2*, for more information on a particular topic. The second book in the Women's Health Series covers breast cancer, fibrocystic breasts, environmental illness, chronic fatigue, fibromyalgia, depression, and osteoporosis.

This icon alerts you to an article published in our bimonthly magazine, *Alternative Medicine*, which is relevant to the topic under discussion.

You Don't Have to Take Drugs

AMERICA HAS CREATED a multibillion dollar synthetic drug market. In 1997 alone, American women bought 33.1 million prescriptions of Premarin (a synthetic estrogen derived from the urine of pregnant horses), making it the nation's best-selling drug. Yet, this estrogen replacement therapy (ERT) may actually be harming the health of the women who take it. Often, too much estrogen in relation to progesterone causes hormonal havoc and leads to symptoms from bloating and headache to major health problems such as gallbladder disease and cancer.

The pharmaceutical companies, however, simply come up with another drug to treat the symptoms the original drug produced. The second drug then creates its own side effects, and so on. In the end, we have come to accept what conventional medicine tells us: we need drugs to control our body functions. We even take drugs to destroy cholesterol which is necessary for the production of essential anti-aging hormones. At the same time, these cholesterol-lowering drugs let loose toxic side effects, which can result in liver problems, depression, immune system dysfunction, and, once again, cancer.

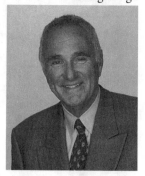

There is, however, an escape from this destructive cycle of drug-taking. That escape is alternative medicine. Instead of treating symptoms with synthetic drugs, alternative medicine goes to the root causes and uses safe, noninvasive methods to address and reverse these causes.

One such natural alternative is enzyme therapy. In this book, Lita Lee, Ph.D., one of the nation's leading enzyme therapists, shows you how to treat 36 health problems without using synthetic drugs. Here, you will read about desperate people who consulted Dr. Lee after going through countless drugs and a lot of money. They came to her, not only with their original symptoms, but often with damage from the drugs they had taken, and she put them back on the path to good health.

Unlike conventional medical practitioners, Dr. Lee does not search for a single cause behind a health problem. Nor does she believe in giving vitamins and supplements to a patient without first addressing the digestive dysfunction which often accompanies chronic illness. For her, that would be like throwing money out the window. Instead, Dr. Lee looks at the whole person. Before she begins any treatment, she gets a complete picture of the individual's symptoms, health history, diet, and possible digestive problems and hormonal imbalances. She then designs a treatment plan tailored to that individual, using a combination of enzyme therapy, dietary recommendations, and thyroid and other hormonal balancing, as appropriate.

This book gives you detailed accounts of over 60 people whose health problems were successfully reversed through these therapies. Dr. Lee's advice is simple: you don't have to take drugs to get well. By treating the underlying causes of your health condition—whether asthma or insomnia—you will improve your overall health, and leave the drugs behind. God bless.

—Burton Goldberg

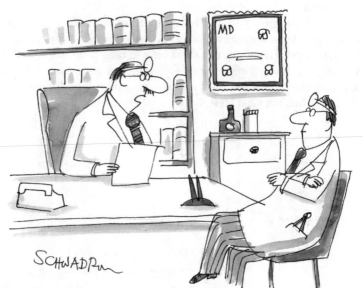

"BEFORE, WE COULD GET BY WITH MEDICAL FIDDLEFLOP. NOW EVERYONE WANTS LAYMEN'S TERMS."

PART ONE

What You Need to Know About Enzymes

CHAPTER 1

Why Enzymes?

ENZYMES are vital to health—to life itself. These special proteins are necessary for every chemical reaction in your body and the normal activity of your cells, tissues, fluids, and organs. Enzymes digest the food you eat and are essential for the production of energy required to run your body. Vitamins, minerals, and hormones can do nothing without enzymes. With all of these functions to perform, there are literally hundreds of thousands of these "Nature's workers" in your body.

Types of Enzymes

Enzymes can be divided into three major categories: metabolic enzymes, pancreatic enzymes, and food or plant enzymes.

Metabolic Enzymes

Hundreds of thousands of metabolic enzymes are made by the human body, and are responsible for running its chemistry. These enzymes are involved in all body processes including breathing, thinking, talking, moving, and immunity. You may be familiar with antioxidant enzymes, one type of metabolic enzyme manufactured by our bodies. Antioxidant enzymes help to quench free radicals, unhealthy compounds which if left unchecked contribute to the development of disease.

Pancreatic Enzymes

In addition to metabolic enzymes, humans (and animals) have digestive enzymes, secreted mainly by the pancreas, but also in the mouth, small intestine, and stomach. These enzymes play a vital role in the digestion of food.

The pancreas is a complex organ, responsible for many functions. A healthy pancreas secretes insulin into the blood, and produces and secretes alkaline fluid (sodium bicarbonate) into the upper portion of the small intestine, which alkalizes the acidic contents that arrive there from the stomach. There are approximately 22 pancreatic enzymes, including amylase, lipase, and proteolytic (breaking down protein) enzymes, such as protease, which continue the digestion of food in the duodenum (the beginning of the small intestine) after plant enzymes have begun the digestive process in the stomach.

Plant (Food) Enzymes

Plant, or food, enzymes are essential in the proper digestion of food. Present in all raw plants (and also available as supplements), plant enzymes include protease (digests protein), amylase (digests carbohydrates), lipase (digests fat), disaccharidases (digest sugar), and cellulase (digests fiber). Unlike pancreatic enzymes, plant enzymes work in the mouth and the stomach where they predigest foods. Plant enzymes also operate in the small intestine, aiding pancreatic enzymes in continuing the digestive process.

Each plant enzyme does its work only at its own specific pH (SEE QUICK DEFINITION) and temperature ranges and in the presence of moisture (water). Outside its pH range, the enzyme is deactivated but not destroyed, while outside of its temperature range, the enzyme is denatured (destroyed). Enzymes, more heat-sensitive than vitamins, are destroyed by cooking temperatures above 118° F, pasteurization, canning, and microwaving.

How Plant Enzymes Work

Plant or food enzymes are responsible for three classes of work: predigestion, nutritional support, and acute or chronic support.

Predigestion

As discussed, plant enzymes initiate predigestion of foods in the upper portion of the stomach. They can eliminate digestive problems leading to food allergies by increasing the supply of the deficient enzyme during this predigestive process.

The main food enzymes which initiate the process of digestion are: protease for protein digestion; lipase for fat digestion; amylase for carbohydrate digestion; disaccharidases for the digestion of disaccharides (sucrose, lactose,

The term **pH**, which means "potential hydrogen," represents a scale for the relative acidity or alkalinity of a solution. Acidity is measured as a pH of 0.1 to 6.9, alkalinity is 7.1 to 14, and neutral pH is 7.0. The numbers refer to how many hydrogen atoms are present compared to an ideal or standard solution. Normally, blood is slightly alkaline, at 7.35 to 7.45. The pH of a 24-hour urine sample can range from 5.5 to 7.4. The optimum range is slightly acidic, at 6.3 to 6.7.

and maltose) into simple sugars; and cellulase for the digestion of the soluble parts of fiber into smaller units. Since cellulase is not made by the human body, it's important to chew all raw foods well in order to release the cellulase enzyme.

Eating a diet rich in raw foods and/or taking plant enzyme supplements will not make your pancreas lazy because pancreatic enzymes don't operate in the stomach. On the contrary, food enzymes—and only food enzymes—spare the pancreas from having to compensate for inadequate predigestion. The pancreas was never meant to be totally responsible for digestion—early humans consumed primarily raw foods.

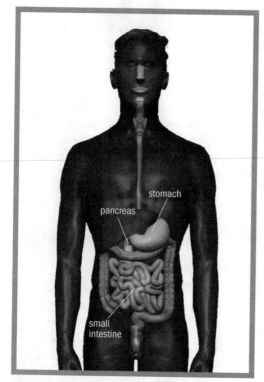

ENZYMES AND THE GASTROINTESTINAL TRACT.
Plant enzymes start digesting food in the mouth and stomach, and they also are active in the small intestine. Pancreatic enzymes (of which there are 22 different kinds) are secreted by the pancreas, located behind the stomach; their work occurs mainly in the small intestine.

Nutritional Support

Food enzymes augment delivery of nutritional support by ensuring digestion of a needed nutrient. Vitamin and mineral deficiencies resulting from a refined-food diet, or the inability to digest whole foods, may be treated by combining small amounts of foods, high in the desired nutrients, with the plant enzymes required to digest them. In this way, the delivery of those nutrients is guaranteed. This is a much better way of relieving nutritional deficiencies than taking isolated vitamins or minerals.

For example, if you have a particular B-vitamin deficiency, taking that one isolated B vitamin will not solve the problem. Instead, taking a combination of brewer's yeast and the right amount of enzymes required to predigest the yeast, provides the lacking B vitamins in proper ratio with the B complex.

Acute or Chronic Support

Taken as a supplement on an empty stomach, plant enzymes enter the bloodstream, where they assist the immune system by digesting and disposing of toxins (any substance that does not belong in the blood) and "eating" the protein coating on certain viruses, enabling immune system workers to then destroy them. Thus, taking enzymes in this way can help reverse inflammation. Each type of enzyme has a specific anti-inflammatory action and will relieve inflammatory conditions related to a deficiency in that enzyme.

Since plant enzymes digest toxins rather than killing them off (as antibiotics do in the case of bacterial infection, for example), the process involves no side effects if the digested toxins can be properly eliminated through the urinary tract, colon, skin, and lungs.

Supplemental plant enzymes can thus be used as therapy in three ways, depending on the particular health condition and needs of the individual: to optimize digestion, absorption, and assimilation of food which in turn keeps a healthy pH balance in the blood; to reverse nutritional deficiencies; and as anti-inflammatories and detoxifying agents.

The Primary Digestive Enzymes

No matter what specific foods we eat, our diets are composed of protein, fat, carbohydrates, sugars (disaccharides), and fiber, and we need the appropriate enzymes (protease, lipase, amylase, disaccharidases, and cellulase) to break them down in digestion. When a person is lacking in one or more of these primary digestive enzymes, the food category associated with that enzyme does not get digested properly and that person is said to be intolerant to that food. For example, without enough protease, a protein-intolerance develops; without sufficient lipase, the individual is fat-intolerant, simply meaning that fat is not being digested properly. When the enzyme deficiency is left untreated, health problems inevitably result. Specific symptoms and conditions tend to develop with each particular enzyme deficiency. Following is a more detailed discussion of the primary digestive enzymes and some of the health problems arising when the enzymes are in short supply.

A Primer on Digestion

Digestion begins in the mouth—*if* you adequately chew your food—with digestive enzymes secreted by the salivary glands. These enzymes include amylase, lipase, and some protease. Also at work in the mouth are the enzymes present in whatever raw foods are being eaten. In addition to amylase, lipase, and protease, plant enzymes include cellulase, which is not made by the human body.

Salivary enzymes combined with plant enzymes (from either raw foods or taken as a supplement) continue the work of digestion in the upper or cardiac portion of the stomach. For example, amylase will digest up to 60% of carbohydrates, protease up to 30% of protein, and lipase up to 10% of fat, *before* HCl (hydrochloric or stomach) acid and pepsin (the main enzyme secreted in the stomach) begin to work on food in the stomach.

After about an hour, stomach cells, called parietal cells, secrete enough HCl from the blood to further acidify the predigested food to a low pH (from 3.0 to 1.5). This acidic pH temporarily deactivates the plant enzymes, and the predigested food passes to the lower or pyloric portion of the stomach, from which chief cells also secrete pepsin. It is here that pepsin continues the digestion of protein. Adequate HCl is required to activate pepsin from its inactive enzyme form pepsinogen inside the chief cells, and to maintain the stomach pH below 3.0, the optimum pH at which pepsin does its work.

In the next stage of digestion, the partially digested food and the deactivated plant (food) enzymes pass through the pyloric valve into the upper part of the small intestine (the duodenum). Here digestion continues, with the help of bile, pancreatic enzymes, and an alkalizing substance (bicarbonate) which reactivates the food enzymes, *if* there is proper alkalinity. Then digestion continues in the jejunum (next section of the small intestine) where disaccharidases (sugar-digesting enzymes) are secreted *if* the jejunum is healthy. From the small intestine, the majority of nutrients from digested food are absorbed into the blood.

Protease (digests protein)

Protease digests protein into smaller units called amino acids (SEE QUICK DEFINITION); not only protein from food, but also other organisms which are composed of protein, such as the coating on certain viruses, toxins from dead bacteria and other microorganisms, and certain harmful substances produced at sites of injury or inflammation.

As mentioned above, someone deficient in protease is protein-intolerant. Although protein-intolerant people may become vegetarians because meat and other high-protein foods don't "agree" with them, that doesn't solve their problem. Their bodies can't digest *any* form of protein, including that found in vegetables. Both the faulty digestive process and the resulting deficiency in protein lead to a deterioration in health.

A protease deficiency compromises the immune system, leaving a person vulnerable to frequent or chronic infections, either bacterial or viral, and more serious conditions, including cancer. Protease deficiency can also lead to edema (fluid retention) anywhere in the body, including swelling of the hands and feet or fluid in the ears. Toxic colon syndrome (a buildup of toxins in the large intestine) is another result of the inability to digest protein. It can lead to various intestinal problems including chronic constipation, appendicitis, and even colon cancer.

In addition, since about half the protein you digest is converted to sugar, protease deficiency and inadequate protein digestion can lead to hypoglycemia (low blood sugar), with such symptoms as moodiness, depression, and irritability.

Protein, when digested properly, supplies acidity to the blood. If protein isn't digested, the blood acquires excess alkaline reserves which must be continuously dumped via the kidneys into the urine. These excess alkaline reserves can produce a state of anxiety, often treated with prescription tranquilizers which do nothing to address this simple underlying imbalance. Since calcium is carried in the blood partly bound to digested protein and partly in ionic (salt) form, inadequate protein digestion, and the resulting excess alkaline reserves, can lead to calcium metabolism problems, such as osteoporosis, osteoarthritis, degenerative disc problems, and bone spurs. Protease also plays an important role in preventing and eliminating blood clots.

Protease supplements can be taken with meals to increase digestion of protein. Between meals, protease helps alleviate infections (bacterial and viral), and enhances the immune system in general. Protease alleviates inflammatory conditions of any kind, especially those associated with soft tissue trauma, as occurs in an accident or surgery. I have also had patients who passed large worms while on high doses of protease (not over-the-counter formulas) followed by total relief of symptoms (rashes, anal irritation, and so on). Some but not all types of kidney problems, such as nephritis and drug-induced kidney damage, can often be relieved with protease.

QUICK DEFINITION

Amino acids are the basic building blocks of the 40,000 different proteins in the body, including enzymes, hormones, and the key brain chemical messenger molecules called neurotransmitters. Eight amino acids cannot be made by the body and must be obtained through the diet; others are produced in the body but not always in sufficient amounts. The body's main "amino acid pool" consists of: alanine, arginine, aspargine, aspartic acid, carnitine, citrulline, cysteine, cystine, GABA, glutamic acid, glutamine, glycine, histidine, isoleucine, leucine, lysine, methionine, ornithine, phenylalanine, proline, serine, taurine, threonine, tryptophan, tyrosine, and valine.

When a person is lacking in one or more of the primary digestive enzymes, the food category associated with that enzyme does not get digested properly and that person is said to be intolerant to that food. When the enzyme deficiency is left untreated, health problems inevitably result.

The only people who cannot tolerate high doses of protease are those who suffer from ulcers, gastritis (inflammation of the stomach), or hiatal (in the stomach) hernia, since damaged mucosal tissue in the stomach cannot handle extra acidity from digested protein. Many people have asked if the protease inhibitors currently being used to treat AIDS patients interfere with plant protease. The answer is no, they can be used simultaneously.

Amylase (digests carbohydrates)

Amylase digests carbohydrates (polysaccharides), breaking them down into smaller units called disaccharides which are later converted into monosaccharides (simple sugars) such as glucose and fructose. People who can't digest fats often eat—and tolerate—large amounts of sugar to make up for the lack of fat in their diet. If their diet is excessive in sugar, they can develop an amylase deficiency in addition to the original lipase deficiency.

Possessing antihistamine properties, amylase can relieve many kinds of skin problems, such as hives and rashes, contact dermatitis, and allergic reactions to bee stings, bug bites, and poison oak or ivy. Amylase, combined with certain herbs, relieves herpes of any kind, including canker sores, genital herpes, shingles, and chicken pox. Combined with certain skin-healing herbs, it can heal acne, eczema, and psoriasis.

Although asthma is a direct result of sugar intolerance, amylase combined with lung-healing herbs helps alleviate the wheezing of asthmatics. This combination acts as a lung expectorant and relieves the coughing accompanying colds and bronchitis. Amylase is useful for athletes because it eases muscle soreness and pain following exercise. It also can treat writer's cramp and joint stiffness that is worse in the morning upon rising or after sitting for long periods.

Amylase is important in preventing the proliferation of dead leukocytes (white blood cells) which manifest as pus. For example, if you have an infected gum area which antibiotics don't heal, it may not be an infection, but rather an abscess—that is, pus with no bacteria.

With adequate amylase, the abscess could disappear or at least be dramatically diminished within 48 hours.

Lipase (digests fats)

Lipase breaks down neutral fats (triglycerides) into glycerol (an alcohol) and fatty acids (SEE QUICK DEFINITION). Before lipase can digest fat, bile, an emulsifier or degreaser, must break the fat down into smaller units. People who are low in HCl cannot make adequate bile. HCl deficiency is caused by protease deficiency (required to provide adequate acidity) and lipase deficiency (required to carry chlorides). Thus lipase deficiency, inadequate HCl, and stagnation of bile are interrelated.

There are two types of lipase-deficient people. The first are those who are truly fat intolerant, get sick when they eat fat, and have gallbladder problems. These people substitute sugar for fat. The second are people who are complex-carbohydrate intolerant and make up for it by eating excessive amounts of fat. These people gradually develop a lipase deficiency.

Lipase is important in maintaining optimum cell permeability, which allows nutrients to flow easily into the cells and wastes to flow out. Two conditions arising from lipase deficiency are diabetes and glucosuria (sugar in the urine without symptoms of diabetes). Most people associate diabetes with sugar intolerance, but fat intolerance is the major enzyme culprit. The inability to digest fat interferes with insulin metabolism and the transport of glucose into the cell by insulin.

Lipase-deficient people may also have one or more of the following conditions or a tendency towards them: high cholesterol and/or high blood triglycerides, high blood pressure, difficulty losing weight, and varicose veins. They may also be deficient in many fat-soluble nutrients, including vitamins A, D, and E.

Disaccharidases (digest sugar)

People who cannot tolerate sugar or disaccharides tend to turn consume more protein. This is a good choice because 46% of digested protein is converted to glucose upon demand and glucose is a major source of energy for the brain and cells. Disaccharidases (sometimes called carbohydrases) break down disaccharides into simple sugars such as glucose and fructose. The three major disaccharides are sucrose (cane sugar), lactose (milk sugar), and maltose (grain sugar). In particular, the digestion of sucrose produces glucose plus fructose; lactose produces glucose plus galactose; and maltose produces two glucose units.

Probably the major cause of sugar intolerance is excessive consumption of refined sugars. Just as an enzyme deficiency can produce intolerance to the food digested by that enzyme, eating too much of that food can result in intolerance to it because the body is unable to keep up with the demand for the enzyme necessary to digest it, and deficiency results.

Thus, eating too much sugar leads to a deficiency in disaccharidases and sugar intolerance develops. For most people in the United States, it is likely that both factors—intitial enzyme deficiency along with excess consumption of sugar—are in operation due to the lack of enzymes in the standard American diet of refined, processed foods and the average per-person consumption of 150 pounds of sugar every year. Before the advent of the processed food industry, Americans consumed an average of only five pounds of sugar per year. This excessive sugar consumption is far beyond the capacity of the small intestine to produce enough disaccharidases to digest all that sugar.

There are physical, mental, and emotional symptoms of a deficiency of disaccharidases and the attendant sugar intolerance. Many of these symptoms also occur in people who have an underactive thyroid gland (hypothyroidism, SEE QUICK DEFINITION). Common physical symptoms include diarrhea, especially from lactose intolerance, but both diarrhea and constipation may result from maltose and sucrose intolerance as well. Lung problems, especially asthma, are common in sugar-intolerant people. People with environmental illness (SEE QUICK DEFINITION) also fall into this category.

Spaciness or dizziness that is worse when bending over is linked to sugar intolerance. If severe enough, a seizure disorder can develop, especially if refined sugar is consumed. Sugar-intolerant people often complain that they fall asleep easily but cannot stay asleep.

Mental and emotional problems include depression, mood swings, angry, aggressive, or violent behavior, severe panic attacks (often requiring prescription medication), manic-depression (bipolar disorders), and hyperactivity/ attention deficit disorder (ADD).

The proliferation of the fungus *Candida albicans* (SEE QUICK DEFINITION), a condition called candidiasis, is also linked to a deficiency of disaccharidases and the sugar intolerance that goes along with it. There are about 2,500 forms of yeast-fungi and all of them live on sugar, especially sucrose. In fact, the fungi make an enzyme that can digest sugar for their use. All of these fungi can be digested by cellulase (described below), but a primary cause of pathogenic yeast overgrowth is excessive sugar consumption coupled with frequent antibiotic use.

Cellulase (digests soluble fiber)

The pancreas can manufacture enzymes similar to all of those found in plants (including protease, amylase, lipase, and disaccharidases) with the exception of cellulase. As mentioned previously, cellulase is not made in the body and can be obtained *only* from food sources or enzyme supplements. Cellulase digests the soluble parts of fiber into smaller units which are eventually converted to glucose. In this process, the beneficial soluble fibers are released. All raw fruits, vegetables, and whole grains contain cellulase.

There are conditions arising from other enzyme deficiencies which are relieved or cured by cellulase. For example, the yeast overgrowth discussed above, caused by sugar intolerance among other factors, can be alleviated by cellulase which digests the yeast-fungi.

Cellulase also digests certain neurotoxins in the colon which cause facial pain or neuralgia and facial paralysis (Bell's palsy). An enzyme formula containing cellulase and antioxidants can bring relief to these conditions within two weeks. Finally, cellulase, along with other enzymes, can alleviate acute food allergies which, again, are created by faulty digestion due to enzyme deficiencies.

A Healthy Diet is the Best Source of Enzymes

To ensure that your body gets the enzymes it needs for optimum digestion, the best approach is to go to the source—your diet. It should be enzyme-rich, with a wide

QUICK DEFINITION

Environmental illness is a multiple-symptom debilitating, chronic disorder involving prolonged, heightened, and often incapacitating allergies or sensitivities to numerous common substances found in one's environment. Symptoms may include headaches, fatigue, muscle pain and/or weakness, coughing or wheezing, asthma, weight loss, infections, and emotional fluctuations, depression, and/or irritability. The illness is sometimes referred to as "20th century disease" because patients become allergic to and functionally incompatible with many products and substances found in the modern world, such as car exhaust, synthetic carpets, plywood and other building materials, cleaning agents, office machines, and plastics, among others.

Candida albicans is a yeast-like fungus found widely in nature, in the soil, on vegetables and fruits, and in the human body. It is frequently present in small quantities in the intestines and in a woman's vagina. When its numbers are few, *Candida* is generally not harmful to the human body. A *Candida* overgrowth, a condition called **candidiasis**, can become pathogenic and cause allergic reactions throughout the body. These reactions can lead to a wide range of symptoms, including depression, fatigue, weight gain, anxiety, rashes, headaches, and muscle cramping.

Guidelines for Healthy Eating

AVOID THESE FOODS	USE THESE FOODS INSTEAD
Refined sugars: white sugar (sucrose), fructose, corn syrup, sorbitol, mannitol. Synthetic sugars: NutraSweet™ and saccharin	Natural sweeteners: fruit juice, raw honey, organic maple syrup, molasses, barley malt, sucanat (organic sugar cane). Avoid if diabetic or sugar intolerant.
Refined flours: white, unbleached, bleached, enriched flour and products containing these flours	Organic whole grains: best are heirloom (genetically unaltered) grains such as kamut, quinoa, amaranth, and spelt. Grain-intolerant people may do well on heirlooms.
Synthetic fats: margarine, partially hydrogenated oils, vegetable shortening, Mocha Mix, Olestra	Butter, preferably raw, organic
Unsaturated oils: (any kind, whether cold-pressed, expeller pressed, or organic, with the exception of extra virgin olive oil) soybean, canola, flaxseed, safflower, corn, and fish oils	Butter, extra virgin olive oil, or coconut oil
Homogenized, pasteurized, nonfat or *acidophilus* milk, and processed cheese	Raw (unpasteurized), whole milk, cultured milk products (kefir, yogurt, buttermilk), and goat's milk; unprocessed cheese. Use in moderation if you are lactose intolerant.
Nuts and seeds: commercial, oiled, sugared, and salted. Beware of aflatoxin mold on old peanuts.	Preferably organic nuts and seeds. Must be soaked (6 hrs) or blanched or roasted to destroy enzyme inhibitors.
Drinks: commercial, sugared fruit juices, juice drinks, and soft drinks (both diet and regular)	Raw juices: juice your own or buy 100% juice, preferably raw, organic. Natural spritzers containing only fruit juice and carbonated water.
Canned coffee and commercial decaffeinated coffee	Grind your own beans, preferably organic. Use only Swiss water-processed decaffeinated beans. Don't exceed more than three cups daily. Try organic black or herbal teas.

AVOID THESE FOODS	USE THESE FOODS INSTEAD
All commercial red meat and poultry	Lamb or organic beef, organic free-range poultry. Fish is fine if it is not from polluted waters; halibut is one of the best.
Commercial eggs or egg substitutes	Organic eggs (no chemicals, drugs, or hormones) from free-range chickens or ducks
Canned, precooked, microwaved, processed, fast foods and junk foods	Buy fresh organic foods first, fresh nonorganic second, frozen third, and canned if that is the only food available.

variety of organic, whole, unprocessed foods. Foods in their whole, unaltered state have the ideal ratio of enzymes needed to digest them. For example, an apple, which is high in carbohydrates, contains more amylase than an avocado, which has a high concentration of fat and is high in lipase.

Most importantly, foods should be eaten raw or, at the most, lightly steamed. There are a few exceptions: seeds, nuts, grains, and beans have enzyme inhibitors which must be deactivated by soaking, cooking, or sprouting. Cruciferous vegetables, such as broccoli, cabbage, cauliflower, and Brussels sprouts, contain compounds that can inhibit the function of the thyroid gland and should not be eaten raw.[1] To ensure optimum health, eat a broad variety of organic raw fruits and vegetables, cooked whole grains, and enough protein from fish, organic meat, poultry, and eggs, and raw or cultured dairy—and your body will take care of the rest.

While eating a healthy diet supplies you with all the enzymes you need, if you have a history of poor diet or are enzyme-deficient for other reasons, your body will need some additional help to reverse the depletion. In that case, plant enzymes in supplement form may be advisable, but always combined with the necessary dietary changes. It is important to understand that enzyme supplements are not a substitute for a healthy diet—taking enzymes while continuing to eat a diet high in processed, refined foods will not resolve your health problems.

CHAPTER 2

Diagnosing Enzyme Defi ciencies

HOW DO YOU KNOW if you're deficient in enzymes? If you have allergies, fatigue, bloating, gas, constipation, indigestion, or any symptom of undigested food, then you most likely have an enzyme deficiency. The question is, which one? Some people can figure it out on their own—you may drink milk and have diarrhea shortly after. Maybe you experience mood swings after eating a chocolate chip cookie or a candy bar, or have nausea and burping after eating French fries or greasy foods.

If you're one of these people, you can find some help with broad-spectrum enzymes from health food stores. Not everyone, however, is aware of the effects foods have on their bodies, and you may be unable to formulate a clear connection between the foods you eat and the way you feel. You might recognize certain pieces of the puzzle, understanding which foods have a profound effect on your health and moods, and you may diligently avoid those foods, but still feel sick.

Here's an example: suppose you know you can't eat candy bars because you have a sugar intolerance, but you still drink milk and eat grains. Milk contains a sugar called lactose and grains contain a sugar called maltose. Since both of these are sugars, no matter how assiduously you avoid white sugar, as long as you're drinking milk and eating certain grains, you'll have a reaction. In this case you need the help of an enzyme "detective" to put together the missing pieces and solve the enzyme puzzle. A qualified enzyme therapist can do a diagnostic workup to find out which foods you can't digest—your food intolerances.

For a list of **enzyme therapists,** see Appendix C.

A food intolerance refers to a food that your body can't digest, which therefore produces adverse effects, ranging from bloating and gas to many other allergic symptoms, such as rashes, hives, nausea, headaches, diarrhea, or constipation. In short, whatever you cannot digest becomes a poison in your body. You may experience food intolerances in a mild form—you can eat small amounts of the offending food, but if you consume large quantities, the digestive capacity of your body is overwhelmed.

The Enzyme Diagnosis: How It Works

The diagnostic workup to determine enzyme deficiencies and offending foods may vary among practitioners. In my practice, I use four detailed questionnaires: a health history, a diet survey, a nutritional deficiencies questionnaire, and an enzyme profile questionnaire. I also perform a 24-hour urinalysis and a palpation test, both developed by enzyme therapy pioneer Howard F. Loomis, D.C., of Madison, Wisconsin. The results of the questionnaires and two tests give me an accurate diagnosis of a client's enzyme deficiencies or food allergies and tell me which enzyme formulas and dietary recommendations are required to correct them.

Patient Health History

This questionnaire (see p. 31) asks for vital statistics (such as childhood diseases and vaccinations), major health complaints (including how long they've existed), and a list of any nutritional supplements and prescription or over-the-counter drugs you are taking. It also includes an environmental toxins survey, and asks you to provide any other facts about your health that you find pertinent. An important corollary of this questionnaire is the oral temperature and resting pulse tests to determine if your thyroid gland is functioning correctly (see pp. 32-33).

Diet Survey

In my practice, I use a nail-you-to-the-wall diet survey (see pp. 34-35). It's not enough to note that you had toast and tea for breakfast. I want to know more. How many times a week do you eat toast? Was it whole grain or white bread? Was it organic? Did you slather it with butter, margarine, or jam? Was your tea caffeinated or decaffeinated? Did you put honey, white sugar, rice syrup, NutraSweet™ (aspartame), or saccharin in your tea? How many

The Loomis test determines enzyme deficiencies and isolates digestive disorders and nutrient deficiencies. This can only be done with a 24-hour urine sample, not a random sample. The fluctuations in the 24-hour urine collection are averaged to give a complete picture of digestive, malabsorptive, and assimilation problems.

cups did you have? Did you lighten it with cream, milk, skim milk, soy milk, or artificial creamer?

The purpose for such questions is to determine what foods you really eat, and if you eat "real" foods. There are many things we put in our mouths—margarine or NutraSweet—that are not real foods at all. I question the quantity and frequency of each food consumed since, as mentioned earlier, some people may be able to tolerate certain foods in small quantities, but have severe reactions to larger quantities. For example, if you have one bagel with a pat of butter for breakfast, you may not experience any symptoms. But if you eat three bagels with a tablespoon of butter on each, your body may not be able to handle it. You simply might not have enough enzymes to digest the wheat in the extra two bagels, or the fat in the extra butter.

I also ask about cooking procedures, since cooking (especially at high temperatures) destroys enzymes and makes foods more difficult to digest, even in the healthiest of people. The average American diet consists of almost 100% cooked foods—with the exception of the occasional salad or piece of fruit. As stressed earlier, microwaving is not a viable food preparation technique; it simply kills digestive enzymes, converts the protein into carcinogens or neuro/kidney toxins, and destroys all the vitamins and minerals.[1]

Nutritional Deficiency and Enzyme Profile Questionnaires

The "Nutritional Deficiency Symptoms" questionnaire (see pp. 36-37) pinpoints the client's current symptoms. Since particular symptoms are associated with depletions in a specific vitamin or mineral, this questionnaire gives me a picture of the person's nutrient status. The "Enzyme Profile" questionnaire (see p. 38) is similar in that it queries the client on symptoms, but symptoms which respond to supplementation with a certain enzyme may not be caused by lack of that

Patient Health History

Vital Statistics
Sex _____ Age _____ Ht _____
Weight _____ B/P _____/_____

Marital History
Married _____(yrs.) Divorced _____(yrs.)
Children _____ Ages _____
Single _____ No. of Pregnancies _____
Deliveries _____ Miscarriages _____
Complications _____ Abortions _____

Childhood Diseases
(circle all you have had): measles, mumps,
chicken pox, diphtheria, whooping cough,
tonsillitis, ear infections; other_____

Childhood vaccinations (list):

Operations (what and when):

Accidents (list):

Family History: Please circle conditions
which your parents, sisters, or brothers have
had: diabetes, cancer, heart disease, asthma,
kidney disease, stomach disorders,
gallbladder disease, arthritis; other_____

Habits: coffee, tea, drugs, sugar,
chocolate, alcohol, cigarettes, laxatives,
recreational drugs
Work _____(hrs/wk)
Sleep _____(hrs/night)
Exercise _____(times/week)

Complaints that brought you here:

Duration:

Method of onset:

How long since you felt well:

Environmental Toxins Survey:
  Do you wear prescription glasses or
  contact lenses?

Are your lenses tinted?

Do you wear sunglasses?

Do you use a computer?

Does it have a shield?

How many hrs/wk on computer?

Commute time per week (hrs)

Do you live within 100 yards of
power lines or high voltage lines?

Are you exposed to any toxic chemicals
in the workplace or elsewhere?

Do you use pesticides/insecticides?

Do you work in an energy-efficient
(airtight) building?

Do you live downwind of a nuclear power
plant?

Do you use a microwave oven/eat in
restaurants that use them?

Circle therapies you have tried:
chiropractic, acupuncture, homeopathy,
osteopathy, herbs, cranio-sacral therapy
List others:

Give any information pertinent to your
health history not covered above:

List all nutritional supplements you take,
including brand names and amounts
taken:

List all prescription drugs you are
currently taking with dosage:

Is Your Thyroid Underactive? Oral Temperature and Resting Pulse Tests Measure Thyroid Function

There is considerable evidence that serum tests for hypothyroidism (low thyroid function) are insensitive and inaccurate. Broda Barnes, M.D., author of *Hypothyroidism, an Unsuspected Illness*, measured the body temperature to determine subclinical hypothyroidism which does not show up in the standard thyroid blood chemistry test. This is based on a test of a basic function of the thyroid: its ability to regulate the metabolic furnace of the body to create heat or control temperature.

Instructions: Use only an oral thermometer, either basal or digital. Before arising each morning, take your oral temperature (compute the average of three days). If you sleep under mulitple blankets or use an electric blanket, get up before you take your morning temperature. It should be 98° F. Women should do this test during menses to avoid the rise in basal temperature during ovulation. An oral temperature of less than 98° F in the morning suggests low thyroid function. During the day (between 10 a.m. and 8 p.m.), your oral temperature should be 98.6°-99° F and not over 100° F. Your oral temperature should be optimum 20-30 minutes after eating. If it's low then, it will get worse as night falls. Forget this test when you are sick, because your thyroid function will decrease. Also, antidepressant drugs and anti-anxiety drugs will cause an abnormal rise in your oral temperature, invalidating this test.

Resting Pulse: Another way to tell if you are hypothyroid is to measure your resting pulse on three days and compute the average. The healthy resting pulse should be about 85 beats per minute (the national average is around 72); but if your pulse is less than 80, you may have an underactive thyroid. Children have a pulse greater than 100 until around the age of eight when the pulse slows down to around 85.

The idea of a slow pulse being healthy is folklore. Studies of healthy people who have no heart disease were found to have an average pulse of 85 beats per minute. Studies of the smartest high school students showed a pulse of 85 versus a pulse of 70 in below average students. On the other hand, some low thyroid people have a high pulse of over 100 beats per minute due to excess adrenaline. These people will have trouble monitoring their temperature because it will not be consistent.

Oral Temperature a.m., before rising
98° F (optimum)

_____   _____

_____

Average Temperature _____

Oral Temperature During Day
between 11 a.m. and 3 p.m.
98.6°-99° F and
not > 100° F (optimum)

_____   _____

_____

Average Temperature _____

Resting Pulse when not eating
85 beats per minute (optimum)

_____   _____

_____

Average Pulse _____

enzyme. For example, candidiasis (yeast overgrowth) responds well to cellulase supplementation, but a cellulase deficiency is not the cause of this weakened immune condition.

Loomis 24-Hour Urinalysis

The diagnostic procedure for enzyme deficiency requires a urinalysis as developed by Dr. Loomis. This test is not to be confused with the typical medical urinalysis which only diagnoses pathology, nor with other urine tests, such as the Reams test, which are based upon random urine samples. The Loomis test determines enzyme deficiencies and isolates digestive disorders and nutrient deficiencies. This can only be done with a 24-hour urine sample, not a random sample.

The procedure is as follows: the client should be following his or her regular diet. In my practice, I ask that my clients abstain from taking vitamins, minerals, enzymes, herbs, or other supplements during

Diet Survey

For each category below, indicate what kinds of foods and drinks you consume and how often
by writing 1 for one day per week, 2 for two days, 3 for three days, and so on, next to the
category. If it's only once a month, put 1/mo. Circle the specific foods or beverages within
each category that you eat or drink and whether organic or commercial, if noted. If you eat
some of each, circle both. If you aren't sure, leave a question mark. Next to each category,
write in any other items you eat or drink which are not listed.

_____Meats (commercial beef, liver, etc.)
_____Meats (organic, free of drugs and hormones; beef, liver, etc.)
_____Meats (lamb)
_____Meats (processed, deli meats, cold cuts, bologna, canned)
_____Pork (ham, bacon, pork chops, sausage)
_____Poultry (commercial, containing antibiotics, treated with additives, hormones, chemi-
        cals, meat tenderizers)
_____Poultry (free-range, no hormones, additives, antibiotics)
_____Fish (shellfish, salmon, cod, halibut or other white fish)
_____High protein drinks (with soy powder, milk, or other protein)
_____Eggs (commercial)
_____Eggs (from free-range chickens)
_____Bread (white, bleached, enriched, commercial, with margarine or other hydrogenated oil)
_____Bread (organic, whole wheat or other whole grain containing no margarine or unsatu-
        rated oils but only butter and a natural sweetener such as honey or molasses)
_____Bread (other whole grains such as corn, rye, sprouted grains, amaranth, spelt, kamut,
        quinoa, with no margarine or unsaturated oils)
_____Pasta (white flour, bleached or unbleached)
_____Pasta (whole wheat or other whole, unrefined grains)
_____Cereal (commercial, with white sugar, fructose, or corn syrup)
_____Cereal (commercial but containing no refined sugar, i.e., Shredded Wheat or Grape
        Nuts or health food store brands)
_____Grains, refined (white flour, white rice)
_____Grains, whole (whole wheat berries, rye berries, oat flakes, millet, rye, brown rice, bar-
        ley, buckwheat)
_____Grains, heirloom (kamut, quinoa, spelt, amaranth)
_____Complex carbohydrates (potatoes, yams, sweet potatoes, corn)
_____Beans (green, red, kidney, pinto, black, lima, pinto, mung, soy)
_____Soy products (unfermented: soymeal, soymilk, tofu, and products containing soy)
_____Soy products (fermented: tempeh, miso, tamari)
_____Vegetables, processed (canned or frozen)
_____Vegetables, fresh, organic or commercial (cruciferous [broccoli, cabbage, cauliflower,
        Brussels sprouts] raw or cooked; asparagus, celery, cucumber, parsnips, squash, peas)
_____Vegetables, root, fresh, organic or commercial (carrots, turnips, beets, burdock, garlic, onions)
_____Vegetables, sea (kelp, dulse, nori)
_____Tomatoes (fresh, organic or commercial)
_____Tomatoes (canned, tomato sauces, commercial catsup)
_____Greens, fresh, organic or commercial (Swiss chard, kale, spinach, arugula, watercress,
        dandelion, turnip greens, bok choy, collards, beet greens, parsley)
_____Lettuce, organic or commercial (head, red leaf, romaine, bib)

_____Salad dressings, commercial (unsaturated oil & vinegar, creamy, blue cheese, ranch)
_____Salad dressings, health food store brands (unsaturated or olive oil)
_____Salad dressings, homemade (with only extra virgin olive oil or coconut oil)
_____Fats (margarine, hydrogenated oils, vegetable shortening)
_____Fats, saturated: coconut oil
_____Butter (commercial, pasteurized)
_____Butter (raw unpasteurized or organic but pasteurized)
_____Oils, commercial unsaturated (flaxseed, soybean, safflower, canola, sesame, corn oil, etc.)
_____Oils, cold or expeller pressed unsaturated (kinds above)
_____Oils: extra virgin or light olive oil
_____Milk, commercial, pasteurized, homogenized (whole, lowfat, nonfat)
_____Milk, raw unpasteurized (whole, lowfat, nonfat)
_____Cheese, processed   _____Cheese, unprocessed but pasteurized
_____Cheese, unprocessed, from raw milk
_____Fruit, fresh organic or commercial (apples, oranges, grapefruit, tangerines, lemons,
     grapes, strawberries, bananas, canteloupe, watermelon, pineapple, blueberries)
_____Fruit, processed (canned, frozen)
_____Juices (canned or frozen)
_____Juices (bottled, from concentrate, with added sugar)
_____Juices (bottled, from concentrate, with no added sugar)
_____Juices (unpasteurized/must be refrigerated)
_____Juices (freshly squeezed, organic or commercial)
_____Nuts (commercial, roasted in oil)
_____Nuts (from bins, dry-roasted, no oil)
_____Nut butters (commercial peanut butter with added sugar/oil)
_____Nut butters (containing only nuts and salt, raw or roasted)
_____Seeds (sunflower, sesame, pumpkin, raw or roasted)
_____Sprouts (alfalfa, clover, mung beans, mixed)
_____Fast foods (hamburgers, fried fish sandwiches, pizza, frozen dinners)
_____Chips (commercial, made with margarine/hydrogenated or unsaturated oils)
_____Chips (made with coconut oil or oil-free)
_____Snacks (corn puffs, rice cakes, lowfat or baked, light salt)
_____Candy (any kind of commercial candy bars)
_____Candy (health food store "energy bars" with all natural ingredients, no margarine or
     hydrogenated oils, no fructose or white or brown sugar)
_____Desserts, commercial (ice cream, pastries, donuts, pies, made with white flour, white
     sugar, corn syrup, etc.)
_____Desserts, health food (sweetened only with fruit juice, honey, or molasses and made
     with whole grains, fruits, etc.)
_____Soft drinks, commercial, non-diet   _____Diet soda
_____Sweeteners (white sugar, commercial honey, fructose, corn syrup, artificial syrup, brown
     sugar, NutraSweet™, saccharin, sorbitol, mannitol, dextrose)
_____Sweeteners (raw honey, organic maple syrup, sucanat, rice syrup)
_____Water, naturally carbonated, no sugar   _____Water, tap untreated
_____Water, spring, distilled, deionized, reverse osmosis
_____Tea (herbal or black)
_____Coffee with caffeine, freshly ground or canned
_____Coffee (commercial decaffeinated or Swiss water-process decaffeinated)
_____Wine (red or white)   _____Hard liquor (any kind)
_____Beer (American or imported; lite beer, dark beer)

Nutritional Deficiency Symptoms

Circle all symptoms and conditions you currently have.

Headaches:
Migraines   Frontal
Back of neck   Sinus
Temples   How often?

Sinus Problems:
Nose: dry, stuffy, congested, runny
Mouth breather
Frequent sinusitis or sinus infections
Sinus headaches

Ears:
Frequent earaches or infections
Fluid in ears
Loss of hearing
Ringing in the ears

Eyes:
Vision getting worse, eye pain
Get headaches when reading
Glaucoma
Cataracts
Macular degeneration

Mouth and Throat:
Sores on tongue or in mouth
Speech problems
Frequent sore or irritated throat
Hard lumps under jawbone (marbles)
Swollen glands

Dental Problems:
Mercury amalgam fillings? How many?
Root canals? How many?
Dentures
Frequent abscesses
Titanium implants

Skin Problems:
Skin: dry, moist, oily

Itching: Where?
Acne, cystic acne
Eczema
Psoriasis
Allergic to bee stings, bug bites
Allergic to poison oak/ivy
Frequent hives or rashes
Frequent skin or nail fungal infections

Cardiovascular System:
Irregular or skipped heartbeats
Heart palpitations
Mitral valve prolapse
Poor circulation
High cholesterol or triglycerides
Chest pain, angina
Congestive heart failure
Heart attacks? How many?
Have you had chelation therapy? If so, when?

Lungs:
Frequent coughing, mucus
Color of mucus?
Shortness of breath
Asthma, wheezing
Frequent lung infections
Bronchitis
Emphysema

Liver:
Can't tolerate vitamins, alcohol, or drugs
Coated tongue
Nausea after high-fat meals
Jaundice
Hepatitis? What kind?

Gallbladder:
Intolerance of fatty or spicy foods
Frequent sour taste in mouth

Frequent regurgitation of food
Can't lie down after eating or regurgitate
Burping, pain, or nausea after meals
Pain under right rib cage after meals
Gallbladder disease/surgery

Stomach:
Frequent stomach pain or bloating
Burning or acid rebound relieved by eating
Ulcers, take antacids
Gastritis, *Helicobacter pylori*
Esophageal reflux
Hiatal hernia
Frequent nausea or vomiting? When?

Urinary Tract:
Frequent bladder infections
Pain when voiding
Burning urination (cystitis)
Frequent urination or urgency
Loss of control or incontinence
Pass small amounts at each voiding
Bedwetting
History of kidney stones/surgery

Intestinal Tract (large and small):
Malabsorption
Constipation
Infrequent bowel movements
Number of daily bowel movements ___
Use laxatives, take enemas
Hemorrhoids
Pain in lower right abdomen
Hard, painful stools

Diarrhea or loose stools
Multiple bowel movements
Constipation alternating with
   diarrhea
Mucus or blood in stools
Rectal pain or bleeding
Pain in lower left abdomen
Diagnosed with: irritable
   bowel syndrome,
   Crohn's disease, colitis,
   diverticulitis,
   diverticulosis, other

Sugar Metabolism Problems:
Hypoglycemia
Diarrhea or loose stools
Seizures
Childhood asthma
Insomnia
Nightmares
Mood swings, irritability
   or anger
Violent behavior
Hyperactivity/attention
   deficit disorder (ADD)
Manic depression (bipolar
   disorder)
Schizophrenia
Panic or anxiety attacks
Glucosuria (sugar in urine)
Diabetes I or II

Calcium Metabolism Problems:
Leg cramps or restless legs at
   night
Night cough
Joint pain or stiffness
Low back pain
Weak joints or ligaments
Fallen arches
Bone spurs
Deep bone pain
Loose teeth or poor fitting
   dentures
Arthritis

Rheumatoid arthritis
Osteoarthritis
Osteoporosis
Gout
Ankylosing spondylitis

Female Problems:
Vaginal discharge
Painful intercourse
Low libido
Hair growth on face
Painful or tender breasts,
   worse at menses
Seizures at menses
Fibrocystic breast disease
Uterine fibroids
Ovarian pain, ovarian cysts
Endometriosis
Infertile, taking fertility drugs
PMS symptoms: cramps,
   irritability, depression,
   moodiness
Acne, worse at menses
Headaches, worse at menses
Vomit during menses
Menses: irregular, scanty,
   excessive, too frequent,
   infrequent, amenorrhea
Surgical menopause:
   hysterectomy,
   oophorectomy
Hot flashes, day or night
Cancer: ovarian, cervical,
   uterine, breast

Male Problems:
Prostatic hypertrophy
Urination difficult or dribbling
Frequent urination
Night urination
Feeling of incomplete bowel
   evacuation
Low libido, impotence
Painful intercourse
Pain in groin or down front
   of legs
Sore genitals
Discharge from genitals
Prostate cancer

Immune System Problems:
Frequent bacterial or viral
   infections/what kind and
   where?
Candida albicans or other
   fungal infections? Where?
Cancer
AIDS
Herpes (oral, genital,
   shingles, CMV,
   Epstein-Barr)

Pain:
Muscular, worse after sitting
   or exercise
TMJ (jaw) pain
Tailbone hurts, tailbone injury
Back pain: neck, upper back,
   mid back, low back, other
Disc problems or surgery
Sciatica
Kidney pain
Joint pain
Knee pain, knee surgery
Hip pain, hip surgery

Miscellaneous Problems:
Dizziness when bending over
Dizziness when moving
Memory loss
Nervousness, panic attacks
Anxiety, frequent sighing, take
   tranquilizers
Depression, take
   antidepressants
Abnormal gait
Numbness or tingling?
   Where?
Tremors or seizures, taking
   medications
Hypertension, taking
   medications
Hypotension

Enzyme Profile

Please circle all symptoms and health problems you currently have.

Conditions that respond to protease:
Anxiety, frequent sighing; taking tranquilizers
Cold hands and feet
Water retention (edema): hands, ankles,
    fluid in ears
Immune system problems: bacterial or
    viral infections, cancer, AIDS
Colon problems: constipation, appendicitis,
    colon cancer
Kidney problems: kidney disease, nephritis
Calcium and bone problems: arthritis,
    osteoporosis, disc problems, gout, bone spurs
Blood clots
Acute pancreatitis
Soft tissue trauma (accidental or surgical)

Conditions that respond to amylase:
Frequent hives or rashes
Eczema, psoriasis
Herpes: canker sores, herpes I or II, shingles,
    chicken pox
Allergies to bee stings, bug bites, poison oak
    or ivy
Abscesses (such as in gums)
Gluten intolerance (celiac disease)
Muscle soreness or pain after exercise
Muscle and joint stiffness, worse in the
    morning or after sitting, writer's cramp

Conditions that respond to lipase:
Low stomach acid (hypochlorohydria)
Frequent sour taste in mouth, burping and/or
    nausea after meals; intolerance of fatty
    or spicy foods
Gallstones; gallbladder surgery
Hidden (recurrent) viruses
High cholesterol and/or triglycerides
Obese, can't lose weight
High blood pressure; taking antihypertension
    medications
Cardiovascular problems; varicose veins
Diabetes I or II/taking insulin or oral
    antidiabetic drug
Dizziness when moving or changing positions

**Conditions that respond to
disaccharidases:**
Physical symptoms:
Diarrhea, abdominal cramps, body odor
Constipation (rare)
Lung problems: asthma, bronchitis
Environmental illness
Spaciness, dizziness, especially when
    bending over
Seizure disorders
Insomnia

Mental/emotional symptoms:
Nightmares
Depression
Mood swings
Irritability or anger
Aggressive or violent behavior
Panic attacks
Manic-depression (bipolar disorder)
Hyperactivity/attention deficit disorder (ADD)

Conditions that respond to cellulase:
Malabsorption syndrome: gas, bloating
Acute food allergies
Fungal/yeast infections, candidiasis
Facial pain or neuralgia
Facial paralysis (Bell's palsy)

**Please list all foods to which you
know you are allergic. These are not
necessarily those identified by blood
allergy tests—list only foods you are
sure produce allergic symptoms.**

**Circle your environmental allergies.
List any others you have to
chemicals, plants, and animals.**
Pollens, molds, smoke, smog, auto fumes,
perfumes, weeds, grasses, flowers, cats, dogs,
horses, detergents, dust, paint, new carpets,
formaldehyde

the testing period and for at least one day before the test. Prescription medications may continue to be used, but I ask my clients to note what drugs they are taking, along with the amounts. A measuring cup and large jar with a lid are required for the test, and both should be sterilized by washing with a mild detergent, rinsing well with hot water and then distilled water, until all traces of the soap are gone. The cup and jug should then be rinsed once more with distilled water.

During 24 hours, the client collects urine in a sterile container, noting the total urine volume eliminated (in cups, or other unit measures) each time. Any symptoms noted during the test should be recorded, along with all foods and liquids consumed. The urine should be refrigerated. After 24 hours, the collection container should be gently inverted (not shaken) several times. The total 24-hour volume should be noted, and a small sample from the entire container poured into the special sterilized two-ounce sample container, which comes with a mailer and blue ice-pack to keep the urine cold. The sample is then sent by overnight delivery or hand-delivered to a practitioner who specializes in the Loomis urinalysis.

Interpreting the Results

The urinalysis provides information on what a person cannot digest, absorb, or assimilate, along with any nutritional deficiencies one might have. This test is prognostic rather than diagnostic (except for the identification of substances, such as glucose, not normally found in the urine and which therefore indicate disease conditions; this is the focus of standard urine tests). In other words, it predicts what lies ahead if you do not clean up your diet and digestion.

The fluctuations in the 24-hour urine collection are averaged to give a complete picture of digestive, malabsorptive, and assimilation problems. Looking at a 24-hour urinalysis is a way of peeking at the blood (the extracellular fluid or ECF). The health of the blood takes precedence in the body and cells will sacrifice nutrients in the service of maintaining the blood's relatively narrow pH range of 7.35 to 7.45 as well as its levels of electrolytes (SEE QUICK DEFINITION), protein, and other nutrients. Thus, the blood takes what it needs from the cells to achieve its necessary balance, or homeostasis.

If a nutrient does not appear in the urine, it means the body is using all there is. For example, there is a healthy

Electrolytes are substances in the blood, tissue fluids, intracellular fluids, or urine which conduct an electrical charge, either plus or minus. Examples include acids, bases, and salts, such as potassium, magnesium, phosphate, sulfate, bicarbonate, sodium, chloride, and calcium. Electrolytes provide inorganic chemicals for cellular reactions and control mechanisms, such as the conduction of electrochemical impulses to nerves and muscles. Electrolytes are also needed for key enzymatic reactions involved in metabolism, or the release of energy from food.

For information about getting a **24-hour urinalysis**, see Appendix C.

A Glossary of 24-Hour Urine Analysis Terms

The following are specific values measured in a 24-hour urine analysis:

Volume—The total urine output, either excessive (polyuria) or inadequate (oliguria), in relationship to the specific gravity indicates how well the kidneys are functioning.

Specific Gravity—This value measures the weight of total dissolved substances (solutes) in the urine against an equal amount of water, such that a normal reading of 1.020 means the urine is 20% heavier than water. Specific gravity shows the general water content (hydration) of the body. The optimum range for specific gravity is 1.018 to 1.022.

Indican—This indicates the degree of toxicity, putrefaction, gas, and fermentation in the intestines. Indican comes from putrefying undigested food in the large intestine which are kicked back into the blood and excreted through the kidneys. Indican is extremely toxic and causes many symptoms; the higher the level, the greater the intestinal toxemia or inflammation in the digestive tract. Readings as close to zero as possible are desirable.

pH—Based on hydrogen ion concentration, this value indicates the degree of urine acidity versus alkalinity on a scale of zero to 14, with optimum urine pH ranging from 6.3 to 6.7.

Chlorides—These are salt residues in the urine and the values give information on salt intake and/or lipase adequacy.

Total Sediment Analysis—This indicates the amount of dissolved organic and mineral substances remaining in the urine after digestion; reading for the three sediment categories (calcium phosphate, uric acid, and calcium oxalate) is 0.4-0.6.

- **Calcium phosphate**—A reading here indicates the status of carbohydrate digestion; a level of 0.4-0.6 signifies normal carbohydrate digestion.

- **Uric acid**—Levels of uric acid signify the status of protein digestion; optimal digestion yields a reading of less than 0.1.

- **Calcium oxalate**—This value indicates the status of fat digestion; a reading of less than 0.1 signifies optimal fat digestion.

Vitamin C—Levels of vitamin C indicate body reserves of this key nutrient; a reading of 1-5 is normal, over 5 deficient.

threshold level of urinary calcium. If the level is below that in the urine test, it indicates that the blood has no calcium to spare and may even be sucking calcium out of the cells and the bone, a condition that leads to osteoporosis. This may be the case even if the blood values for calcium are in the normal range.

On the other hand, levels of nutrients in the urine may be higher than what is considered normal. This means the blood is dumping excess nutrients into the urine. For example, the urine test can show too much calcium or the electrolyte chloride (salt). High chloride levels can mean you are eating too much salt or have a lipase deficiency.

(See "A Glossary of 24-Hour Urine Analysis Terms" for explanations of the terms used throughout this discussion.)

An overly acidic urine pH means that the blood is dumping excess acid reserves into the urine in order to maintain its optimum pH. An overly alkaline urine pH means the reverse—the blood is dumping excess alkaline reserves into the urine.

The 24-hour urine test also shows whether a person has normal kidney function or whether there is kidney-lymphatic stress. The lymphatic system (see "The Lymph System At a Glance," p. 42) becomes exhausted by working overtime to neutralize allergens (substances which produce an allergic reaction) and environmental toxins. When this occurs, allergens and toxins build up in the bloodstream. The kidneys then become exhausted from trying to cleanse the blood. Signs of kidney-lymphatic stress include: allergies, dark circles under the eyes, swollen lymph glands, kidney pain, low blood sugar, and nausea and sometimes vomiting, worse in women during menstruation and pregnancy.

Urine volume (the total output over the 24-hour period) in relationship to its specific gravity (density of the urine compared to water) shows whether the person is suffering from kidney-lymphatic stress. A normal or low urine volume with a low specific gravity indicates a kidney-lymphatic stress pattern.

If the urine volume is normal or high and the specific gravity is also high, it means there are substances in the urine which should not be there. A chemstrip (strip of plastic also used in standard urine tests which is segmented into different test tabs, one for each possible abnormality) identifies the specific substances. Examples of these are: glucose which indicates glucosuria (sugar in the urine without symptoms of diabetes) or diabetes; bilirubin (the pigment in bile) or urobilinogen (a bilirubin derivative) which indicates liver or gallbladder disease; nitrite (a salt of nitrous acid) or leukocytes (pus), indicating an infection or inflammatory condition in the genitourinary tract; and blood, indicating kidney stones, kidney disease, or other problems.

Another function of the urine test is to determine what you cannot digest or are eating in excess. This is revealed by the total sediment analysis which consists of the measures of calcium phosphate, calcium oxalate, and uric acid. Low phosphates indicate sugar intolerance or excess. High uric acid indicates protein intolerance or excessive consumption of sugar. High calcium oxalate indicates fat intolerance or excess. It can also result from excess ingestion of coffee, tea, and cola (all high in oxalates) or ascorbic acid (marketed as a vitamin C supplement).[2]

The Lymph System At a Glance

The human body has three circulatory systems—blood, nerve impulses, and lymph. The lymphatic system, largely ignored by mainstream medicine, includes: a vast network of capillaries which transport the lymph; a series of nodes throughout the body (primarily in the neck, groin, and armpits) which collect the lymph; and three organs, namely, the tonsils, spleen, and thymus gland, which produce white blood cells (called lymphocytes) vital to the immune system.

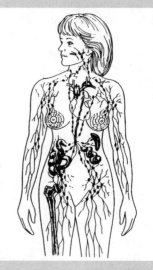

The space between cells occupies about 18% of the body. Fluid in this space, containing plasma proteins, foreign particles, and bacteria which accumulate between cells, is called lymph. Thus the purpose of the lymphatic system is to collect the lymph and to return its contents to the bloodstream. More specifically, the lymph system collects waste products and cellular debris from the tissues.

The lymph flows slowly upward through the body to the chest (at the rate of three quarts per 24 hours) where it drains into the bloodstream through two large ducts. Lymph also flows down from the head and neck into this drainage site. Unlike the heart, the lymphatic system does not have a pump to move it along; rather, its movement depends on such factors as muscle contraction or manual manipulation. The lymph circulation is also a one-way circulation: it only returns fluid to the bloodstream. The lymph system becomes particularly active during times of illness (such as the flu), when the nodes (especially at the throat) visibly swell with collected waste products.

Finally, the indican value indicates colon toxicity and the degree to which digestion is malfunctioning. Indican is a group of toxic compounds which are formed when undigested protein is decomposed by "unfriendly" bacteria in the small intestine. These unfriendly bacteria feed on undigested protein, especially when refined carbohydrates are consumed at the same meal, or when undigested fats coat the food and prevent penetration by the digestive enzymes. Thus, the level of urinary indican is a general indicator of the inability to digest food. The higher the level of indican, the greater the digestive problem. There is one exception to this. Undigested sugar interferes with the indican test, so zero indican does not indicate good digestion but, rather, severe sugar intolerance.

Indican that is not excreted in the feces is absorbed into the blood, detoxified by the liver, returned to the blood, and passed through the kidneys to be eliminated in the urine. This process causes particular stress to the bowels and liver but can affect almost any tissue, and is associated with dozens of pathological conditions, from acne to cancer.

Improving digestion and the elimination of waste materials through diet and multiple enzyme digestive formulas normalizes both indican and sediment. There are, however, patterns that indicate the need for certain intestinal cleansing formulas. For example, a high indican or a zero indican level with a low sediment level indicates the need for Thera-zyme SmI. This formula digests pathogenic yeast (*Candida albicans* and other fungi) and is excellent for constipation, diarrhea, or both (alternating), and certain parasites. On the other hand, a high indican level combined with a high sediment indicates the need for Thera-zyme Challenge Food Powder, a mixture of five different seeds. This is a colon cleansing formula that normalizes bowel function and is also specific for parasites.

Palpation Test

Along with the urine analysis, an important information-gathering procedure in enzyme therapy is the palpation test. Palpation literally means to elicit information by touch. It has been in use since the 1950s when chiropractors began correlating muscle palpation with subluxations (vertebral misalignments). Pain and visceral (internal organ) dysfunction are always accompanied by muscle contraction and indicate stress in the body, which is caused by changes in either structure (subluxations) or function (physiology). The enzyme therapist uses palpation to identify places of muscle contraction which in turn are reliable indicators of particular deviations in the normal homeostasis and health of the body.

Dr. Loomis developed a palpation test in which each positive palpation point (meaning there is a muscle contraction) corresponds to a deviation in structure (subluxation) which in turn corresponds to an undernourished organ.[3] Changes in normal function (acute or chronic conditions) can also be determined. Each palpation point also corresponds to one of his enzyme formulations, so palpation serves as both diagnosis and guideline for treatment.

Patients must fast for at least two hours before the test. They should then lie face-up on a chiropractic table. The practitioner first observes the position of the hips and the feet. In most people, one hip is higher or lower than the other, and sometimes one leg is longer or shorter than the other. This baseline position is noted. Then, the practitioner tests each palpation point by touch and observes any shift in the position of the hips or leg lengths following palpation.

Any observed shift (for example, the hips which were uneven become even) indicates a positive palpation, which means that the person may need the enzyme formulation corresponding to this palpation point. This phase of the test also reveals nutritional deficiencies and acute conditions such as viral or bacterial infections.

Then, the client either eats a meal or consumes a tablespoon of Thera-zyme Challenge Food Powder, which is equal to a complete meal. After 45 minutes, the palpation test is repeated. Positive palpation points now indicate what the body cannot digest. They also indicate acute and chronic conditions, including inflammation, kidney or urinary tract problems, soft tissue trauma, allergies, and colon problems.

The palpation area may be non-tender, tender, sore, or painful. The degree of pain or tenderness sometimes, but not always, correlates with the seriousness of the condition. From the palpation test, 24-hour urinalysis, and a complete patient history, it is clear what kind of enzyme therapy is required for the individual.

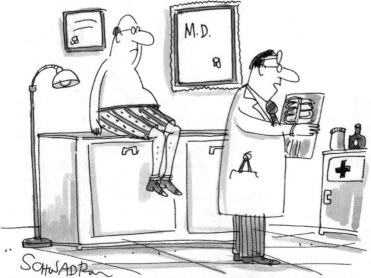

"THERE'S NOTHING WRONG WITH YOU THAT THROWING-A-LOT-OF-MONEY-AT-IT WON'T CURE."

CHAPTER

3

What Causes Enzyme Deficiencies?

ITTLE MORE than a century ago food was unprocessed and unrefined, grown on clean, living soil, with fresh air and pure water. It contained no preservatives, chemicals, or pesticides. Cooking techniques were simple, and the microwave oven nonexistent. Today, agribusiness chemicals and pesticides destroy living soil, which should be teeming with millions of living organisms—not just earthworms, but beneficial microorganisms essential in maintaining health and preventing disease. Dead soil creates dead food deficient in enzymes, nutrients, and soil-based organisms (beneficial microbes) which help prevent proliferation of intestinal toxins.

This already serious enzyme depletion of our food is then accentuated by the way most Americans eat. We gulp down pesticide-laden coffee and pastries concocted of refined flour, sugar, and margarine for breakfast, rush by fast-food restaurants for lunch, and grab canned or frozen sauces and soups, chemically treated vegetables, hormone-laden meats, and hybridized grains to microwave for dinner. Meanwhile, in the constant quest for flatter stomachs and trimmer thighs, we consume artificial sweeteners and fake fats by the pound.

In addition to these agricultural and dietary factors, there are a number of other sources of enzyme depletion integral to modern living, from the poisoning of enzymes by chemical exposure to the common dental practice of root canals.

Pesticides and Chemicals

Over 400 pesticides are currently licensed for use on America's foods, and in 1995, 1.2 billion pounds were dumped on crop lands, forests, lawns, and fields.[1] Unfortunately, we're not informed about which pesticides have been used to produce the food we buy at our local supermarkets.

So what do pesticides have to do with enzymes? All poisons, including pesticides, work by poisoning (destroying) enzymes in both plants and animals—and since enzymes are the life source of your body, any substance that kills enzymes is a threat to your health.

All synthetic chemicals, including pesticides and herbicides, poison one or more of the thousands of metabolic enzymes created from the raw materials of digested foods and genetic material—that is, DNA and RNA. DNA, or deoxyribonucleic acid, is located in the nucleus of the cell. It's responsible for hereditary influences as well as the overall function of cells. DNA also controls the formation of another nucleic acid, RNA (ribonucleic acid), which is responsible for the formation of proteins, the majority of which are enzymes.

Causes of Enzyme Depletion

- Pesticides and chemicals
- Hybridization and genetic engineering
- Bovine growth hormone (BGH)
- Pasteurization
- Irradiated food
- Excess intake of unsaturated and hydrogenated fats
- Cooking at high temperatures
- Microwaving
- Radiation and electromagnetic fields
- Geopathic stress zones
- Fluoridated water
- Heavy metals
- Mercury amalgam dental fillings
- Root canals

Research has documented the damage of pesticides to enzymes. In one five-year study of the impact of three major classes of pesticides (carbamates, organophosphates, and halogenated pesticides) on over 8,000 people, the effects included the following:

For more about **soil-based organisms,** see "Success Story: Treating Crohn's Disease With Soil-Based Organisms," Gastrointestinal Disorders, pp. 140-141.

- Carbamates, the active ingredients in ant, fly, and roach killers, poison enzymes that control essential cell functions.

- Organophosphates, used to control insects in agriculture, block enzymes that control nervous system activity.

- Halogenated pesticides, also used to control insects in agriculture, poison enzymes that run the functions of the cells.

According to Russell Jaffee, M.D., the research director, the "study shows clearly that even small amounts of pesticides are dangerous to

Genetic engineering breaks down fundamental genetic barriers and permanently alters the genetic code of plants and animals by combining the genes of dissimilar and unrelated species into novel organisms which will pass their genetic changes on to their offspring. One of the most worrisome consequences of genetically altered foods is their effect on enzymes.

For more information about **pesticide use,** see the *Journal of Pesticide Reform,* published by the Northwest Coalition for Alternatives to Pesticides (NCAP), P.O. Box 1393, Eugene, OR 97440.

sensitive people. This includes even the common household pesticides."[2]

The spraying of pesticides is conducted without notice to the public, and almost all of the 20,000 pesticides used in the United States contain ingredients the government terms "inert," which is supposed to mean they are not biologically active. Inert ingredients are used to make pesticides more potent or easier to apply. Contrary to the claim, they are active biologically, chemically, and physiologically.[3] Many "inerts" are extremely toxic, but since their identity is a manufacturer's "trade secret," they are rarely disclosed and the U.S. Environmental Protection Agency (EPA) does not require their testing. Further, by its own report, the EPA lacks information to ascertain the toxicity of more than 75% of chemicals used as inert substances.[4]

If we don't know what's in pesticides and don't know where they are sprayed, how can we protect ourselves? By buying and eating only organic food, we can at least limit the amount we ingest.

Hybridization and Genetic Engineering

While the agribusiness industry, with its reliance on toxic farm chemicals and pesticides, creates low- or no-enzyme foods, hybridization and genetic engineering create foods that are guaranteed to cause allergies. In hybridized wheat—that is, wheat in which two parent strains are crossed—the gluten content is much higher than in the so-called "ancient" or heirloom (nonhybridized) grains such as amaranth, kamut, spelt, and quinoa. Gluten is a component of the protein in wheat—the part that makes bread dough rise. Unfortunately, many people are allergic to gluten. In a study of gluten-intolerant people, it was found that 70% could tolerate kamut, with its lower gluten content and untampered genes.[5]

The proliferation of what are known as "Frankenfoods" is another example of the devastating effect agribusiness has had on our food supply. Frankenfoods are foods that, like the fictional laboratory-generated monster Frankenstein for which they are named, have been genetically engineered. Genetic engineering breaks down fundamental genetic barriers and permanently alters the genetic code of plants and animals by combining the genes of dissimilar and unrelated species into novel organisms which will pass their genetic changes on to their offspring.

One of the most worrisome consequences of genetically altered foods is their effect on enzymes. All foreign substances (including Frankenfoods) in the body must be eliminated or neutralized—a process requiring enzymes—to prevent allergic reactions. After a prolonged period of trying to digest foreign substances, the body becomes severely enzyme depleted and the lymphatic system exhausted, which leads to an increase in allergic symptoms.

Scores of companies are now using the new gene-splicing technology to produce never-before-seen combinations of vegetables, fruits, fish, poultry, and farm animals. Over 90% of current genetic research in agriculture is for the purpose of creating plants that are cheaper to grow and cheaper to transport, and have an indefinite shelf life without losing the appearance of freshness—in other words, for bigger profits.[6]

Bovine Growth Hormone

Recombinant bovine growth hormone, or BGH, is a genetically engineered, synthetic version of a hormone naturally produced by cows. Its purpose is to increase a cow's milk production by as much as 25%. This is economically absurd, since American dairy farmers already produce such a surplus of dairy products that taxpayers spend billions of dollars to buy excess production through government dairy price supports.

BGH can completely deplete your body of enzymes as your immune system tries to counteract the immune-suppressing impact of the hormone. However, it's difficult to avoid BGH unless you buy organic dairy and beef because the Food and Drug Administration (FDA) does not require labeling of BGH-laced products, despite surveys showing that the majority of consumers favor labeling. Again, the only way to be sure you are not ingesting BGH is to buy organic dairy products and beef.

Pasteurization

In the pasteurization process, milk is heated at high temperatures—much higher than necessary to kill bacteria. In the process,
all the enzymes are destroyed. In fact, that's how pasteurized milk
is tested: when all the enzymes are dead, the milk is considered
fully pasteurized.

What's wrong with pasteurized milk? First, let's look at what's
right with raw, unpasteurized milk. Raw milk is a living food containing many enzymes, beneficial bacteria (lactic acid *Bacillus*), vitamins,
minerals, fats, proteins, and lactose (milk sugars). If you leave raw milk
at room temperature, the lactic acid *Bacillus* will convert (ferment) the
sugars into lactic acid. This is called sour milk, and it's even more
nutritious than sweet milk, because it's partly digested.

In addition to killing the enzymes, pasteurization kills the lactic
acid *Bacillus* which turns milk sour, and alters the proteins, fats, and
sugars in milk, leaving the digestion of these nutrients entirely dependent on the person, which puts a severe stress on the pancreas. Few
people would be allergic to milk if they drank raw milk in which
there's exactly enough lactase to digest the lactose, protease for the
protein (casein), and lipase for the fat. In addition, some of these
enzymes are essential for calcium absorption and the assimilation of
other minerals. Further, raw milk contains enzymes and antibodies
that destroy certain pathogenic bacteria.

The claim that pasteurized milk is safer than raw milk is simply
wrong. Raw and pasteurized milk are equally susceptible to human
contamination. The only way to make milk safe is to keep it clean—
that means scrupulously clean cows, clean dairies, and clean workers,
which takes a great deal of effort, time, and money.[7]

Irradiated Food

The practice of using radioactive waste material to keep food "fresh"
and kill harmful organisms has been approved by both the FDA and
U.S. Department of Agriculture (USDA) for pork, poultry, beef,
spices, grains, fruits, and vegetables. Many of these foods are sold
without special labeling, and when they are marked it is with an
innocent-looking flower symbol called the "radura." Labeling is not
required at all in food mixtures, meaning that about 80% of irradiated foods will never be labeled. For example, if you bought a can of
potato soup containing irradiated potatoes, you wouldn't know it.
Should food irradiation become a widespread or mandatory prac-

tice, even people who buy organic food may not be able to avoid it.

While proponents of food irradiation extol its supposed benefits, here are a few facts they do not tell consumers:

■ Along with bugs and bacteria, food irradiation destroys important nutrients including vitamins A, E, K, and B complexes, essential amino acids, fats, and enzymes. With irradiation, not a single component of the original whole food remains chemically unchanged.[8]

■ Food irradiation kills some, but not all, harmful bacteria. Aflatoxin, a carcinogenic substance which develops from food molds, is produced in greater quantities in irradiated food. The bacteria which causes botulism, the most fatal form of food poisoning, is not killed, but its natural enemies are. Thanks to food irradiation, there will be no characteristic warning smell when botulism is present.

Despite public protest, the government is still trying to require food irradiation. A bill introduced in September, 1997, in the U.S. House of Representatives would require the irradiation of beef. This is in response to recent numerous outbreaks of *E. coli* poisoning among meat consumers and the discovery of contaminated products in several meat-packing facilities with unsanitary handling practices.[9]

To keep informed about the **hazards of food irradiation, pesticides, and genetic engineering,** see the journal *Safe Food News,* published by Food & Water, RR1, Box 68D, Walden, VT 05873; tel: 802-563-3300; fax: 802-563-3310.

Excess Intake of
Unsaturated and Hydrogenated Fats

Most people are aware of the detrimental health effects of hydrogenated oils, such as margarine, but few know about the toxic effects of a diet high in unsaturated oils (excluding extra virgin olive oil which is high in monounsaturated fats). In fact, Americans have been led to believe that unsaturated oils are superior to saturated fats. Since all plants, seeds, nuts, beans, corn, grains, and cold water fish contain these unsaturated oils, it is virtually impossible to avoid them or to be deficient in them. Most commercial animals are fed soybeans and corn, both high in unsaturated fats, so even the so-called saturated fat in meat is highly unsaturated.

Here is a brief summary of the toxic effects of excess unsaturated oils, including polyunsaturated fatty acids (PUFAs):

■ Unsaturated oils can impair all body systems, mainly

EDITOR'S NOTE

The position on unsaturated fats presented here is a controversial one. Many physicians advocate the dietary use and supplementation of essential fatty acids in the form of fish, primrose, borage, and flaxseed oils, among others, in the unsaturated category. There is research to support both positions.

A Profile of Fats

The terms "fats" and "oils" are generally, if erroneously, used interchangeably. In the strictest sense, fat denotes lipids (fats) that are solid at room temperature, while oil means lipids that are liquid at room temperature. Fats and oils are made of building blocks called fatty acids. Structurally, a fatty acid is made of a chain of carbon atoms with hydrogen atoms attached, and an acid group of atoms at the end able to combine with glycerol. When three fatty acids attach to one molecule of glycerol, this makes a simple fat called a triglyceride. The chain of carbon atoms can be short (2-6 atoms), medium (8-10), or long (12-30). Butyric acid, found in milk fat, butter, and cream, is a short-chain fatty acid.

A fatty acid that has its full quota of hydrogen atoms is a *saturated* fatty acid; saturated fats, which include animal fats, butter, and coconut oil, tend to be solid at room temperature (lower than about 75° F).

A fatty acid with less than its full allotment of hydrogen atoms is an *unsaturated* fatty acid. Unsaturated oils come from seeds, nuts, beans, and fish. They are liquid at room temperature and include soybean, safflower, sesame, canola, flaxseed, corn, salmon, cod liver, borage, and evening primrose oils, among others. When a fatty acid lacks only two hydrogen atoms, it is a *monounsaturated* fatty acid. Monounsaturated oils, such as extra virgin olive oil, contain mostly saturated fats. A fatty acid lacking four or more hydrogen atoms is a *polyunsaturated* fatty acid or PUFA. Linoleic acid, found in corn, beans, and some nuts and seeds, is a PUFA.

Partially hydrogenated oils, such as margarine, are formulated by a process called hydrogenation, which involves the chemical addition of hydrogen to cause the oil to become solid.

by inhibiting enzymes essential to digestive and metabolic processes required for health and immune protection; unsaturated oils can directly kill white blood cells.[10]

■ Unsaturated oils inhibit protease enzymes and this interferes with many important enzyme processes, including the digestion of dietary protein, the elimination of clots, and the healthy function of the thyroid gland.[11]

■ Circulating unsaturated oils can lead to insulin resistance, and a diet high in safflower oil may cause diabetes.[12]

■ Unsaturated oils inhibit thyroid function and vitamin E metabolism, promote age spots and clot formation, and aggravate seizures.[13]

■ Unsaturated oils are so immunosuppressive that they are now advocated as a way to prevent graft rejection.[14]

■ Excess unsaturated fats are cardiotoxic, especially when combined with low thyroid function.[15]

■ Unsaturated oils are essential for the growth of tumors, and are present in high concentrations in cancer cells.[16] In addition, tumor cells secrete a chemical that allows unsaturated fats to be released from the tissues, thus guaranteeing their supply until the fat tissues are depleted.[17]

■ Unsaturated fats cause both skin aging and an increased sensitivity to ultraviolet damage. Unsaturated fats and their oxidized products are involved in the process that causes ultraviolet light-induced skin cancer.[18]

■ The USDA has issued a recommendation against the use of soy oil in infant formulas because of studies showing that unsaturated oils interfere with learning and behavior. Yet, soybean oil is still present in soymilk formulas.[19]

Good Fats

Due to the harmful effects of unsaturated oils, I recommend only three types of fats or oils: extra virgin olive oil; organic, preferably raw, butter; and coconut oil. Many understand the first two, but cringe at the thought of eating coconut oil, due to undeserved media criticism.

Coconut oil has been used as a cooking oil for thousands of years. Coconut oil is so stable that, even after one year at room temperature, it shows no evidence of rancidity.[20] Unsaturated oils in cooked foods become rancid in a few hours, even in the refrigerator—one reason for the stale taste of leftovers.

Over the past 40 years, Americans have increased their consumption of unsaturated fats and partially hydrogenated fats and have decreased their consumption of saturated fatty acids. With coconut oil one of the casualties of this switch, people are no longer reaping its many health benefits, which include the following:

■ Coconut oil has antiseptic properties.[21] In particular, it contains 40% lauric acid, a potent antibacterial also present in breast milk.[22] The body converts lauric acid to a substance that protects infants from infections. A number of studies have confirmed the protective qualities of lauric acid against bacteria, viruses, yeasts, and fungi.[23] With the demise of coconut oil as the main oil used in cooking, lauric acid is rarely present in the American diet.

■ Coconut oil lowers cholesterol, a direct result of its thyroid-stimulating properties.[24] In the presence of adequate thyroid hormone, cholesterol (SEE QUICK DEFINITION) is converted by enzymatic

Pregnenolone repairs certain enzymes, helps restore hormones which decline during aging, protects from cortisone toxicity, relieves anxiety and panic attacks, enhances memory, improves concentration, reduces mental fatigue, and generally keeps the brain functioning at peak capacity.

processes to the vitally necessary anti-aging steroids, pregnenolone, progesterone, and DHEA (SEE QUICK DEFINITIONS).[25] These substances are required to help prevent heart disease, senility, obesity, cancer and other conditions associated with aging and chronic degenerative diseases.

■ Coconut oil has properties that stimulate weight loss—another result of its thyroid-stimulating attributes. Farmers discovered this when they used coconut oil to fatten their animals but found instead that it made them lean, active, and hungrier. That's why they switched to soybeans and corn which are high in unsaturated oils. It was a cheap way to fatten their animals.[26]

■ Coconut oil may help ward off cancer. Since the 1920s, studies have shown an association between consumption of unsaturated oils and an increased incidence of cancer.[27] In cancers of the colon and breast chemically induced in rats, coconut oil was by far more protective than unsaturated oils. For example, 32% of corn-oil eaters got colon cancer, compared to only 3% of coconut-oil eaters.[28]

Cooking at High Temperatures

Even if you scrupulously buy organic whole foods, they must be prepared with care to preserve their enzyme content. Cooking at temperatures higher than 118° F—much lower than the normal cooking temperature for preparing soups or baking casseroles, for example—destroys enzymes. One of the primary signals of enzyme deficiency due to cooking is a condition called digestive leukocytosis. *Leukocytosis* simply means that there is an increase in the number of white blood cells circulating in the blood, a sign that the immune system is mobilizing. It accompanies many adverse conditions, including infections and food poisoning.

Digestive leukocytosis occurs about 30 minutes after eating cooked or processed foods. While it may seem strange that your immune system mobilizes every time you pop cooked food into your mouth, the process is actually simple. When you eat cooked or refined foods, your white blood cell count rises dramatically within half an hour because enzymes are carried on white blood cells. If the body is lacking in enzymes to digest food, white blood cells come to the rescue. This continuous mobilization of your immune system will eventually weaken it.

The preparation of your food is also a crucial factor in how many white blood cells have to troop out to help with the digestive process. In general:

- Raw organic foods produce no increase in white blood cell count.
- Common stovetop or oven-cooked foods cause a mild leukocytosis.
- Pressure-cooked or canned foods produce moderate leukocytosis.
- Processed foods and beverages, including candy, refined carbohydrates (such as white flour and sugar), and soft drinks produce severe leukocytosis. Processed meats, such as all deli meats, can cause a rise in the white blood cell count equivalent to that observed in cases of food poisoning. Microwaved foods (discussed below) fit into this category as well, since microwaving dramatically alters the molecular structure of the food and destroys enzymes.

Remember, however, that a few foods, including seeds, nuts, grains, and beans, contain enzyme inhibitors and must be cooked, soaked, or sprouted before eating. Cruciferous vegetables (cabbage, broccoli, cauliflower, and Brussels sprouts) contain thyroid inhibitors and should be steamed before eating.[29] Meat should also be cooked, due

QUICK DEFINITION

Progesterone is a female sex hormone (produced in the *corpus luteum* of the ovaries) which prepares the uterus for a fertilized egg and then stops the cell proliferation in the uterus if pregnancy does not occur. When estrogen is high, during days seven to 14 of a woman's cycle, the level of progesterone is at its lowest. Its levels climb to a peak from around days 14 to 24, and then dramatically drop off again just before the start of menstruation. When the cells stop producing progesterone, it's a signal to the uterus to let go of all the new cells produced during the month and to start afresh. In a sense, menstruation is progesterone withdrawal. Starting at age 35, a woman's progesterone production begins to decline.

DHEA (dehydroepiandrosterone) is naturally produced by the human adrenal glands and gonads with optimal levels occurring around age 20 for women and age 25 for men. After those ages, DHEA levels gradually decline. DHEA is an antioxidant, hormone regulator, and the building block from which estrogen and testosterone are produced. Low DHEA levels have been associated with cancer, diabetes, multiple sclerosis, hypertension, obesity, AIDS, heart disease, Alzheimer's, and immune dysfunction illnesses. Excess DHEA (more than 15 mg daily) in the body can convert to estrogen and thus contribute to hormonal imbalance. The safest way to raise DHEA levels is by supplementing with its precursor, the hormone pregnenolone.

to the unsanitary practices in meat and poultry processing plants. Other than these exceptions, I advise that you "eat it raw."

Microwaving

Microwave ovens affect your health in two ways: by emitting electromagnetic radiation into your immediate environment, and by destroying not only the enzymes in food, but the nutritional value of the food itself.

The first of these dangers consists of two types of radiation: the microwaves or high-frequency radio waves, and the magnetic fields common to other home appliances. The oven door is the most dangerous place for microwave leakage but magnetic fields can occur all around the oven. This is especially dangerous for children who like to watch the food bubbling inside, and restaurant workers, who are often stationed nearby.

While people may worry about whether their microwave ovens leak, few consider the effects of microwaves on the food itself. These include: destruction of enzymes and nutrients, transformation of nutrients into toxic substances and/or carcinogens, and leakage of toxic chemicals from the packaging into the food.[30]

Radiation and Electromagnetic Fields

In addition to microwave ovens, other sources of radiation in our environment can deplete enzymes from our bodies. These include ionizing radiation, such as that emitted by nuclear reactors, and nonionizing radiation, such as the electromagnetic fields (EMFs) of common electrical appliances and geopathic zones (see below).

EMFs contain both electric and magnetic components; the magnetic component is believed to cause the most damage to the body. EMFs come from all electronic devices including battery-powered appliances, microwave ovens, microwave transmitting towers, radar (including police radar guns), radio frequencies, televisions, video display terminals (VDTs), power lines, and cellular telephones, among other sources.

Such devices can be especially dangerous since we use them and work with them on a daily basis, and sleep near them at night. Radiation weakens the immune system, causes free radical proliferation in the body, and leads to a variety of catastrophic illnesses, including cancer. Damage can occur to whatever parts of the body are exposed to

You can **test the magnetic fields** in your home when the power is on and at peak times of power output by using a simple device called a Trifield Meter. For information, contact: BEFIT Enterprises, P.O. Box 2143, Southampton, NY 11969; tel: 800-497-9516 or 516-287-3813.

radiation. For example, people who use cellular telephones might develop brain tumors. Male police officers who use radar speed detectors may get testicular cancer. VDT users can harm their head, face, and upper body, and a child who sits closer than six feet from the television is exposed to a harmful level of EMFs.[31]

Geopathic Stress Zones

Another source of non-ionizing radiation comes from geopathic stress zones. These zones are long, narrow bands of radiation coming from the earth itself. While the exact origin of geopathic stress zones is uncertain, they seem to be associated with geological fractures and subterranean water veins. When situated below a home, this magnetic radiation can have harmful health effects, including immune suppression and respiratory difficulties, on the occupants. Since the zones are often very small areas, shifting a bed just a few feet in a geopathically troubled bedroom could make a great difference in a person's health.[32]

Any form of radiation, including geopathic zones, directly affects the enzymes in the cells by causing mutations in the cell which can, in time, lead to illness, including cancer. Long-term exposure to geopathic radiation can damage DNA which weakens the immune system and lays the groundwork for chronic degenerative diseases.

In one study of 500 people with benign and malignant tumors, all of them slept over geopathic radiation zones. Another study showed that 95% of 3,000 learning-disabled children were exposed to geopathic radiation. This form of radiation has also been strongly associated with numerous degenerative illnesses, including heart disease, multiple sclerosis, asthma, arthritis, and cataracts.[33]

Fluoridated Water

Before you turn on the tap to fill a cooking pot with water, remember this: unless you are using pure water, you are steaming organic vegetables and boiling whole-grain rice in contaminated fluid.

Tap water is filled with dozens of unsavory substances. One of the most harmful may be fluoride which is added to our water because it supposedly prevents tooth decay. However, a study of more than 39,000 schoolchildren, five to 17 years old, in 84 geographical areas across the U.S., showed no relationship between tooth decay rates and fluoridation. In fact, the lowest tooth-decay rate reported occurred in

Any form of radiation, including geopathic zones, directly affects the enzymes in the cells by causing mutations in the cell which can, in time, lead to illness, including cancer. Long-term exposure can damage DNA which weakens the immune system and lays the groundwork for chronic degenerative diseases.

a nonfluoridated area.[34]

Not only does fluoride have no effect on preventing cavities, it is harmful to your health. Fluoride poisons enzymes, inhibits the thyroid gland, damages the immune system, makes minerals such as calcium and magnesium unavailable to the body, increases the risk of bone cancer and other bone problems such as osteoporosis, and, in some people, can cause seizures. Fluoride also increases the risk of autoimmune diseases, such as lupus and rheumatoid arthritis, and the incidence of Down's syndrome and sudden infant death syndrome (SIDS) in newborns.[35]

To avoid the hazards of fluoride, the best solution is to buy bottled spring water or use a high-quality water purification system in your home. Unfortunately, carbon filters—the most popular filters on the market—remove some of the odor, chlorine, bacteria, and particulates, but they don't remove fluoride. The more expensive reverse osmosis filters and ion-exchange systems can. Be alerted, however, that fluoride is not just in tap water, but is used to grow crops and in the preparation of processed foods, soft drinks, and beer.

Heavy Metals

Heavy metals are also prolific in our tap water as well as in our commercial food supply. Loosely defined as minerals, which at certain levels interfere with the vital functions of the body, heavy metals inhibit the actions of enzymes. Several of these metals (aluminum, cadmium, lead, and mercury) have no known biological role. Others, such as nickel, are believed to be essential at very low concentrations but toxic at high concentrations. Iron and copper have known biological functions, but are toxic at certain levels.

Toxic levels of heavy metals end up in drinking water primarily due to industrial chemical plants that discharge wastes into water, and from pesticides and herbicides used in commercial agriculture, which then seep into the ground water supply. Other sources of heavy metals are paints, ceramics, dental fillings (see below), and

Environmental Hazard Questionnaire

No matter how healthy your diet is, you may be subjected to environmental or other influences which can deplete enzymes. Put a check mark next to each of the following questions to which you can answer 'yes'. If you have more than several check marks, environmental hazards may be contributing to enzyme deficiencies, depending upon your degree of exposure.

_____Is untreated tap water your major source of water?

_____Is your drinking water fluoridated?

_____Do you have mercury amalgam fillings?

_____Do you have root canals?

_____Do you use a toothpaste containing fluoride, or do you get fluoride treatments at your dental office?

_____Do you microwave your foods, or frequently eat at restaurants where microwave ovens are in use?

_____Do you use a computer more than ten hours a week?

_____Are you living within 100 feet of high-power lines?

_____Do you drive more than one hour per day?

_____Do you smoke?

_____Do you work in a building that is energy-efficient, such as a high-rise with no open windows?

_____Are you exposed to toxic chemicals in your workplace?

_____Do you wear sunglasses or tinted contact lenses?

_____Do you live near or downwind of a nuclear plant, toxic waste dump, or garbage incinerator?

certain drugs. All heavy metals can cause severe reactions, depending upon the degree of exposure, and can be fatal if ingested at their toxic levels.

To purify your tap water, reverse osmosis filters, ion-exchange systems, and some carbon filters are reasonably effective at removing heavy metals. A note of caution: heavy metals readily collect in carbon filters and contaminate them, so it's crucial to change the filter frequently or you will be getting an even more concentrated amount of metals in your water.

Mercury Amalgam Dental Fillings

Mercury amalgam fillings have been the subject of much contro-

Why are root canals dangerous? Mainly because they create an infection in the body that must be combated by enzymes—thereby depleting precious enzyme reserves.

versy in the past two decades. Countless clinical studies have shown their deleterious effects. Problems are caused by the mercury contained in the filling material—sometimes as much as 50% of a filling is composed of mercury—as well as other toxic metals in the amalgam, which can leak into the body and wreak havoc.

The American Dental Association claims that mercury does not leak out of fillings into the body, but research contradicts that position. A recent study found evidence of mercury uptake from the teeth into the lungs, the gastrointestinal tract, and jaw tissue, after less than a month. Once absorbed at these sites, high concentrations of mercury rapidly localize in the kidneys and the liver.[36]

Other research indicates that mercury can transform a normal bacterial organism into one that is resistant to antibiotics. Also, there is evidence of a direct effect of mercury amalgams on the suppression of protective white blood cells.[37]

The pathology of mercury poisoning is complicated because mercury binds to many different sites in the body. For example, mercury is especially attracted to sulfur and there are a number of "sulfur sites" in the body. Sulfur is found in red blood cells, heart muscle, and in portions of the cells that control genetic reproduction. Mercury will poison any enzymes containing sulfur, including those involved in the formation of insulin, the ability of blood to clot, and processes related to DNA.

For information about **mercury detoxification**, see *Alternative Medicine Guide to Chronic Fatigue, Fibromyalgia, and Environmental Illness* (Future Medicine Publishing, 1998; ISBN 1-887299-11-4); to order, call 800-333-HEAL.

Additionally, mercury suppresses thyroid function by poisoning the enzyme required to produce the active form of the thyroid hormone (T3) from the inactive form (T4). Mercury poisoning has the curious talent of being able to mimic certain diseases, including multiple sclerosis, rheumatoid arthritis, arthritis, scleroderma, and lupus.

Root Canals

Dental root canals were found to be extremely toxic as long as 100 years ago. Even so, in 1994, dentists placed 24 million root canals into the mouths of Americans to save their diseased teeth. It was Weston Price, D.D.S., who discovered the root canal/disease connection after performing hundreds of root canals on patients and noticing that nearly three-quarters of these clients began to develop illnesses and disease after the procedure. He also found that the health of nearly all of his patients improved after root canals were removed.

Why are root canals dangerous? Mainly because they create an infection in the body that must be combated by enzymes—thereby depleting precious enzyme reserves. Dr. Price postulates that a person can have an infection in one location in the body, and the bacteria involved can subsequently be transported through the bloodstream to another gland or tissue to create a new infection. He found that 95% of infections started in the teeth and the tonsils, and showed how bacteria trapped in the tonsils and teeth change form, multiply, and infect other organs of the body, including the eyes, heart, kidneys, lungs, and stomach—much like the metastasis of cancer from one part of the body to another.

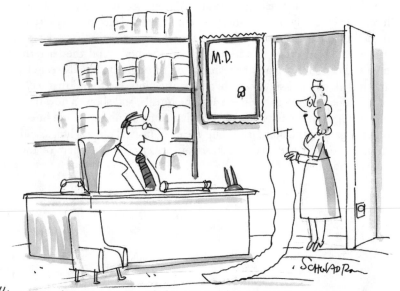

"TELL MRS. ADDAMS TO MAKE AN APPOINTMENT AND TO STOP FAXING US HER SYMPTOMS."

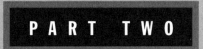

PART TWO

An A-Z of Health Conditions

with Enzyme Therapy Success Stories

AN A-Z OF HEALTH CONDITIONS
with Enzyme Therapy Success Stories

I n this guide to health conditions, I describe specific problems along with the enzymes and other supplements used to treat them. Conditions are illustrated by patient success stories from my many years of clinical practice as an enzyme therapist. All patient histories are documented and, of course, patient names have been changed to protect privacy.

These case histories clearly show the importance of enzymes in digestion, in supporting the immune system, and in nourishing the body in general. While the Thera-zyme line of enzyme formulas I use in treating these conditions is available only to health-care professionals, corresponding formulas in a consumer line of enzyme formulas for those who prefer the self-care approach can be found in Appendix B.

For complete information on the **products** mentioned throughout the A-Z section of health conditions, see Appendix D. For details on **enzyme formulations** used as treatment, see Appendix B. For details on **24-hour urine analysis and other tests** performed by an enzyme therapist, see Chapter 2: Diagnosing Enzyme Deficiencies.

A word of caution: don't assume that if you have a health problem similar to one in a patient history, that the same enzymes prescribed will be right for you. Symptoms can indicate a number of conditions. For example, bloating and gas are not always indicative of candidiasis—they also occur in people with digestive problems. One enzyme formula is appropriate for candidiasis, another for whatever specific digestive problem you might have. In order to determine the best enzyme formulas for your particular condition, it is important to have a 24-hour urine analysis performed by a professional enzyme therapist (see Appendix C for a list of practitioners).

ALLERGIES

An allergy is an adverse immune system reaction to an undigested food or to an environmental substance that cannot be neutralized (detoxified) by the lymphatic system. In other words, whatever cannot be digested or detoxified becomes a poison. Environmental allergies encompass just about any substance in the environment, from the pollen of flowers, trees, weeds, and grasses, to air pollution, auto exhaust, household or industrial chemicals, paint fumes, smoke, dust, and animals.

Allergic reactions go beyond the familiar sneezing, watery eyes, stuffy nose, and dark circles under the eyes associated with allergies. An allergy, whether to food or to something in the environment, can produce a wide array of symptoms, including flatulence, burping, headache, stomachache, nausea, vomiting, intestinal irritation or swelling, rashes or hives, fatigue, and dizziness.

Allergies can also cause more serious reactions such as asthma attacks, seizures, and life-threatening anaphylactic shock (a severe and sometimes fatal allergic reaction, characterized by a sharp drop in blood pressure, hives, and breathing difficulties). The allergic reaction may not be immediate, making it difficult to identify the allergen (the substance causing the reaction). In fact, many people are not even aware that they have an allergy.

What Causes Allergies?

Generally, whether a reaction comes from something you eat, breathe, or absorb through the skin, allergies arise from enzyme deficiencies, either inherent or aggravated by dietary excess. Constant exposure to allergens, whether undigested food or environmental substances, weakens the body and lays the groundwork for diseases of all kinds. First, the body is undernourished, since food is not being properly digested. Second, digestive enzyme deficiencies put stress on the pancreas which tries to make up for the lack and the inadequate digestion. Third, enzyme deficiencies tax the immune system, which attempts to get rid of the undigested food that has leaked from the intestines into the bloodstream and is now viewed by the body as a toxin.

For information on the **enzymes** for this health condition, see Appendix B.

A number of factors can cause digestive enzyme depletion. The most obvious ones are: eating too much of one

Generally, whether a reaction comes from something you eat, breathe, or absorb through the skin, allergies arise from enzyme deficiencies, either inherent or aggravated by dietary excess.

For more about **substances that poison enzymes,** see Chapter 3: What Causes Enzyme Deficiencies?

kind of food; and eating foods in which the digestive enzymes have been destroyed by cooking, refining, or processing. There are also substances that poison, inhibit, or destroy one or more of the thousands of metabolic enzymes made by the body. These include most conventional drugs (such as antibiotics and vaccinations), agricultural chemicals (found in pesticides, herbicides, and synthetic fertilizers), and environmental poisons (such as fluoride in tap water or carbon monoxide in the air).

Success Story: Ending Five Years of Infections, Antibiotics, and Severe Allergies

Debbie, 10, had become increasingly sick since the age of five, with the onset of severe food allergies which led to headaches, stomachaches, and nausea. She also had frequent infections which were treated with repeated courses of antibiotics. In the year prior to consulting me, she had missed 47 days of school because of illness. In the month prior, she had been sick for almost three weeks. Debbie had undergone numerous tests, including for mononucleosis, parasites, and urinary tract infections, all of which produced negative results.

Debbie was so allergic to fruit that even smelling an apple would cause a severe allergic reaction. Two minutes after eating one, her cheeks would flush, her eyes would glaze over, her tongue would swell up, and she would get a severe headache and stomachache, and occasionally vomiting. Her known allergies included all fruits, especially citrus, salicylates (in aspirin, dyes, and skin cleansers), cream of tartar (in baking powder and hard candy), malic acid (in apples, grapes, and rhubarb), food colorings, most preservatives, almonds, peanuts, celery, cucumbers, beans, salad dressings, olive oil, and tomatoes.

An extensive health evaluation revealed that Debbie had a history of consuming highly processed foods. In addition, her symptoms had become extreme after she received her second set of vaccinations when she was five years old. Immediately following the shots, which included diphtheria, pertussis, tetanus, polio, measles, mumps, rubella, tuberculosis, and the haemophilus B polysaccharide vaccine, Debbie nearly passed out and then became ill. The 24-hour urine analysis revealed a severe vitamin C deficiency as well as fat, sugar, and protein intolerance. Further testing showed liver problems. In short, Debbie was severely enzyme depleted and could not tolerate even healthy, unprocessed foods.

I prescribed an organic, whole-foods diet for Debbie and cautioned her to avoid refined, processed foods. Along with these dietary changes, I recommended the following enzyme formulas:

- Thera-zyme HCL: multiple digestive formula for fat, sugar, and protein intolerance
- Thera-zyme Opt: for vitamin C deficiency
- Thera-zyme Kdy: for allergies
- Thera-zyme Lvr: to support the liver

After one month, her mother reported great improvement in Debbie's condition—she felt much better, had grown half an inch taller, and had regained her spunk and vitality. Debbie's case illustrates some of the possible deleterious effects of processed foods, vaccinations, and overuse of conventional drugs, such as antibiotics.

Success Story: Stopping Stevens-Johnson Syndrome

When she walked into my office, Eileen, 45, looked like a burn victim. She had a high fever, a full body rash, and ongoing eye infections—all the classic symptoms of Stevens-Johnson syndrome, a severe and often fatal allergic reaction to a common synthetic drug or chemical, characterized by rash and blisters. Eileen, on a visit from her native Ireland, had taken the antibiotic Septra® to get rid of a lung infection before her trip. Although a fever and rash had developed after the first round, her doctor prescribed a second round, and she had just finished it when she arrived in the United States.

Her urine test indicated the need for Thera-zyme Bil (multiple digestive formula for fat intolerance and gallbladder problems), Thera-zyme MSCLR (natural antihistamine), Thera-zyme Lvr (to cleanse her liver), Thera-zyme TRMA (the major immune system formula used for any sort of infection or skin trauma), and Thera-zyme Kdy (to help relieve her allergic symptoms).

In the normal course of Stevens-Johnson syndrome, blisters develop after the fever and rash; this never happened to Eileen, probably because she started taking enzymes early enough. By the time her visit was over, her condition had stabilized and she was able to travel home without further incidence.

Vitamin and mineral deficiencies develop in a relatively short period of time—60 to 90 days—but enzyme deficiencies take longer to develop. When an allergic reaction occurs, an enzyme deficiency has likely existed for months or even years prior to its onset.

Success Story: Controlling a Bug-Bite Allergy

The antihistamine effect of amylase (the enzyme that digests carbo-hydrates) is excellent for a reaction to any type of bug bite or bee sting. Normally, I do not use this treatment as a preventive measure, but one patient's allergy was severe enough to warrant it.

Sally, 13, was terrified of bugs, including mosquitoes, because each bite would produce a severe lesion with scabbing and scarring. Her mother requested help for an upcoming family trip to South America. I gave Sally a bottle of Thera-zyme MSCLR, a natural antihistamine which is high in amylase (three capsules, three times daily), along with Thera-zyme Lvr for cleansing her liver (two cap-sules, three times daily). She took both formulas with her to South America and returned home with no sores or scars.

Prevention and Elimination of Allergies

The following are recommendations for preventing and treating allergies. They will vary according to the specific enzyme and dietary deficiencies of the sufferer.

Enzyme Therapy

A common misconception is that vitamin and mineral supplements will make up for dietary deficiencies. The fact is, without enzymes, nothing works in the body, no matter how well formulated the sup-plement might be. If food is not completely digested, the body does not get the full complement of nutrients it needs. That's why people with food allergies often have accompanying vitamin and mineral deficiencies. Enzymes, ingested either in the form of raw, whole organic foods or supplements, optimize digestion, and not only can the allergy disappear, but the accompanying vitamin and mineral deficiency as well.

Vitamin and mineral deficiencies develop in a relatively short period of time—60 to 90 days of depleted dietary intake—but enzyme deficiencies take longer to develop, simply because the body has so many compensation mechanisms. When an allergic reaction occurs, an enzyme deficiency has likely existed for months or even years prior to its onset.

Under the guidance of an enzyme therapist, find out what digestive problems—that is, enzyme deficiencies—you have. Determine which foods are hardest for you to digest: proteins, fats, carbohydrates, sugars, or fibers. Then, limit these foods in your diet, while taking the food enzymes required to digest them.

One of the main enzyme therapies I use addresses the kidney-lymphatic system, because chronic allergies, with their attendant toxins, put stress on it. Fortunately, enzyme formulas can help the kidneys get rid of circulating immune complexes (CICs, SEE QUICK DEFINITION) which form when food is not completely digested. Eliminating CICs reduces kidney-lymphatic stress and does away with the pain resulting from a chronically overloaded kidney.

Thera-zyme Kdy contains enzymes plus herbs with antiseptic, blood-cleansing, and lymphatic-cleansing properties. People requiring this type of nutritional support may have environmental allergies characterized by sneezing, nasal congestion, itching or watery eyes, sinus problems with a clear, watery discharge, and swollen lymph glands. They may also have one or more of the following symptoms: frontal headaches, low back or kidney pain, low blood sugar, and sometimes nausea and vomiting. When the CICs are cleared from the blood and lymphatics, these symptoms are also cleared.

Not only children and adults, but also nursing babies with severe environmental allergies manifesting as swollen, red, watery eyes and noses, show a remarkable reduction of these symptoms within hours of ingesting this formula. Symptoms can be held in check with a minimum maintenance program.

An enzyme therapist can determine the need for kidney support by comparing the volume and specific gravity of a 24-hour collection of urine. The specific gravity indicates the amount (concentration) of dissolved materials (solutes) in the urine. Ordinarily, the specific gravity increases with low fluid intake and decreases with high fluid intake.

People who need the kidney formula may exhibit either a normal (four to nine cups) or low (less than four

QUICK DEFINITION

Circulating immune complexes (CICs) form in the body when poor digestion results in undigested foods "leaking" through the intestinal wall and into the bloodstream. The immune system treats these foreign substances or antigens as invaders, causing antibodies to form and couple with them. This antigen and antibody combination is known as a CIC. In a healthy person, CICs are neutralized, but in someone with a compromised immune system, they tend to accumulate in the blood where they burden the detoxification pathways or initiate an allergic reaction. If too many CICs accumulate, the kidneys cannot excrete enough of them via the urine. The CICs are then stored in soft tissues, causing inflammation and bringing stress to the immune system. The overload can lead to a variety of chronic health conditions.

cups) 24-hour urine volume with a low specific gravity. This is a sign that the kidneys are not cleansing the blood properly, an indication of kidney-lymphatic stress. Urine analysis does not indicate the extent or longevity of this condition. However, the longer it has been occurring, the more likely the person is to exhibit symptoms.

Common symptoms of needing Kdy include swollen glands, nausea, and rashes; when Thera-zyme TRMA is indicated, symptoms include a fever and rashes. I have seen all of these symptoms disappear within 30 minutes to a few hours of taking the enzyme formula.

Most patients need enzymatic "drainage" formulas, which include Kdy and sometimes TRMA. Taken on an empty stomach, enzymes digest toxins in the blood. When an enzyme digests "junk" (undigested foods, CICs, bacterial debris, or certain viruses) in your blood, you must be able to eliminate the digested junk via your kidneys or colon. If not, it will manifest as a skin rash, fever, or other unpleasant symptom. Many of these symptoms can be relieved with either Kdy or TRMA; both of these formulas help the body to eliminate toxins of any kind.

The usual dose of Kdy is three capsules between meals, three times daily; of TRMA, four capsules between meals, three times daily. TRMA is contraindicated in people with gastric problems, such as ulcers.

Finally, in very severe cases of allergies, Thera-zyme MSCLR which is high in amylase (digests carbohydrates), can be taken along with the Kdy formula. MSCLR is a potent, natural antihistamine. The usual dosage is three capsules, three times daily between meals.

Dietary Recommendations

For more **dietary rec-ommendations**, see "Guidelines for Healthy Eating," Chapter 1: Why Enzymes?, pp. 26-27.

Eat a wide variety of organic, whole, unprocessed foods, including fresh fruits and vegetables, whole grains, beans, organic eggs, organic poultry or beef, and raw, unpasteurized milk and dairy products.

APPENDICITIS

Appendicitis is an acute or chronic inflammation (presence of leukocytes, or pus) with or without infection (presence of bacteria) of the appendix, medically termed the vermiform appendix and located at the cecal end of the large intestine, or colon.

Chronic appendicitis seems to be a common condition, even among young children. Symptoms vary widely and often go unrecognized. They may range from vague complaints such as mild nausea or stomachache, slight headache, and a general feeling of malaise, to severe abdominal pains without fever, severe nausea or vomiting, and chronic vomiting episodes without fever or pain. While acute appendicitis symptoms include nausea and vomiting, it is usually, but not always, accompanied by fever and extreme pain. Another difference between the two conditions is that in chronic appendicitis symptoms disappear between episodes. In acute appendicitis, the symptoms do not disappear and the condition can be fatal without surgery.

CAUTION

Please remember that unattended acute appendicitis is highly dangerous. For acute appendicitis, which includes symptoms of nausea, vomiting, extreme pain, and, most importantly, fever, get emergency help.

In much of Europe, chronic appendicitis is a recognized health condition and is often treated with both antibiotics and nutritional remedies. Surgery is avoided unless the condition is judged to be life threatening. In America, most doctors do not recognize chronic appendicitis and the general opinion is that all cases of appendicitis are acute, requiring surgery. However, there are American health practitioners who believe chronic appendicitis can be reversed with diet and nutritional therapy. Unfortunately, most people who have chronic appendicitis don't realize it until it has developed into a life-threatening condition.

For information on the **enzymes** for this health condition, see Appendix B.

What Causes Chronic Appendicitis?

Appendicitis, whether chronic or acute, can be caused by a low-fiber, junk-food diet, a toxic colon from long-standing poor digestion, or chronic constipation. It can also follow a viral or bacterial infection.

Success Story: Two Years of Pain and Chronic Nausea Reversed

Emma, 40, consulted me for help with kidney stones, severe fatigue, bone pain, and constipation, along with a weight gain of 60 pounds over a five-year period. However, her most disturbing symptom was chronic vomiting lasting two to three hours once a week, which had persisted for almost two years. She had no pain, abdominal cramping, or fever—only disorientation, weakness, and nausea prior to each episode. She could not correlate these symptoms with anything; they occurred whether she ate or fasted.

When first tested, Emma was in such overall pain that it was difficult to prioritize her needs. During her third visit, I suspected that she might have chronic appendicitis. It was the medical "jump start" test for appendicitis that alerted me to her condition. This test consists of palpating the lower right abdominal area and then quickly withdrawing the fingers. If it hurts more when the fingers are pulled away than when they are pressed into this area, it is a good indication of appendicitis, whether chronic or acute. When I performed this test on Emma, she nearly leapt from the table and said that it felt like I'd just "ripped out" her organs.

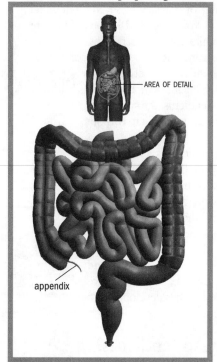

AREA OF DETAIL

appendix

THE APPENDIX. The appendix, located at the cecal end of the large intestine, or colon, can develop an acute or chronic inflammation, producing pain, nausea, vomiting, or fever. While acute appendicitis requires immediate medical intervention, chronic appendicitis may be treated with alternative methods including enzymes.

Confirming the palpation test results, Emma's urine analysis indicated chronic appendicitis, along with severe stomach irritation, possibly an ulcer, and severe kidney-lymphatic stress (allergies). These were Emma's most immediate problems and, since pathology rules, I could not treat her other problems, such as bone pain, weight gain, and nutritional deficiencies, until I had dealt with them.

I gave her Thera-zyme Stm, a multiple digestive enzyme formula for people who have stomach problems and cannot tolerate protease, which Emma's test also revealed was the case with her.

Maintain optimum digestion with a multiple digestive enzyme formula that addresses your particular digestive weaknesses: protein, fat, carbohydrate, sugar, or fiber intolerance. Whatever you don't digest can cause constipation, diarrhea, and other toxic colon problems.

(Stm is the only multiple digestive enzyme formula devoid of protease.) Emma needed TRMA for her immune system and to combat any infection arising from the appendicitis, but since she could not tolerate its high level of protease, I instead gave her Citricidal, a nontoxic antimicrobial extract of grapefruit seed and pulp.

To help treat her intestinal problems, Emma took Thera-zyme SmI, which helps relieve a toxic colon as well as constipation or diarrhea (or both) and parasites. For her kidney-lymphatic stress, I gave her Thera-zyme Kdy.

Emma improved her diet and took her remedies faithfully. Her vomiting stopped almost immediately. She also started to lose weight, even though she was not dieting. The enzyme therapies and switch to a wholefoods diet completely alleviated her two-year history of pain and nausea.

Prevention and Elimination of Chronic Appendicitis

The following are general guidelines for preventing appendicitis and for reversing chronic cases.

Enzyme Therapy

Maintain optimum digestion with a multiple digestive enzyme formula that addresses your particular digestive weaknesses: protein, fat, carbohydrate, sugar, or fiber intolerance—or a combination of these. Whatever you don't digest can cause constipation, diarrhea, and other toxic colon problems. In addition to your special multiple digestive enzyme formula, I recommend the following major enzyme formulas to prevent appendicitis, as well as colon problems:

■ Thera-zyme SmI (small intestine): for toxic colon, diarrhea, constipation or both (alternating), parasites, and yeast/fungal infections including candidiasis

■ Thera-zyme LgI (large intestine): mainly for constipation

■ Thera-zyme TRMA (trauma): an immune-system formula, for bacterial/viral infections and parasites

Thyroid Support

Make sure your thyroid gland is functioning well. An underactive thyroid gland (hypothyroidism) causes many colon problems, including constipation and a toxic colon, which, as mentioned, can lead to appendicitis. If testing determines that your thyroid function is low, seek the advice of a health professional. If treatment is needed, I recommend a thyroid glandular extract. (See Appendix A.)

Soil-based organisms (SBOs) are beneficial microbes, or probiotics, found in soil. Before chemical farming, the earth was rich in these organisms which naturally destroyed molds, yeast, fungi, and viruses in the soil. Transmitted in the food supply to humans, SBOs perform the same function in the human body, working with the "friendly" bacteria (such as *Lactobacillus acidophilus* and *Bifidobacterium bifidum*) inhabiting the gastrointestinal tract to maintain balance in the intestinal flora and thus ensure a healthy digestive system. Since soil has become depleted of SBOs, the ratio of good to bad bacteria in the intestines has become skewed and a host of health problems, including allergies, candidiasis, hormonal dysfunction, and Crohn's disease, among other gastrointestinal conditions, are the result.

Dietary Recommendations

Eat an organic, whole-foods diet. This provides adequate fiber to maintain a healthy colon and to prevent constipation which can arise from a no- or low-fiber diet. Do not think you can eat junk foods and make up for it by taking a fiber formula. Eating fibers such as brans, isolated from wheat or oats, is very different from eating whole foods containing these fibers and, in fact, can irritate the colon. Raw carrots should be eaten on a daily basis. If you can't eat them raw (an indication of enzyme deficiencies), cook them. Carrot fiber binds many intestinal toxins that, left in the colon, can lead to appendicitis and other diseases.

Nutritional Supplements

■ Citricidal (grapefruit seed and pulp extract): nontoxic antimicrobial with the advantage that very few people are allergic to it

■ Soil-based organisms (SEE QUICK DEFINITION): an intestinal formula of beneficial bacteria from soil which helps prevent proliferation of intestinal toxins

ARTHRITIS

Arthritis is inflammation of a joint, often accompanied by swelling and pain. There are a variety of arthritic conditions, with the two most common being osteoarthritis and rheumatoid arthritis.

Osteoarthritis is a degenerative disease of the large weight-bearing joints, often associated with aging, in which small bony growths, calcium spurs, and occasional soft cysts appear on bones and in the joints. Symptoms include mild early-morning stiffness, stiffness following periods of rest, pain that worsens with joint use, loss of joint function, local tenderness, soft tissue swelling, creaking and cracking of joints on movement, and restricted mobility.

Rheumatoid arthritis, while less common than osteoarthritis, is a serious and painful joint disease, frequently resulting in crippling disability. It typically occurs in middle age, but the juvenile form tends to appear in children before the age of 16. Rheumatoid arthritis incapacitates the synovial tissue, the membrane which lines joints and secretes the lubricant allowing bones to move painlessly against each other. The joints—most commonly the small joints of the hand—then become tender and swollen, even deformed. Night sweats, fever, depression, fatigue, and lethargy are among the other symptoms.

What Causes Arthritis?

Conventional wisdom holds that arthritis is a natural result of the aging process. This equates aging with disease, an inaccurate assumption. Like any other chronic degenerative disease, osteoarthritis has its roots in genetic, dietary, enzymatic, hormonal, and environmental factors. In particular, osteoarthritis can result from a lifetime of eating refined foods (which contain no enzymes), repeated athletic injury, especially of the knees, and an underactive thyroid gland (hypothyroidism).[1] In menopausal women with low thyroid function, the resulting decrease in progesterone can cause osteoarthritis, in addition to other common menopausal symptoms such as hot flashes and weight gain.[2]

Rheumatoid arthritis is often classified as an autoimmune disease in which the body attacks its own tissues. From an enzymatic point of view, the body does not attack itself, but reacts to undigested foods which enter the bloodstream from the intestines; this condition of intestinal per-

For information on the **enzymes** for this health condition, see Appendix B.

Postponing the operation, Dr. Loomis focused on developing an enzyme formula that could truly relieve his arthritis. After a number of formulations, he perfected Thera-zyme OSTEO. After taking Thera-zyme OSTEO for three days, all of his pain disappeared.

meability is commonly called "leaky gut" syndrome. Any undigested food can cause an inflammatory reaction because the immune system creates circulating immune complexes (CICs, SEE QUICK DEFINITION) in response to these "foreign" invaders.

Other causes of rheumatoid arthritis include genetic susceptibility, lifestyle factors, nutritional factors, microorganisms, hypothyroidism leading to estrogen dominance, and certain vaccinations such as DPT (diphtheria, pertussis, and tetanus).

Success Story: A Doctor Heals Himself

Howard Loomis, D.C., an enzyme therapy pioneer, began to experience knee problems at the age of 14 after he was tripped while running down the court during a basketball game. He landed on his knees and skidded six feet across the hardwood floor, seriously injuring both knees. However, he continued to play basketball and baseball through college and chiropractic school, putting his knees under constant stress. During these years, he also sprained his ankles at least ten times each. Dr. Loomis played these sports well into his thirties.

As the years passed, he noticed more and more arthritic pain in his legs, feet, and, especially, knees. By the time he was 58, the pain was so severe in his knees that he scheduled orthopedic surgery—one knee at a time. Following surgery on his left knee, Dr. Loomis took Thera-zyme TRMA, his major enzyme formula for relieving postsurgical pain, swelling, and bruising (hematoma). Even so, three months passed before the pain subsided and he was able to work again.

At this point, Dr. Loomis' legs and feet had become so painful that it was difficult for him to walk without limping. He dreaded the second knee surgery and the debilitating months of recovery. Postponing the operation, he focused on developing an enzyme formula that could truly relieve his arthritis. After a number of formulations, he perfected Thera-zyme OSTEO. After taking Thera-zyme OSTEO for three days, all of his pain disappeared. Not only his knees, but his feet and legs were free of pain—even when walking. Occasionally, some stiffness reappears—a reminder that he has forgotten to take his arthritis formula.

Success Story: Crippling Arthritis Reversed

Heather received a routine DPT shot (vaccine for diphtheria-pertussis-tetanus) at the age of 12. Until that day, she had been an energetic, athletic young girl. Immediately after the shot, she became ill. Her initial problems included flu-like symptoms, a constant sore throat, chronic sinus infections, and severe fatigue. She took so many different antibiotics that she became immune to them.

Heather began to spend more and more time lying on the couch, as painful arthritic symptoms appeared. Over the next five years she was given high doses of methotrexate (used to treat rheumatoid arthritis and cancer), as well as cortisone shots, prednisone (synthetic cortisone), and nonsteroidal anti-inflammatory drugs (NSAIDs). Yet, the drugs did nothing for her symptoms and, as time passed, Heather became nearly immobilized by her arthritis. She could no longer lift her arms, her feet were severely crippled, and she walked stooped over from the pain.

Finally, at the age of 17, Heather decided to take control of her health. She stopped taking all of the drugs and consulted a naturopathic doctor who started her on a cleansing program of fresh fruits, vegetables, and high-protein foods. "This was a turning point," recounts Heather. But she still had a long way to go. That same year Heather's mother, a registered dietitian, began studying enzyme therapy. When Heather turned 18, she began an enzyme treatment program under her mother's supervision. At this point, Heather had dark circles under her eyes and was jaundiced (her skin had a yellow hue, a sign of jaundice which is an excess of bilirubin, the pigment in bile, in the blood as a result of blood or liver dysfunction). She still had only limited motion in her arms and walked bent over in severe pain.

Heather's mother gave her the following formulas:

■ Thera-zyme PAN: for sugar intolerance
■ Thera-zyme Kdy: for allergies
■ Thera-zyme TRMA: for the immune system
■ Thera-zyme Lvr: an enzymatic liver formula

In two weeks, Heather's jaundice was gone, her dark circles had disappeared, and she felt much better—but she still walked with difficulty and pain. To help her posture, she was fitted with arch supports. She put them in her shoes and stood up straight for the first time in years. The only pain now remaining was an aching in her joints, for which she took Thera-zyme OSTEO. In less than two weeks, Heather felt less overall pain. Within three months, she no longer felt pain when sitting. Now, some six months later, she still feels some pain in her left ankle when she walks, but this too is decreasing. Heather is back in school and full of energy again.

Prevention and Elimination of Arthritis

The following are guidelines useful for preventing and alleviating arthritis.

Enzyme Therapy

Each individual has specific enzyme needs, but the following formulas are generally recommended for arthritis:

- A multiple digestive enzyme formula: the major enzyme deficiency in arthritics is protease so a formula high in protease (Thera-zyme Bil or HCL) is commonly indicated; other digestive enzyme formulas such as Thera-zyme SvG, PAN, or Adr may be needed to address sugar digestion
- Thera-zyme OSTEO: for arthritic pain relief; contains pain-relieving herbs along with glucosamine and methylsulfonylmethane (MSM, an organic sulfur), essential components of connective tissue which can help reduce inflammation
- Thera-zyme Kdy: to support the immune system of people with allergies
- Thera-zyme TRMA: for immune system problems
- Thera-zyme Lvr: for liver problems

Thyroid Support

If testing determines that your thyroid function is low, seek the advice of a health professional. If treatment is needed, I recommend a thyroid glandular extract.

A glandular extract is a purified nutritional and therapeutic product derived from one of several animal glands including the adrenal, thymus, thyroid, ovaries, testes, pancreas, pineal, and pituitary. It is prescribed by a physician for a person whose corresponding gland is underfunctioning and not producing enough of its own hormone. The various glands are part of the endocrine system which, along with the nervous system, coordinates the functioning of all of the body's systems. (See Appendix A.)

Dietary Recommendations

■ Eat a whole-foods diet, with as many foods as possible in their raw state, including raw (unpasteurized) dairy products. Studies carried out in the 1930s found that there is an unidentified substance in raw butter that helps prevent arthritis.[3]

■ Eliminate NutraSweet™ from your diet. This synthetic sweetener can contribute to arthritic symptoms. When NutraSweet is eliminated, joint pain often stops.

■ Eliminate processed and canned foods as much as possible. In particular, avoid white sugar, white flour, margarine, other hydrogenated oils such as shortening, and low-fiber foods. These can hardly be considered foods at all. They don't nourish the body, but rather create severe nutritional deficiencies which lead to disease.

■ Be aware of foods that can cause problems for you. For example, some arthritics are intolerant to the nightshade plant family which includes tomatoes, green peppers, eggplant, and white potatoes. Food enzymes can be effective in alleviating or eliminating such allergies.

ASTHMA

Asthma is characterized by a narrowing of the bronchial passages and can manifest in many symptoms, ranging from minor difficulty in breathing to severe wheezing and coughing with an excessive excretion of mucus. These symptoms can accelerate rapidly, even in children and newborns. Between asthma attacks, an asthmatic may be perfectly healthy, but a severe attack can be life threatening.

As of 1994, an estimated 14.6 million Americans had asthma, a 33% increase from 1990.[4] Of these, 4.8 million were children (under age 18).[5] Asthma appears to be turning into a childhood epidemic; it is now the leading cause of disease and disability in children and teens from two to 17 years old.[6]

Over 450,000 annual hospital admissions are for asthma.[7] In the past, asthma was not considered a potentially fatal disease, but the death rate from asthma has increased by 67% from 1979 to 1991. Estimated medical costs are $6.2 billion per year, including $1.1 billion for medicines, $295 million in emergency room visits, and $345 million in lost work time.[8]

Corticosteroids (such as prednisone) were originally the drugs of choice for asthma. Then the adrenaline mimics, called beta agonists, appeared on the market. The most common beta agonist used in the United States is albuterol (brand names Proventil® and Ventolin®). Beta agonists are also available in over-the-counter aerosol canisters, such as Primatine Mist.

Although corticosteroids have terrible side effects, including seizures, diabetes, and osteoporosis, those of the newer beta agonists are far worse and have been statistically linked to increased deaths among asthmatics.

For information on the **enzymes** for this health condition, see Appendix B.

One study found that the risk of death among asthmatics nearly doubled with each canister of albuterol spray they used per month. The researchers point to two possible causes for this dramatic rise: the beta agonists may cause harm to the lungs and heart or mask fatally severe asthma.[9]

Do not attempt to discontinue your asthma medication without the guidance of a qualified medical professional.

What Causes Asthma?

Factors contributing to asthma include dietary intolerances, an underactive thyroid (hypothyroidism), environmental factors, and emotional problems. Childhood asthma is almost always associated with sugar intolerance, allergies, and low thyroid function.

Sugar Intolerance

According to Dr. Loomis, asthmatic children are sugar intolerant. This is not surprising, in view of the increased sucrose consumption in the U.S. from five pounds per person annually in 1922 to 135 pounds in 1990, and the fact that most people who eat excessive amounts of sugar become intolerant to it. Sugar intolerance includes more than sucrose (cane sugar), lactose (milk sugar), and maltose (grain sugar). It encompasses all sugars, including fructose, corn syrup, honey and other sweeteners, as well as synthetic sweeteners such as Nutrasweet, saccharin, sorbitol, and mannitol. All of these sugars must be strictly avoided by sugar-intolerant people. Sugars present in organic fruits are generally tolerated.

Other Dietary Intolerances

Asthma attacks can also be triggered by food additives, most commonly sodium metabisulfite and related sulfite derivatives used as preservatives in processed, canned, and bottled foods or, in restaurants, sprayed onto salad greens to keep them crisp. Bisulfite sprays have caused serious and

sometimes fatal respiratory distress in asthmatics who unwittingly ate from a salad bar where sulfites were used.

Excessive consumption of protein powders containing isolated amino acids can also trigger an asthma attack by creating an acid stress on the body. This means that excess acid reserves are created, which the kidneys must continuously dump into the urine to keep the blood pH stable and slightly alkaline (7.34-7.45). I have known bodybuilding athletes who started wheezing as a result of drinking these isolated amino acid (protein) drinks. I have also

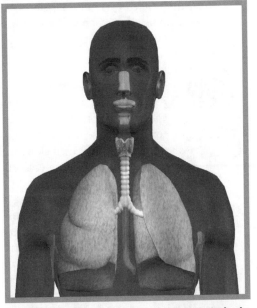

ASTHMA AND THE LUNGS. Asthma is characterized by a narrowing of the bronchial passages of the lungs and can produce symptoms including breathing difficulties, severe wheezing, and coughing with mucus excretion.

known asthmatics who had to make an emergency room trip after taking acidifying supplements often prescribed as a digestive aid. These include betaine HCl and other formulas containing hydrochloric acid (HCl, a component of digestive juices in the stomach).

Hypothyroidism
Chronic infections are common in people who have an underactive thyroid, because hypothyroidism can lead to immune system suppression; these infections can include chronic lung conditions such as asthma, pneumonia, and bronchitis. (See Appendix A.)

Environmental Factors
On the long list of environmental factors that can cause asthma are pollens, spores, danders, dusts, cigarette smoke, fireplace smoke, and chemicals polluting the air. In addition, common chemicals such as PVC film can cause "meat wrappers" asthma when the film is heated during packaging.

An often unrecognized contributing factor to asthma is geopathic stress, the result of natural radiation from the earth.[10] When situated below a home, this magnetic radiation can, over time, have harmful health effects on the occupants, including immune suppression and respiratory difficulties.

For more about **geopathic stress**, see Chapter 3: What Causes Enzyme Deficiencies?, p. 57.

Emotional Factors
Any emotional stress can trigger asthma. Sometimes the simple recognition of repressed emotions can alleviate an attack or prevent one from occurring. To treat stress, homeopathic remedies can be used along with an enzyme herbal formula, Thera-zyme Adr; for nervousness, CLM.

Success Story: The Man Who Couldn't Breathe for Six Decades
David, 75, had suffered from asthma for 61 years and had to use an inhaler (with Proventil) up to six times daily. He also had arthritis which woke him at night with throbbing pain and, for the last four years, had suffered from painful herpes on his legs, arms, and the back of his neck.

Diagnostic tests, including urine analysis, showed that David's system was too acidic and that he was deficient in calcium and magnesium. He also had both poor digestion and assimilation; in particular, he had trouble digesting fats and was intolerant of sugars. I started David on the following program:

- Thera-zyme PAN: a multiple digestive enzyme formula for sugar

intolerance

■ Thera-zyme Rsp: an enzymatic respiratory formula for wheezing and coughing

■ Thera-zyme Rbs: for his herpes

■ Thera-zyme Mal: for his arthritis

■ *Coleus forskohlii*: an herb from Ayurvedic medicine (SEE QUICK DEFINITION) used for asthma

■ Raw thyroid glandular extract for his underactive thyroid, common in asthmatics and arthritics

David also underwent chiropractic and acupuncture treatments. He had suffered from asthma for so long I assumed it would take quite a while for him to be able to reduce his inhaler dosage. But only two days after he started the enzyme program, David called me and announced that he had "tossed" his inhaler. Three weeks later, his arthritis and herpes were so much improved that he was no longer awakened at night by pain from them. One small remaining area of herpes was shrinking.

Within a short time, David was able to reduce the intake of his respiratory formula without experiencing a relapse. He only needed an inhaler once in three weeks and then only because he had forgotten to take his enzymes.

David's case shows that seemingly unrelated health conditions can be cleared up when you provide the correct enzyme supplementation.

Ayurveda is the traditional medicine of India, based on many centuries of empirical use. Its name means "end of the Vedas" (which were India's sacred scripts), implying that a holistic medicine may be founded on spiritual principles. Ayurveda describes three metabolic, constitutional, and body types (doshas), in association with the basic elements of Nature in combination. These are *vata* (air and ether, rooted in intestines), *pitta* (fire and water/stomach), and *kapha* (water and earth/lungs). Ayurvedic physicians use these categories (which also have psychological aspects) as the basis for prescribing individualized formulas of herbs, diet, massage, breathing, meditation, exercise and yoga postures, and detoxification techniques.

Success Story: Calming Eric's Asthma

When his parents brought Eric, 8, to see me, he was small for his age and suffering from asthma attacks which seemed to be triggered mainly by emotional upsets, but also by excessive sugar consumption and exposure to smoke. Eric had an asthma attack whenever he was upset, whether it came from teasing at school, a difficult relationship, or fear of not succeeding. In my opinion, asthma attacks triggered by emotions are the most frightening because they are the least predictable.

Eric's first onset of asthma had occurred when he was five years old, following exposure to pesticides and excessive cigarette smoke. At that time, his parents used only homeopathic remedies to control his condition. When I first treated him, he lived in a relatively pesticide-free environment and his major environmental trigger was smoke of any kind, including that of cigarettes and fireplaces. These were relatively easy to recognize and avoid.

I recommended a strict diet of organic meat, poultry, or eggs, organic, raw dairy products, and organic vegetables and fruits. Since sugar intolerance is characteristic of asthma, Eric was to avoid refined sugar, candy, junk foods, and soda.

For enzymes, he took Thera-zyme PAN (a multiple digestive enzyme formula for asthmatics), Thera-zyme Rsp (a lung formula for coughing and wheezing), and Thera-zyme Kdy for allergies. I also suggested thyroid therapy, and counseled his parents to become aware of upsetting situations in their son's life so they could help him deal with the emotions before they produced an asthma attack.

Today, at age 19, Eric is 5'11" and still growing. He is increasingly aware of his asthma triggers. Now, when he has difficulty breathing, he completely avoids sugar, gets more rest, and takes whatever enzymes are indicated in addition to his regular multiple digestive formula (Thera-zyme PAN). For example, when exposed to allergens, he adds Thera-zyme Kdy, and for wheezing and other breathing problems, he takes Thera-zyme Rsp. In addition, he gets regular chiropractic treatment to correct structural misalignments contributing to his condition.

Success Story: A Holiday Asthma Crisis

The anxious parents of 19-month-old Victor called me from the hospital where their son was in intensive care. He was being treated with a battery of toxic synthetic drugs for a severe asthma attack. I was surprised, since the baby, who had been diagnosed as asthmatic at the age of one, had been doing well on the enzyme formulas Thera-Zyme PAN (for sugar intolerance and asthma) and Thera-zyme Rsp (a respiratory formula), and I had strictly warned his parents not to give the child sugar.

However, the Christmas season with all its sweets had proven too much for them. Victor, who was suffering from a cold at the time, was given candy. This combination, a simple cold followed by candy, was enough to trigger the severe asthma attack. His condition quickly worsened and he ended up in the emergency room. Eleven days and $10,000 later, Victor went home. I placed him back on his earlier enzyme therapies for sugar intolerance and respiratory problems and didn't need to repeat my warnings about sugar. He soon improved and now, a year later, Victor is doing fine on the enzyme program and a sugar-free diet.

Asthma Elimination Program

Many asthmatics using steroids or beta agonists can either reduce or entirely eliminate these toxic drugs by employing enzyme therapy and other appropriate natural therapies. The age of the person or the length of time on drugs does not seem to matter. What does matter is determining the cause and treating it appropriately. I generally use enzymes along with thyroid therapy, herbal medicine, and aromatherapy.

Asthmatic children often respond to a change in diet, with avoidance of all refined sugars, plus a multiple digestive formula (Thera-zyme PAN) which includes the sugar-digesting enzymes or disaccharidases. Since sugar consumption is difficult to control in children, other formulas are often needed, such as the respiratory formula (Thera-zyme Rsp), which helps relieve wheezing and coughing. If environmental allergies are a trigger, you can relieve them by using the allergy formula, Thera-zyme Kdy. In severe allergy cases, add Thera-zyme MSCLR, a formula high in amylase (digests carbohydrates). If emotional factors are the trigger, be aware of what upsets your child so you can help him or her deal with the emotions involved and possibly deter an attack.

Enzyme Therapy

Please note that not everyone with asthma needs all of the following formulas. Treatment protocols are tailored to the individual.

- Thera-zyme PAN: a multiple digestive enzyme formula, containing the four food enzymes plus disaccharidases (note: most asthmatics do well on Thera-zyme PAN *if* they avoid refined and artificial sugars, including Nutrasweet, saccharin, fructose, sucrose, corn syrup, honey, maple syrup, and other sweeteners); for severe sugar intolerance, I sometimes add Thera-zyme SvG and Adr
- Thera-zyme Rsp: a respiratory formula which nourishes the lungs, helps expectorate mucus, and relieves coughing and wheezing
- Thera-zyme Kdy: for relief of allergic reactions that can cause an asthma attack; can be used in the case of exposure to allergens that trigger asthma
- Thera-zyme CLM: nutritional support for the nervous system

Thyroid Support

If testing determines that your thyroid function is low, seek the advice of a health professional. If treatment is needed, I recommend a thyroid glandular extract. (See Appendix A.)

Herbal Medicine

The following herbs can be taken one at a time or in combination. Seek professional help to decide which ones are right for you.

- *Coleus forskohlii:* Ayurvedic herb useful in lung, heart, and skin problems

For more about **aromatherapy**, see Cancer, p. 93.

■ Ephedra (*Ephedra*) or *ma-huang*: stimulates the adrenals; some people cannot tolerate it and it's generally contraindicated for people with high blood pressure

■ Lobelia (*Lobelia inflata*): excellent asthma remedy; use with caution—too much causes vomiting

■ Licorice (*Glycyrrhiza glabra*): relaxing expectorant and adrenal supporter

■ Coltsfoot (*Tussilago farfara*): relaxing expectorant; cough reliever, helps soothe dry, irritated airways

■ Grindelia (*Grindelia camporum*): relaxing expectorant and antispasmodic (useful for bronchial spasms of asthma); helps ease dry, irritable cough

Aromatherapy/Essential Oils

Two aromatherapy oils specifically for asthma and lung problems are RC and Raven. They should be used daily, two or three drops each, alternating on the soles of the feet and the chest. Other aromatic oils for lung problems include: hyssop, ravensara, frankincense, oregano, peppermint, thyme, cypress, eucalyptus, sandalwood, cedarwood, and chamomile. One or more of these additional oils may be used along with RC and Raven in the same application and dosage as above.

CANCER

Cancer is a disease in which healthy cells stop functioning and maturing properly. As the normal cycle of cell creation and death is interrupted, these newly "mutated" cancer cells begin multiplying uncontrollably. This process, if unchecked, will eventually lead to the formation of a cancerous tumor. Cancer cells become parasitic, and can develop their own network of blood vessels to siphon nourishment away from the body's blood supply. As the abnormal cells circulate within the bloodstream, the cancer can spread to other parts of the body. When this happens, it is said to have metastasized.

For information on the **enzymes** for this health condition, see Appendix B.

What Causes Cancer?

Cancer can be caused by a wide range of factors, usually acting in combination to create an overload in the body. These factors, among many others, include poor diet and nutrition, stress and related psychological conditions, heredity, free radical (SEE QUICK DEFINITION) overload, and toxic accumulation from air pollution, tobacco smoke, radiation, chemicals and pesticides, and poisons in the water we drink.

In addition, some prescription drugs and hormones have been reported to contribute to cancer. Of these, the most common is synthetic estrogen found in oral contraceptives and conventional hormone replacement therapies, widely prescribed for perimenopausal (nearing menopause) and menopausal women. The natural estrogen estradiol can also contribute to cancer when its level in a woman's body is chronically too high in relation to her progesterone level, a condition called estrogen dominance. Environmental estrogens, which mimic the action of estrogen in the body, also contribute to estrogen dominance and therefore to cancer.

Success Story: Overcoming Breast Cancer

Diana, 45, found a suspicious lump in her breast and a needle biopsy revealed it to be cancerous. She had a lumpectomy in her doctor's office, but refused the lymph gland surgery which her doctor recommended to make sure the

QUICK DEFINITION

A **free radical** is an unstable, toxic molecule of oxygen with an unpaired electron that steals an electron from another molecule and produces harmful effects. Free radicals are formed when molecules within cells react with oxygen (oxidize) as part of normal metabolic processes. Free radicals then begin to break down cells, especially the cell membranes, often in a matter of minutes to an hour. A single free radical can destroy a cell. Their work is enhanced if there are not enough free radical–quenching nutrients, such as vitamins C and E, in the cell. While free radicals are normal products of metabolism, uncontrolled free–radical production plays a major role in the development of degenerative disease, including cancer and heart disease. Free radicals harmfully alter important molecules, such as proteins, enzymes, fats, even DNA. Other sources of free radicals include pesticides, industrial pollutants, smoking, alcohol, viruses, most infections, allergies, stress, even certain foods and excessive exercise.

For information on the **temperature and pulse thyroid tests**, see "Is Your Thyroid Underactive?" Chapter 2: Diagnosing Enzyme Deficiencies, pp. 32-33. For more about the **damaging effects of estrogen dominance**, see "Factors to Consider Before Using Estrogen Replacement Therapy," Menopausal Symptoms, pp. 179-181, and "Comparison of Progesterone and Estrogen," Appendix A, p. 260.

For more on **cancer and its causes**, see *Alternative Medicine Definitive Guide to Cancer* (Future Medicine Publishing, 1997; ISBN 1-887299-01-7); to order, call 800-333-HEAL.

QUICK DEFINITION

A **cancer marker** refers to any of a variety of blood tests which measure the level of a protein material or other chemical produced by cancer cells. These numbers become elevated in the presence of a cancer or tumor. There are different cancer markers for different kinds of cancer; CEA (carcinoembryonic antigen) test for colon cancer, AFP (alpha-fetoprotein) test for liver cancer (primary hepatocellular carcinoma), PSA (prostate specific antigen) for prostate cancer, CA (carcinoma) 15-3 or 27.29 for breast cancer, and CA 125 for ovarian cancer, to name a few.

cancer had not spread to her lymph nodes. Diana also refused chemotherapy and radiation. Instead, she decided to go on a strict enzyme treatment program and came to me for a urinalysis to determine her enzyme deficiencies.

Diana's previous health history included an underactive thyroid (hypothyroidism), a toxic colon condition characterized by constipation (this condition is often related to hypothyroidism which slows body functions), and severe skin problems. Her urine test showed sugar intolerance, a vitamin C deficiency, low calcium, and allergies.

I gave Diana the following enzyme, hormonal, and herbal therapy:

- Thera-zyme VSCLR: a digestive formula
- Thera-zyme Spl: an oxygenating, immune support formula
- Thera-zyme SvG: for sugar intolerance
- Thera-zyme Kdy: for allergies
- Thera-zyme TRMA: for all immune system problems, including cancer
- Thyroid glandular extract: Diana regularly monitored her oral temperature and resting pulse to make sure she was getting the proper glandular dosage
- 10% natural progesterone in vitamin E oil
- *Coleus forskohlii:* Ayurvedic herb believed to enhance thyroid function and help prevent the metastasis of cancer

Diana's diet of organic whole foods was satisfactory, although low in protein, which I urged her to increase. Adequate protein is essential for the liver to convert the inactive form of thyroid hormone, T4 (thyroxine), to the active form, T3 (tri-iodothyronine).

Five years later, Diana is still doing fine and has no signs of cancer. She has frequent medical tests which show a strong immune system and a normal blood profile.

Prevention and Treatment of Cancer

My recommendations for cancer treatment vary, depending on what other treatments the person is undergoing as well as factors such as diet and general vitality. During treatment, I follow blood cholesterol levels and various cancer markers

(SEE QUICK DEFINITION). Cholesterol falls as the immune system weakens (a healthy cholesterol level is 160-200 mg/dl). Ideally, cholesterol levels should rise and the cancer marker numbers should decrease with healing.

Enzyme Therapy

I always recommend the following three enzyme formulas for people with cancer. The dosages listed are general guidelines only.

■ Thera-zyme VSCLR: a digestive formula; for sugar intolerance, Thera-zyme SvG can be used in addition (two capsules of each formula with each meal)

■ Thera-zyme Spl: for the spleen and the immune system; also helps increase oxygen in the body (two capsules with each meal)

■ Thera-zyme TRMA: immune support (four capsules, 3-5 times a day between meals—30 to 60 minutes before, or two hours after, eating). For people with cancer, AIDS, or severe infections, I recommend five doses daily; more is not necessary. It is important to take this on an empty stomach to speed transport directly into the blood and to the site of the trauma. People with gastric irritation can usually tolerate the protease TRMA contains if they open up the capsules, stir the contents into water, and drink immediately. These people should use Thera-zyme Stm as their multiple digestive enzyme formula.

Additional formulas may be required, depending on the urinalysis. Among the most commonly needed are the following:

■ Thera-zyme Opt: vitamin C formula which supports the immune system, useful for all health conditions

■ Thera-zyme Nsl: vitamin C antioxidant/enzyme formula. Since free-radical pathology accompanies all diseases, this formula can be used for any illness.

■ Thera-zyme Kdy: kidney-lymphatic formula which helps the kidneys cleanse the blood and thus relieves kidney stress and pain which result from an exhausted lymphatic system. Symptoms of the need for Thera-zyme Kdy include allergies of all kinds, frontal headaches, swollen glands, painful kidneys, and nausea.

■ Thera-zyme SmI (small intestine): potent probiotic (friendly bacteria, SEE QUICK DEFINITION) formula containing cellulase. This should be used only in people with candidiasis, parasites, or severe constipation or diarrhea resulting from antibiotics.

QUICK DEFINITION

Friendly bacteria, or probiotics, refer to beneficial microbes inhabiting the human gastrointestinal tract where they are essential for proper nutrient assimilation. The human body contains an estimated several trillion beneficial bacteria comprising over 400 species, all necessary for health. Among the more well known of these are *Lactobacillus acidophilus* and *Bifidobacterium bifidum*. Overly acidic bodily conditions, chronic constipation or diarrhea, dietary imbalances, consumption of highly processed foods, and the excessive use of antibiotics and hormonal drugs can interfere with probiotic function and even reduce the number of these microbes, setting up conditions for illness.

Thyroid Support

Most immune-suppressed people have sluggish thyroid function, and can be helped with a good thyroid glandular extract. If testing determines that your thyroid function is low, seek the advice of a health professional. (See Appendix A.)

Hormonal Balancing

■ Natural progesterone (10% oil in vitamin E): Since progesterone is an antitumor hormone, this is an important treatment for people with cancer. I suggest five doses of three drops daily. Using the tip of your finger rub it onto your gums. The oil or 3% natural progesterone cream can also be rubbed directly on the tumor. Applying a thin coat of olive oil helps the skin to absorb the progesterone oil.

■ Pregnenolone Powder: I generally recommend $^1/_{16}$ teaspoon of this formula daily, for both men and women. Pregnenolone is converted by the body into progesterone and DHEA only as it is needed. I do not advise the use of supplemental DHEA. Although DHEA has anticancer properties, it is a precursor to both estrogen and testosterone. The peak output of DHEA is 12 mg to 15 mg at about age 25, then decreasing with age. Many people take far in excess of this—as much as 100 mg daily. There is reported evidence that taking more than 12 mg of DHEA daily, and especially taking it without pregnenolone and progesterone, may actually promote tumor growth, because the DHEA can convert to estrogen.[11]

For a more about the antitumor effects of progesterone, see Appendix A, pp. 256-261.

Dietary Recommendations

The following antitumor or radioprotective foods have special properties that may help prevent cancer or provide support to the immune system. "Radioprotective" refers to a substance that helps protect against the damage of radiation, one cause of cancer.

■ Cultured (fermented) milk products such as yogurt, kefir, buttermilk, and unprocessed cheese. By yogurt, I do not mean most commercially available yogurt containing sugar, potato starch, artificial colors and flavors, and a few half-dead bacteria, but real yogurt made from fresh, raw, unhomogenized milk with billions of live friendly bacteria, a minimum of honey, and perhaps some real fruit. Many people who are lactose intolerant can handle cultured milk products, in which the lactose has been converted to lactic acid.

■ Sauerkraut and other fermented vegetables. These contain the friendly bacteria *Lactobacilli* which convert carbohydrates to lactic acid. Research has shown that *Lactobacilli* (and other milk-fermenting bacteria) have antitumor activity.[12]

■ Cruciferous vegetables (cabbage, broccoli, cauliflower). These vegetables appear to have anticancer value beyond their vitamin A and C content, containing substances which may inhibit cancer cell growth. Cruciferous vegetables should always be steamed because they contain thyroid inhibitors which are destroyed in cooking.[13]

■ Vegetables and fruits containing beta carotene: dark-green leafy vegetables, broccoli, spinach, kale, Swiss chard, chicory, escarole, watercress, collard greens, mustard greens, dark-yellow and orange vegetables, carrots, sweet potatoes, yams, pumpkins, winter squash, cantaloupe, apricots, peaches, papayas, and watermelon. Carrots, preferably raw, are efficient colon cleansers and bind bowel toxins and carcinogens.

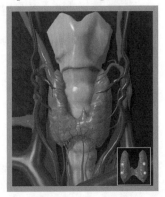

■ High-fiber foods: whole grains, fruits, and vegetables. A high-fiber diet can protect against colon cancer for several reasons. It dilutes bowel carcinogens, decreases colon transit time, and changes the composition and metabolic activity of the fecal flora and certain carcinogenic substances in the colon. It's always healthier to eat whole grains containing the bran and the fiber, along with whole fruits and vegetables, instead of their processed counterparts.

■ Miso: a paste made from fermented soybeans, sometimes with grains such as rice or barley. A superior source of usable whole protein, miso aids digestion and assimilation, is low in fat, and may help to neutralize environmental pollution, including radiation. It is believed that miso's anticancer substances are a result of the fermentation process. Thus, raw or unfer-

The **thyroid gland**, one of the body's seven endocrine glands, is located just below the larynx in the throat, with interconnecting lobes on either side of the trachea. The thyroid is the body's metabolic thermostat, controlling body temperature, energy use, and, in children, the body's growth rate. The thyroid controls the *rate* at which organs function and the *speed* with which the body uses food; it affects the operation of all body processes and organs. Of the hormones the thyroid synthesizes and releases, T_3 (tri-iodothyronine) accounts for 7% and T_4 (thyroxine) almost 93%; T_4 is converted into T_3 outside the thyroid gland. Iodine is essential to forming normal amounts of thyroxine. The secretion of both these hormones is regulated by thyroid-stimulating hormone, or TSH, secreted by the pituitary gland in the brain. The thyroid also secretes calcitonin, a hormone required for calcium metabolism.

For information on **Dr. Livingston's cancer research and treatment protocol**, see *Alternative Medicine Definitive Guide to Cancer* (Future Medicine Publishing, 1997; ISBN 1-887299-01-7); to order, call 800-333-HEAL.

mented soybeans do not share these properties. To prevent destruction of enzymes, miso should not be boiled, but added to soup or other already cooked food.

■ Foods containing abscisic acid: a component of vitamin A that stops cancer cells from multiplying, according to cancer researcher Virginia Livingston, M.D. These include grasses (green kamut, wheat grass juice, etc.), pea shoots, lima beans, potatoes, yams, sweet potatoes, asparagus, tomatoes, onions, spinach, grapes, avocados, pears, oranges, apples, and green leafy vegetables.

Herbal Remedies

By cleansing the liver, kidneys, colon, and lymphatics, herbal remedies support the body's effort to initiate healing. A detailed discussion of herbal remedies is beyond the scope of this book, so the herbs included here are only some of the many you can use.

■ Burdock (*Arctium lappa*): to cleanse the blood and the liver; has a reputation as an antitumor herb, although it is unclear if that property is the result of its cleansing and detoxifying action rather than a direct effect on the tumor itself

■ Essiac tea: herbal tea (containing burdock root, slippery elm, Indian rhubarb, and sheep sorrel, among others) formulated by the late Rene Caisse, a Canadian nurse who used it to treat thousands of cancer patients from the 1920s until her death in 1978

■ Cleavers (*Galium aparine*): one of the best lymphatic drainage remedies available, which may be why it has a history of use in the treatment of tumors and ulcers

■ Echinacea (*Echinacea angustifolia*): antimicrobial and immune support

■ Mistletoe (*Viscum album*): a nervine (acts on the nervous system); has antitumor properties, according to cancer research

■ Red clover (*Trifolium pratense*): used mainly in respiratory and skin disorders; research demonstrates antitumor action in animals

■ Sweet violet (*Viola odorata*): used as an expectorant and in urinary infections; also reported to be an anticancer herb

■ Saffron (*Crocus sativus*) tea: contains colchicine, a substance which has been used in the treatment of leukemia

■ Cat's claw (*Uncaria tomentosa*): a powerful immune enhancer; dosage varies from three to 12 capsules daily depending on the severity of the condition

■ *Coleus forskohlii:* Ayurvedic herb with antimetastasis properties

Aromatherapy/Essential Oils

I suggest the following essential oils for people with cancer:
- Immupower, Thieves: to enhance the immune system
- Clove, Tarragon, Melrose: developed for certain kinds of cancer
- Frankincense, Rose, Hope, Forgiveness, Joy, and Ravensara: for the emotional stress that accompanies cancer

It is best to choose one or two essential oils to use at a time rather than all of them, perhaps one for the immune system and another for emotional stress. Choose based on which odors most appeal to you or how they make you feel. Aromatherapy oils can be used in various ways: put 3-6 drops in bath water; use an aromatherapy diffuser to fill the air with the scent; apply 1-6 drops directly onto the feet (the skin of the feet absorbs oils quickly) or any area of concern; or dilute with massage oil by 15% to 30% and use in massage.[14]

CANDIDIASIS

Candida albicans is a yeast-like fungus found widely in nature, in the soil, on vegetables and fruits, and in the human body. In small quantities it is a normal flora of the skin, mouth, intestinal tract, and vagina. However, a *Candida* overgrowth, a condition called candidiasis, can become pathogenic and cause allergic reactions throughout the body. These reactions can lead to a wide range of symptoms, including depression, anxiety, fatigue, skin problems, weight gain or loss, headaches, muscle cramping, and gastrointestinal problems such as bloating, gas, indigestion, constipation, and diarrhea.

For information on the **enzymes** for this health condition, see Appendix B.

For more on **candidiasis**, see *Alternative Medicine Guide to Chronic Fatigue, Fibromyalgia, and Environmental Illness*, (Future Medicine Publishing, 1997; ISBN 1-887299-11-4); to order, call 800-333-HEAL.

What Causes Candidiasis?

Many clients come to me convinced that they have candidiasis and that it is the cause of all their health problems. I reserve that diagnosis until I've conducted a thorough medical history, since the symptoms of candidiasis overlap with many other conditions, especially severe digestive problems caused by enzyme deficiencies. Predisposing factors for candidiasis include: the use of steroid hormone medications such as cortisone or corticosteroids, which are often prescribed for skin problems; prolonged or repeated use of antibiotics; oral contraceptive use; estrogen therapy; and a diet high in sugar. Certain illnesses, such as AIDS, cancer, and diabetes, which are accompanied by extreme immune suppression, can also increase susceptibility to *Candida* overgrowth.

Success Story: The Man Who Couldn't Drink Wine

Carl, 25, had symptoms of digestive problems and a long history of treatment for candidiasis. He was currently taking nystatin, an anti-fungal drug commonly given for *Candida*. His urine analysis indicated that he was sugar intolerant and had an allergic pattern. A palpation test showed immune system and liver problems, but no yeast overgrowth. Carl's most recent complaint was that he could no longer tolerate drinking wine with dinner. His symptoms included those of common liver problems: when he drank wine, he felt queasy, sleepy, and as though he had been "drugged." He thought that this was due to his candidiasis, so he had increased his daily dose of nystatin, which worsened his symptoms.

I recommended the following enzyme formulas:
- Thera-zyme PAN: a multiple digestive formula for sugar and wheat intolerance
- Thera-zyme Lvr: an enzymatic liver formula
- Thera-zyme TRMA: for immune support
- Thera-zyme Kdy: for allergies

Carl took these formulas for six months by which time his digestive problems had cleared up and he was once again able to enjoy wine with his dinner.

Prevention and Elimination of Candidiasis

The following nontoxic enzyme and nutritional therapies are general recommendations to rid the body of pathogenic yeast and improve the immune system, however, as with all health conditions, treatment must be tailored to the individual.

Enzyme Therapy
- A multiple digestive enzyme formula: determined by urinalysis, to address the foods the person has difficulty digesting or eats in excess
- Thera-zyme SmI: contains a form of cellulase that breaks down pathogenic yeast into nontoxic particles which are then eliminated through the urine and feces; contains *L. acidophilus* and *B. bifidum* which reestablish friendly bowel flora, thus lessening the likelihood of yeast overgrowth in the future
- Thera-zyme TRMA: for immune support; used for any kind of infection
- Thera-zyme Kdy: kidney-lymphatic formula which helps relieve many symptoms, mainly allergies, but also kidney pain and low blood sugar, among others

Nutritional Supplements
- Citricidal (grapefruit seed and pulp extract): nontoxic antibacterial, antiparasitic, antifungal, and antiviral; kills 11 fungi, including *Candida albicans*; dosage is 1-2 tablets (tablets contain four drops each), three times a day.
- Soil-based organisms (SEE QUICK DEFINITION): an intestinal formula of beneficial bacteria from soil which kill pathological microbes

QUICK DEFINITION

Soil-based organisms (SBOs) are beneficial microbes, or probiotics, found in soil. Before chemical farming, the earth was rich in these organisms which naturally destroyed molds, yeast, fungi, and viruses in the soil. Transmitted in the food supply to humans, SBOs perform the same function in the human body, working with the "friendly" bacteria (such as *Lactobacillus acidophilus* and *Bifidobacterium bifidum*) inhabiting the gastrointestinal tract to maintain balance in the intestinal flora and thus ensure a healthy digestive system. Since soil has become depleted of SBOs, the ratio of good to bad bacteria in the intestines has become skewed and a host of health problems, including allergies, candidiasis, hormonal dysfunction, and Crohn's disease among other gastrointestinal conditions, are the result.

and help prevent proliferation of toxins in the intestines; usual dosage is one capsule daily, increasing by one capsule per week up to six capsules daily in divided doses.

Dietary Recommendations

■ Avoid sugar in all its forms, including sucrose (cane sugar), lactose (milk sugar), maltose (grain sugar), fructose, corn syrup, and honey as well as synthetic sweeteners.

■ Eat an organic, whole foods diet. Limit or avoid those foods that you have trouble digesting or that cause allergic symptoms. Anti-*Candida* diets often automatically eliminate the consumption of nutritional yeast and fermented foods, but these foods need not be avoided if they do not produce allergic symptoms in you. Excessive consumption of alcohol should be avoided.

CARDIOVASCULAR DISEASE

Among the conditions included in the category of cardiovascular disease are coronary heart disease (decreased blood flow to the heart), congestive heart failure (cardiomyopathy), heart attack (myocardial infarction), stroke, chest pain (angina pectoris), high blood pressure (hypertension), arrhythmia (irregular heartbeat), rheumatic heart disease, and hardening of the arteries (arteriosclerosis).

For information on the **enzymes** for this health condition, see Appendix B.

What Causes Cardiovascular Disease?

A common precursor of many cardiovascular problems is a form of arteriosclerosis called atherosclerosis, in which the inner arterial walls harden and thicken due to deposits of fatty substances. These substances form a plaque that, with buildup, causes a narrowing of the arteries. Over time, plaque can block the arteries and interrupt blood flow to the organs they supply, including the heart and brain (see illustration, next page).

High cholesterol (SEE QUICK DEFINITION) is commonly cited as the culprit behind plaque formation and, therefore, atherosclerosis. This misguided explanation not only ignores some important facts about cholesterol, including that it is vital to crucial body processes such as the manufacture of hormones, but dangerously overlooks numerous contributing factors to cardiovascular disease. Those factors are discussed below but, first, here are some things you should know about cholesterol.

In Defense of Cholesterol

The renowned and extensive Framingham study, begun in the 1950s, shows that 50% of people who die of heart disease do not have high cholesterol. Further, researchers in this study could find no relationship between dietary cholesterol and serum cholesterol levels. Regardless of the cholesterol intake, levels in the blood varied from low to moderate to high. Despite this and the fact that only 10% of

Cholesterol is an essential component in cell membranes needed by the body to make bile salts, which help absorb the fat-soluble vitamins (A, D, E, K) and essential fatty acids from the small intestine. Cholesterol, a steroid, is also at the beginning of the pathway that manufactures steroidal hormones and male and female sex hormones, including pregnenolone, testosterone, estradiol, estrone, progesterone, DHEA, and cortisol. These are critical for the health of the immune system, the mineral-regulating functions of the kidneys, and the smooth running of the hormonal systems in men and women. Cholesterol is not only obtained through the diet, but produced by the liver, which synthesizes about 3,000 mg of new cholesterol in any 24-hour period, a quantity equivalent to the amount contained in ten eggs. This new cholesterol is used to repair cells; when cholesterol levels get too low, depression, lung disease, and even cancer can result.

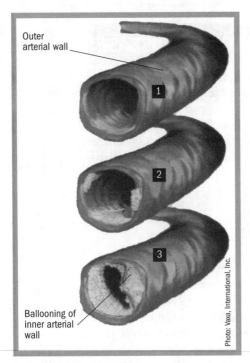

Outer arterial wall

Ballooning of inner arterial wall

Photo: Vaxa, International, Inc.

HOW ARTERIES THICKEN
1. A normal, healthy artery with open and clear passages.
2. The beginning of cholesterol plaque buildup within the artery. The inner arterial wall is also beginning to weaken and bulge with cholesterol and toxic deposits.
3. Severely restricted artery with cholesterol plaque filling the majority of the passage. Note further breakdown and ballooning of inner arterial wall.

cholesterol is in our blood while the balance is in our tissues, medical focus has been on blood levels of cholesterol. In an April 1990 article in *Townsend Letter for Doctors*, entitled "Cholesterol Mania," Rosetta Shuman notes that "cholesterol, from having been merely vilified 30 years ago, has become the sole indicator of one's lifeline." She too cites evidence of the lack of correlation between dietary cholesterol and heart disease.

Since cholesterol is vital for life processes, the body has a protective feedback mechanism in which endogenous cholesterol (that is, cholesterol manufactured by the liver) increases as dietary cholesterol decreases. That's why dietary restriction of cholesterol only reduces the serum levels by 15% at best.[15]

In general, your cholesterol level—whether high or low—will not be a factor in heart disease or other diseases *if* your thyroid functions properly and *if* your diet is healthy. (In addition, as discussed below, it is not cholesterol itself, but *oxidized* cholesterol, that leads to atherosclerosis.)

A healthy diet means that in addition to eating organic whole foods, you must: avoid thyroid toxins and inhibitors which can hinder the conversion of cholesterol into hormones, resulting in increased cholesterol; choose foods that stimulate thyroid function; and avoid excess cholesterol-lowering foods (mainly starches). Maintaining a total cholesterol level between 160 and 230 (mg/dl) ensures that there will be enough cholesterol for the production of the anti-aging hormones.

How to Avoid Excessive Cholesterol—While some cholesterol is needed by your body, *excess* cholesterol is indeed unhealthy, especially if you have certain health conditions (such as an underactive thyroid gland) which compromise your body's ability to process cholesterol. Attending to the following will help keep your cholesterol level from rising too high:

For more about the **cholesterol**, see *Alternative Medicine Guide to Heart Disease* (Future Medicine Publishing, 1997; ISBN 1-887299-10-6); to order, call 800-333-HEAL.

■ Check your thyroid function. Avoid thyroid toxins and inhibitors including: excess polyunsaturated fats (including soybean, safflower, canola, flaxseed, and fish oils); raw cruciferous vegetables (broccoli, cauliflower, and cabbage; lightly steaming them destroys the thyroid inhibiting substances they contain); excess estrogen (from birth control pills, herbal estrogens such as black cohosh, and pesticides which are estrogenic); fluoride; and the mercury in silver amalgam fillings.[16] Also note that a low-protein diet promotes hypothyroidism.

■ Control your weight. Obesity interferes with the normal assimilation of fats, causing a tendency toward increased cholesterol and triglycerides (lipids or fats formed from fatty acids and glycerol; they travel in the blood along with cholesterol).

■ Avoid stress. It increases cholesterol, which may be nature's way of increasing the pathways to the stress hormones such as cortisol.

■ Avoid synthetic fats (such as margarine) produced from the hydrogenation of vegetable oils, which cause increased cholesterol.

■ Eat foods high in fiber. Low-fiber diets promote high cholesterol. Water-soluble fiber—found in fruits, vegetables, grains, and legumes—binds intestinal cholesterol and inhibits its intestinal reabsorption. It is far better to get your fiber from whole foods than from supplements.

■ Get sufficient food enzymes. Enzyme-deficient diets lead to increased cholesterol and triglycerides. The need for lipase, the fat-digesting enzyme, is obvious.

■ Eat whole foods rich in vitamins and minerals. Nutrient deficiencies associated with high cholesterol include vitamin C, the B-complex vitamins (especially B6 and B3), and certain minerals, such as chromium, zinc, and magnesium. Note that taking supplements while continuing to eat a junk-food diet will not address these nutritional deficiencies. A junk-food diet leaves you enzyme-deficient; without enzymes (as are found in whole foods), vitamin and mineral supple-

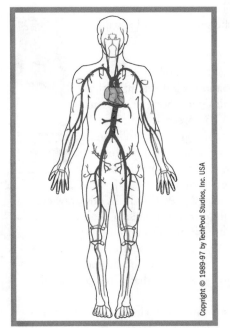

THE CIRCULATORY SYSTEM. A network of arteries (shown here) carries oxygenated blood from the heart to all parts of the body. A system of veins carries blood back to the heart.

Copyright © 1989-97 by TechPool Studios, Inc. USA

ments cannot be utilized by the body and are therefore wasted.

Raising Deficient Cholesterol— Like excessive cholesterol, an abnormally *low* cholesterol level (below 160) can compromise your body's functioning, particularly by not providing enough of the building blocks for the production of hormones. Here are some tips for raising your cholesterol to a healthy level:

■ Try to correct any condition, such as excessive starch consumption or immune suppression, that might be lowering your cholesterol.

■ Heal your thyroid gland if it is sluggish. Eat thyroid-stimulating foods (adequate fruit, protein, organic salt, and coconut oil), avoid thyroid inhibitors (listed above), and take adequate thyroid glandular extract. Proloid, a synthetic mixture of thyroid hormones, is a good substitute for vegans. Pregnenolone, from wild yam (*Dioscorea*), also helps heal the thyroid gland, and natural progesterone stimulates release of thyroid hormone. Other thyroid-stimulating herbs include *Coleus forskohlii* and *Gugulipid*, both Ayurvedic herbs.

■ If you eat excessive starch, cut down and balance it with extra fruit and protein. Fresh organic fruit—especially citrus and tropical—can raise low cholesterol due to its sugar (fructose) content, which stimulates the liver to produce cholesterol. At the same time, fresh fruit will not cause a normal cholesterol level to become abnormal. In people with adequate sucrase (enzyme that digests sucrose), sucrose in the fruit is split into two units, a glucose and a fructose unit. The fructose half is involved in cholesterol synthesis. In other words, the sugar in fruit stimulates cholesterol formation. However, I do not recommend eating any type of refined or synthetic sugars.

■ If you do eat sucrose, eat only organic, unrefined sugar cane, raw honey, or organic maple syrup which contains cardioprotective

Hypothyroidism is a primary factor in heart disease for a number of reasons. Low thyroid function can interfere with the body's ability to process cholesterol. When thyroid hormone is deficient, the body cannot convert cholesterol into the key steroidal (anti-aging) hormones, resulting in high cholesterol levels.

nutrients such as vitamin B6 and magnesium.

Hypothyroidism

Low thyroid function is a primary factor in heart disease for a number of reasons. As mentioned above, hypothyroidism can interfere with the body's ability to process cholesterol. When thyroid hormone is deficient, the body cannot convert cholesterol into the key steroidal (anti-aging) hormones, including pregnenolone, progesterone, and DHEA, resulting in high cholesterol levels. Second, the excess adrenaline produced in hypothyroid people appears to cause chronic degeneration of the aorta (the main arterial trunk). Third, hypothyroidism and heart disease are causally related to excess consumption of polyunsaturated oils (PUFAs), including soybean, safflower, canola, flaxseed, fish, borage, and evening primrose oils—all oils, with the exception of extra virgin olive oil, that are liquid at room temperature. These unsaturated oils are quickly oxidized, leaving behind a substance called age pigment (lipofuscin). In heart attack patients, age pigment has been identified in arterial lesions in quantities that correspond to the severity of the lesion.[17]

Estrogen Dominance

Women suffering from hypothyroidism often have excess or unopposed estrogen, meaning in relation to progesterone levels, a condition called estrogen dominance. Again, low thyroid function means that you cannot convert cholesterol into pregnenolone, progesterone, and DHEA. When the body cannot produce enough progesterone, estrogen becomes dominant. Hormonal balance depends on the ratio of progesterone to estrogen. In women, the optimum ratio is ten to one, whether the estrogen level is normal, low, or high.[18] Estrogen dominance is associated with thrombosis (formation of a blood clot), embolism (blood vessel blockage), stroke, hypoxia (oxygen deficiency), edema (fluid retention), and heart attack.[19] (See Appendix A.)

Oxidized Cholesterol (Oxysterols)

Cholesterol is harmless until it is oxidized by combining with oxygen. The resulting oxysterols can initiate arterial plaque formation, which in turn can lead to atherosclerosis and ultimately to heart attacks and strokes. Heart researcher Kilmer S. McCully, M.D., found that most people who die of heart attacks have low or normal cholesterol and that the severity of acquired atherosclerosis correlates, *not* with high cholesterol, but with the concentration of oxysterols in the blood and in plaques.[20]

Oxysterols can be generated internally by chemicals that oxidize cholesterol. These include chlorine and fluoride, both of which are common in public water supplies. Oxysterols can also enter the body through processed, cholesterol-containing foods; high-temperature processing in the presence of oxygen converts the cholesterol to oxysterols. The most common food sources of oxysterols are the powdered egg yolks, milk, and buttermilk used in hundreds of products, including baked goods, dessert mixes, pies, pastries, salad dressing mixes, and dried soups.

Electromagnetic stress (overexposure to electromagnetic fields, such as those emitted by power lines, household appliances, and computers) is another common source of oxysterols.

The Homocysteine-Oxysterol Connection

There is growing evidence that a major culprit responsible for oxidizing cholesterol and producing atherosclerosis, and, therefore, heart disease, is homocysteine, a substance naturally found in the body.[21]

Homocysteine is a by-product of protein metabolism (specifically, of the amino acid methionine, found mainly in

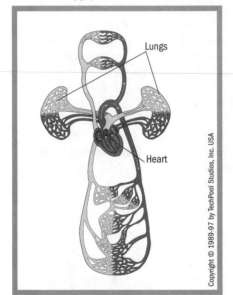

Copyright © 1989-97 by TechPool Studios, Inc. USA

BLOOD FLOW THROUGH THE BODY. The heart pumps blood rich with oxygen (the darker shade) through the arteries to the tissues of the body; blood from the body (the lighter shade) moves through the veins back to the heart and on to the lungs to be reoxygenated.

red meat and milk products). Homocysteine increases oxysterol formation inside the body, particularly in the absence of adequate B-complex vitamins. A well-nourished body contains enough B complex—notably B6, folic acid, riboflavin (B2), and cobalamin (B12)—to convert homocysteine either to a nontoxic product (cystathionine) or back to methionine.

Thus, B complex is essential in the prevention of oxysterol proliferation. Junk-food eaters, smokers, alcoholics, and women taking birth control pills are all likely to have decreased B6 levels in the blood and, therefore, increased cardiovascular risk. In addition, many common synthetic drugs, such as nitrous oxide (laughing gas, used as a dental anesthetic) and methotrexate (used in chemotherapy) destroy the B complex and lead to increased homocysteine.[22]

Elevated Triglycerides

A Swedish study found that increased triglycerides are an independent risk factor for heart disease.[23] Triglycerides, lipids (fats) formed from fatty acids and glycerol, travel in the blood with cholesterol. Triglycerides are often elevated in obese people and in those who consume excess refined sugars, alcohol, and starches.

Imbalanced Calcium/Phosphorus Ratio

The healthy ratio in the blood is 2.5 times more calcium than phosphorus (an ideal level of 10 mg/dl calcium to 4 mg/dl phosphorus). The main disturbers of the calcium/phosphorus ratio are white sugar and other sweeteners, such as corn syrup and fructose. Sugar depletes phosphorus which is required for its utilization. As phosphorus decreases, the blood dumps calcium to maintain the proper ratio. This calcium is then excreted into the urine and feces or into the soft tissue (all body tissues other than teeth and bone). When deposited in the arterial walls, this can cause atherosclerosis.[24]

Excess Iron

In excess, iron can become a cardiovascular risk factor. A 1992 Finnish study showed a statistical correlation with high iron levels and increased risk of heart disease.[25] Excess dietary iron is deposited in heart muscle which has a higher affinity for iron than other muscles of the body.[26]

It is difficult to avoid excess consumption of iron since the FDA requires that it be added to nearly all processed foods. Other sources of iron overload include tap water, iron pots and skillets, and supplements containing iron.

Loss of iron during menses may protect women from heart disease during their fertile years, since after menopause or following a hysterectomy, women experience the same risk of heart disease as men. I do not recommend iron supplements for anyone unless they are anemic from blood loss or illness, and then only herbal forms of iron such as that found in Thera-zyme Spl.

Asthma Drugs

During the last decade, adrenaline mimics, called beta agonists, have become the drugs of choice to control asthma. At the same time, there has been a sharp increase in the death rate from cardiovascular failure in asthmatics using these drugs. Adrenaline and its synthetic drug–mimics seem to cause chronic degeneration of the aorta. In addition, adrenaline mimics damage heart mitochondria (SEE QUICK DEFINITION), the "energy factories" of cells.

Anti-Cholesterol Drugs

According to a Finnish study, a group of men taking cholesterol-reducing drugs (such as Mevacor®, cholestyramine, and clofibrate) suffered a statistically higher number of deaths from cancer, stroke, suicide, and even accidents. In the study of 2,400 clinically healthy middle-aged male business executives with one or more cardiovascular risk factors, total deaths were 46% higher and cardiac mortality 163% higher in those treated with anticholesterol drugs than in the control group.[27]

Success Story: Lowering High Blood Pressure and Cholesterol

Barry, 50, presented with high blood pressure (185/105) along with high cholesterol (255). He was worried about losing his health insurance, which could be canceled if he didn't reduce his cholesterol level. His doctor had prescribed Mevacor (an anticholesterol drug) to bring down his cholesterol level, but Barry had become depressed and suspected the drug to be the cause. When I examined him, I found liver dysfunction (one of the side effects of Mevacor, as reported in the *Physicians' Desk Reference*) and a problem with his thyroid gland which I treated with the following:

- Thera-zyme VSCLR: multiple digestive formula for hypertension
- Thera-zyme Lvr: for liver support

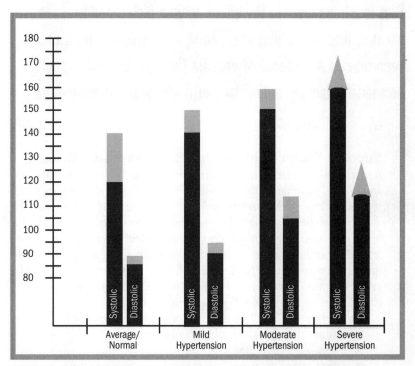

BLOOD PRESSURE RANGES. Hypertension is usually measured as a range of the systolic (when the heart contracts) and diastolic (when the heart rests, filling with more blood) values.

■ *Coleus forskohlii:* Ayurvedic herb for hypertension and cardiovascular problems

■ Thyroid glandular extract

Gradually, over several months on this treatment, Barry not only felt better, but he also lost weight. He stopped taking his Mevacor at the beginning of treatment. At his next check-up, his doctor was surprised at Barry's improved blood results, finding it hard to believe that Barry had lowered his cholesterol without taking Mevacor. This reduction was due to the thyroid hormone, which is needed for the conversion of cholesterol to the anti-aging hormones (pregnenolone, progesterone, and DHEA), thus lowering cholesterol to healthy levels.

Correcting thyroid dysfunction also lowers adrenaline and cortisol (hormones released during a stress reaction) to normal levels, a factor in lowering blood pressure. This, combined with the Thera-zyme VSCLR and the *Coleus forskohlii*, gradually decreased his blood pres-

Diet is a key player in the effort against high blood pressure, stroke, and heart disease. Along with proper nutrition, I recommend a protocol of enzyme therapy, thyroid support, hormonal balancing, antioxidant nutrients, and herbal remedies.

sure to a healthy level (120/80).

Success Story: Quitting High Blood Pressure Drugs

Barbara, 60, needed help in controlling her high blood pressure, for which she was taking three antihypertension drugs. She also complained of an inability to lose weight, a chronic cough (she smoked), and muscle spasms (a possible side effect of the drugs). Barbara had a history of lung and kidney problems, along with lifelong sinus problems. Her urine analysis showed fat and sugar intolerance, low calcium, an anxiety pattern (indicated by low calcium with alkaline pH), and a vitamin C deficiency. In addition, she had an underactive thyroid. I placed her on the following treatment:

- Thera-zyme VSCLR: multiple digestive formula for high blood pressure and other cardiovascular problems
- Thera-zyme SvG: for sugar intolerance
- Thera-zyme Para: for low calcium, which sometimes leads to muscle spasms
- Thera-zyme Rsp: for her cough
- Thera-zyme Nsl: a vitamin C/antioxidant formula, for her sinus problems
- Thera-zyme TRMA: for anxiety and the immune system
- Thera-zyme Kdy: for kidney-lymphatic stress
- *Coleus forskohlii:* Ayurvedic herb to help lower blood pressure
- Thyroid glandular extract
- 10% natural progesterone in vitamin E oil

After two months of enzyme therapy and hormonal balancing, Barbara was able to stop taking two of her prescription drugs for hypertension, and she began to lose weight. Her muscle spasms ceased when she stopped the drugs. Her cough is intermittent because she has not quit smoking, but now, at age 66, she is considering it.

Success Story: The Anorexic Hypertensive Woman

Isabelle, 57, was 5'2" tall but weighed only 77 pounds when she first visited my office. She had a history of hypertension as well as heart and gallbladder problems, and had suffered from two strokes, four episodes of Bell's palsy (partial facial paralysis), and two nervous breakdowns. Isabelle's history also included severe abuse as a child. Currently, her face was distorted from the Bell's palsy, and she had problems sleeping. Her goals were to gain weight, lower her blood pressure, prevent further strokes, and improve her digestion of food.

Isabelle blamed much of her ill-health on the drugs prescribed to help her. She said that seven months earlier she had stopped taking all of the prescription drugs for her various maladies, and swore that she would never touch them again. Even when on antihypertensive drugs, her blood pressure was 180/90. When she was hospitalized with the strokes (and still taking her drugs), it went up to 250/100.

Isabelle had no major source of protein in her diet—no meat, poultry, fish, eggs, milk, or cheese. She lived on a no-salt regimen of vegetables, grains, nuts, and legumes—not a healthy diet for anyone, especially an underweight, hypertensive woman with a history of strokes and, probably, an underactive thyroid. Isabelle had numerous symptoms of low thyroid function including weight change (in her case, weight loss), hair loss, dry skin, slow pulse, irregular heart beat, severe fatigue, panic attacks, cold hands and feet, chronic infections, attention deficit disorder (ADD) and, her major complaint, hypertension.

Isabelle's urinalysis indicated severe sugar intolerance, fat intolerance, malabsorption syndrome, low calcium, and kidney-lymphatic stress. She also had low progesterone which, along with the fat intolerance, could explain her gallbladder problems. Low progesterone is also associated with hypothyroidism in women.

My first effort was to change Isabelle's diet by recommending that she increase her protein, fruit, and salt consumption. I told her to eat protein at least once a day and not be afraid of salt. Salt helps mobilize blood sugar, which is necessary to keep adrenaline and cortisol (the stress hormones) at normal levels. Due to this, salt is essential in preventing, edema, hypertension, hardening of the arteries, and, in women, hot flashes.[28]

I also told Isabelle to eat raw carrots every day, since carrot fiber is probably the best colon cleansing fiber available. It binds colon carcinogens and toxins, some of which are associated with anorexia. I suggested that she add butter, coconut oil, and extra virgin olive oil in small amounts to her diet, and to see if she could digest raw milk, raw cheese, or cultured milk products, such as yogurt. Finally, I instructed her to drink carbonated water daily. The carbon dioxide in carbonated water helps regulate sodium and calcium, prevent edema, and increase tissue oxygenation, important for stroke recovery.[29]

Isabelle's treatment was as follows:

- Thera-zyme HCL: digestive formula for fat, protein, and sugar intolerance; its high lipase content is important in addressing high blood pressure
- Thera-zyme Para: for low calcium
- Thera-zyme Kdy: for kidney/lymphatic stress
- Thera-zyme Nsl: vitamin C/antioxidant formula which would also help relieve her Bell's palsy
- Thera-zyme TRMA: immune system formula which also relieves anxiety; its high protease content helps prevent strokes and blood clots
- *Coleus forskohlii:* Ayurvedic herb for hypertension and heart problems in general
- *Ginkgo biloba:* herb helpful for vascular insufficiency (circulation problems) associated with stroke
- Thyroid glandular extract
- 10% natural progesterone in vitamin E oil

With her new diet and the above treatment, Isabelle gradually started to feel better. She increased her thyroid glandular extract and progesterone very slowly to avoid possible surges in blood pressure, due to increased circulation and higher sensitivity to adrenaline.

After five months of treatment, her blood pressure began a steady downward trend, her oral temperature and pulse increased (a sign that her thyroid function was improving), and she gained seven pounds. Her breasts started to fill out, her face became more symmetrical, her energy level rose, and her sleep improved. Isabelle reported that her overall health was "amazingly better" than before treatment. Now, although her thyroid gland is still not functioning perfectly, she can see her progress and is full of hope and optimism for the future.

Prevention and Elimination of Cardiovascular Disease

As seen in the success stories above, diet is a key player in the effort against high blood pressure, stroke, and heart disease. Along with proper nutrition, I recommend a protocol of enzyme therapy, thyroid support, hormonal balancing, antioxidant nutrients, and herbal remedies.

Enzyme Therapy

The following enzyme supplements modulate blood fats and decrease cardiovascular risk. I choose one multiple digestive enzyme formula, determined by a 24-hour urinalysis and palpation test. In addition to food enzymes, I suggest antioxidant enzymes, since a deficiency of these can cause free-radical activity and the formation of oxidized cholesterol and other toxic substances.

- Thera-zyme VSCLR: high-lipase multiple digestive formula needed by people who eat excess fat and who may be fiber intolerant; helps hypertension
- Thera-zyme HCL: multiple digestive formula for fat and sugar intolerance, which also improves protein digestion
- Thera-zyme Stm: multiple digestive for people with ulcers and gastritis who cannot tolerate high levels of protease because it aggravates their condition
- Thera-zyme Circ: formula designed to increase circulation, strengthen the heart, and nourish the cardiovascular system in general; beneficial for people with a history of heart disease, irregular or skipped heart beats, pain under the breast bone upon exertion, and hypertension; also relieves hemorrhoids and varicose veins
- Antioxidant Enzymes: catalase is the only antioxidant enzyme that can be cultured in a stable form; its major function is to convert hydrogen peroxide into water and oxygen, a reaction that occurs in every cell (catalase-containing Thera-zyme formulas are Stm and TRMA)

Hormonal Balancing

Since adequate thyroid function is essential for a healthy heart, the thyroid should be checked and thyroid glandular therapy used if necessary. In addition, hypothyroid women need natural progesterone therapy because a chronically underactive thyroid gland leads to a deficiency of progesterone. (See Appendix A.)

Dietary Recommendations

While all organic, whole foods contain cardioprotective nutrients, certain foods have specific cardiovascular benefits. Here are a few examples:

- Soluble fiber increases fecal excretion of cholesterol and triglycerides, decreasing their level in the blood. Also, soluble fiber has a modulating effect on blood glucose levels.
- Garlic and onions help lower cholesterol, bring down blood pressure, and decrease platelet adhesiveness (the likelihood that platelet cells in the blood cells will adhere to arterial walls, contribut-

ing to cardiovascular disease).

■ Ginger decreases platelet adhesiveness and stimulates circulation.

■ Silicon-rich foods, such as brown rice, oats, and other whole-grain cereals, water-soluble fiber (pectin), and horsetail herb are good for the heart. Silicon acts as a binder in connective tissue and helps lower cholesterol.

Nutritional Supplements

Antioxidant nutrients such as vitamins A, E, C, and B complex and the minerals zinc and selenium can help promote cardiovascular health.

■ Vitamin C: Thera-zyme Opt or Nsl

■ Vitamin E: Thera-zyme Rbs (food sources of vitamin E include vegetables and whole grains)

■ Vitamin B complex: Thera-zyme Adr (most whole foods contain B complex in the correct proportions); Adr also helps relieve stress

■ Minerals: Heart-healthy minerals include chromium, zinc, magnesium, and potassium but they should not be taken as isolated supplements. Both Thera-zyme TRMA and Thy contain minerals from kelp. It is important not to take too much kelp because it can suppress thyroid function. Brewer's yeast contains chromium (other dietary sources include meat, whole grains, vegetables, and fruits). Fruits juices and alfalfa as a juiced grass or tea are good sources of calcium and magnesium. I do not recommend chelated colloidal minerals because they may contain toxins such as aluminum, cadmium, arsenic, fluoride, and iron.[30] Instead I recommend organic, non-iodized sea salt and purified sea water as good mineral supplements.

Herbal Remedies

There are numerous herbs that strengthen the cardiovascular system. This is only a partial list and excludes those that should be avoided during pregnancy. These products are available at health food stores; follow the recommended dosages on the labels.

■ Hawthorn (*Crataegus oxyacantha*): for high blood pressure

■ Rosemary (*Rosmarinus officinalis*): for low blood pressure

■ Cayenne (*Capsicum annuum*) and ginger (*Zingiber officinalis*): for poor circulation

■ *Ginkgo biloba*: for all cardiovascular problems, including hardening of the arteries, poor circulation, and stroke

■ *Coleus forskohlii*: for hypertension, congestive heart failure, and angina; has also been shown to stimulate the release of thyroid hormone[31]

CHILDREN'S HEALTH PROBLEMS

The following health conditions (bed-wetting, infant colic, and hyperactivity/ADD) are found either solely or predominantly in children. For other problems common to both children and adults, please refer to the specific condition.

BED-WETTING

Involuntary wetting of the bed is a complex childhood phenomenon which is often a sign of one or more underlying problems.

What Causes Bed-Wetting?

An underactive thyroid, structural problems, nutritional deficiencies, allergies, and psychological problems can all contribute to bed-wetting.

For information on the **enzymes** for this health condition, see Appendix B.

Hypothyroidism

One of the most common underlying factors in this childhood ailment is hypothyroidism, or low thyroid function. Hypothyroidism can lead to bed-wetting by suppressing the sympathetic nervous system (a branch of the autonomic nervous system, SEE QUICK DEFINITION). This leads to dominance by the parasympathetic nervous system which is responsible for increasing glandular and gastrointestinal activity. Bed-wetting can be the result.

Adults who have an underactive thyroid are generally not bed-wetters because they have trained themselves to wake up and are more sensitive to visceral irritations, including a full bladder. The lack of sex hormones in children may also account for the difference between children and adults.[32] Estrogen and testosterone are brain excitants—in fact, one function of estrogen may be to make women with children wake up easily. (See Appendix A.)

Structural Problems

One possible structural cause of incontinence (inability to control urination) is phrenic reflex disorder, a respiratory problem in which the diaphragm is not able to move properly (the

The **autonomic nervous system** (ANS) can be likened to your body's automatic pilot. It keeps you alive through breathing, heart rate, and digestion, without your being aware of it or participating in its activities. The ANS has two divisions: the sympathetic, which expends body energy; and the parasympathetic, which conserves body energy. The sympathetic nervous system is associated with arousal and stress; it prepares us physically when we perceive a threat or challenge by increasing our heart rate, blood pressure, and muscle tension. The parasympathetic nervous system slows heart rate and increases intestinal and most gland activity.

phrenic nerve is a motor nerve to the diaphragm). When the diaphragm is "locked" in inhalation mode, the patient's sympathetic nervous system becomes dominant. On the other hand, when the diaphragm is "locked" in the exhalation mode, the patient becomes parasympathetic dominant, which as discussed above, can lead to bed-wetting.

Another structural problem that can contribute to bed-wetting is a misalignment of the vertebral column in the pelvic area (the vertebrae from the eighth thoracic to the third lumbar).

Nutritional Deficiencies/Allergies

See **Allergies**, pp. 65-70.

Diets deficient in enzymes, especially protease (digests protein), may contribute to bed-wetting by causing allergies; bed-wetting is one of the many symptoms of allergies. Another nutritional deficiency which may lead to bed-wetting is iron deficiency.[33]

Psychological Problems

Emotional stress, whether from family, school, or friends, can be a cause of a child's bed-wetting. These problems, if recognized, can be addressed accordingly. Another factor could almost be called "spiritual." Some children are simply not "in their bodies" enough to control their functions during sleep. This is not a physical problem and self-corrects over time, as children become more conscious of their physical nature.

Success Story: Healing Lucy's
Bed-Wetting, Thyroid, and Digestion

Lucy, 7, suffered from both daytime and nighttime incontinence. When she first presented, she had a goiter, puffy face, round belly, and knock-knees—all signs of hypothyroidism. Lucy's average body temperature was only 96° F, another indication of an underactive thyroid. She had allergies to dust, cats, and certain foods, including dairy, chocolate, strawberries, raspberries, and peppermint. She also complained of upper respiratory congestion throughout the year.

Lucy's urinalysis indicated a toxic colon, poor sugar metabolism, and excess fat intake, as well as vitamin C and calcium deficiencies. Her physical exam indicated a parasympathetic dominance (see above), lung problems, and fat intolerance, and confirmed the toxic colon. I recommended a natural thyroid glandular extract along with the following enzyme formulas:

- Thera-zyme HCL: multiple digestive enzyme formula for fat and sugar intolerance
- Thera-zyme Rsp: for respiratory problems and adjusting

parasympathetic dominance

■ Thera-zyme SmI: cellulase formula, high in *acidophilus* to help restore balance of intestinal flora

■ Thera-zyme Challenge Food Powder: for toxic colon and parasites

I also recommended avoidance of all processed foods which, for Lucy, at that time included white flour, margarine, frozen juices, and commercial sugars and sweeteners. When Lucy returned six weeks later, her whole body had changed from the round, chubby shape I had first observed to a thinner, less bloated, more natural looking form. Her bed-wetting problems had diminished and continued to subside as her thyroid function healed.

Prevention and Elimination of Bed-Wetting

The following are guidelines useful for eliminating a child's bed-wetting.

Enzyme Therapy

There is no specific enzyme therapy for bed-wetters. In general, I give a multiple digestive formula which addresses the individual's specific digestive needs. Here are a few examples.

■ Thera-zyme PAN: for sugar intolerant and environmentally sensitive people

■ Thera-zyme Bil: for fat intolerant people who may have gall-bladder problems

■ Thera-zyme HCL: for fat and sugar intolerance and also to help digest protein; contains no hydrochloric acid

■ Thera-zyme Stm: for people who have stomach problems (ulcer, hiatal hernia, or gastritis) and who cannot tolerate the protease in the above formulas

The following formulas are also sometimes indicated:

■ Thera-zyme Spl: contains organic (herbal) iron; used for iron-deficient people

■ Thera-zyme Kdy: for people who have environmental allergies

If other conditions, such as candidiasis, liver dysfunction, or colon problems, are present, they must be addressed with the appropriate enzyme formulas.

Thyroid Support

If your child's bed-wetting is due to an underactive thyroid, he or she can be helped with a good thyroid glandular extract. (See Appendix A.)

Chiropractic Treatment

If incontinence is due to structural problems such as the vertebral misalignment discussed previously, chiropractic adjustments can often correct the condition and bring relief.

Herbal Remedies

■ Dandelion (*Taraxacum officinale*): diuretic (the French word for dandelion, *pissenlit*, literally means "piss-in-bed"). Some doctors recommend giving an infusion of dandelion early in the day to help readjust the child's circadian rhythm (cycle of biological activities in sleep and waking).

■ St. John's wort (*Hypericum perforatum*): used for many symptoms of nervous tension, including anxiety, colic, irritable bowel, and bed-wetting.[34] If there is lack of nervous control of the bladder, try an infusion of one part each of St. John's wort, cornstalk, horsetail, wild oat, and lemon balm ($\frac{1}{2}$ cup, three times a day).

■ An herbal tea made of three parts horsetail, one part agrimony, and one part sweet sumac: for lack of tone in the sphincter muscle of the bladder or in the case of general muscle or nervous debility.

INFANT COLIC

Infant colic refers to spasmodic abdominal pain, accompanied by irritability, crying, and/or vomiting. Although colic is more common among bottle-fed infants, breast-fed babies can also suffer from the condition.

What Causes Infant Colic?

Infant colic, and the projectile vomiting that sometimes ensues, is caused by poor digestion. In bottle-fed babies, pasteurized cow's milk and infant formulas are often the culprit.[35] Breast-fed babies may have colic due to a digestive problem in the mother.

Prevention and Elimination of Infant Colic

If you are breast-feeding and your baby has colic, consider taking multiple digestive enzymes with each meal. The specific enzymes you need can be determined by a urinalysis and detailed health history. If the problem continues, I suggest giving your baby Thera-zyme

DGST, a pediatric multiple digestive enzyme formula. One-half capsule of DGST three times daily should relieve colic within a day. This is much safer than treating your child with the addictive tranquilizer Valium, which is one conventional medical prescription for colic.

HYPERACTIVITY/ATTENTION DEFICIT DISORDER

A child who is inattentive, overly talkative, impulsive, excessively irritable, or is simply unable to sit still is often labeled as hyperactive or as having attention deficit disorder (ADD).

What Causes Hyperactivity?

Hyperactivity has two major causes: low thyroid function and sugar intolerance. Hypothyroid function has a direct effect on the frontal lobe of the brain, which appears to be responsible for the ability to sustain prolonged mental attention. The frontal lobe has a high energy (glucose) requirement, and it follows that when it receives inadequate glucose, there is an inability to focus and concentrate—a major symptom of ADD.

Thyroid hormone is essential for providing the necessary glucose to the brain and to the body. When thyroid hormone is deficient, the body produces excess adrenaline to keep itself going. The result is hyperactivity (from excess adrenaline) and tension, with tiredness at the same time. A drug such as Ritalin is often prescribed since, by temporarily stimulating the brain, it produces more attention and focus in those who take it. However, the *Physicians' Desk Reference* reports that Ritalin can provoke numerous adverse reactions, including nervousness, insomnia, skin rashes, nausea, dizziness, abdominal pain, and weight loss—this last effect being especially troublesome in a growing child.

As an alternative to Ritalin, a number of physicians are using thyroid glandular therapy, not only to quiet hyperactive children, but also to increase energy in lethargic ones, or for those with "growing pains."[36]

Sugar intolerance—the second major cause of ADD—is easy to correct by removing all refined, processed sugars from the diet and giving a multiple digestive enzyme formula which includes the sugar-digesting enzymes (disaccharidases).

Success Story: Saying No to Ritalin

Nick, 4, was intelligent and creative, but could not sit still long enough

Hyperactivity has two major causes: low thyroid function and sugar intolerance. As an alternative to Ritalin, a number of physicians are using thyroid glandular therapy to quiet hyperactive children and to increase energy in lethargic ones. Sugar intolerance is easy to correct by removing all refined, processed sugars from the diet and giving a multiple digestive enzyme formula.

to learn. He was diagnosed with ADD and sent home from preschool with the suggestion that he start taking Ritalin. His mother, not wanting Nick on the drug but needing to do something about his disruptive behavior, called me for advice.

Nick's physical examination and medical history revealed multiple allergies, a chronic skin rash, sores on his tongue, headaches, and an inability to gain weight. A urinalysis indicated sugar intolerance. It also showed the allergy pattern plus low calcium, severe vitamin C deficiency, and a toxic colon. His oral temperature was low, indicating an underactive thyroid which could explain his ADD state. In fact, Nick's mother could predict his body temperature by simply observing her son's behavior. When his temperature decreased, he became agitated and hyperactive. When it reached a more normal range, he calmed down.

I recommended the following enzyme and thyroid treatment for Nick:

■ Thera-zyme DGST: multiple digestive enzyme formula which includes the disaccharidases (digest sugar)

■ Thera-zyme Nsl: antioxidant/vitamin C enzyme formula especially good for acute allergies and nasal problems

■ Thera-zyme Kdy: enzyme/herbal formula for allergies

■ Thyroid glandular extract: I suggested a very small dose, less than ¼ grain, which was gradually increased until Nick's temperature and pulse rose to normal

Nick's mother carefully monitored his temperature and observed his behavior. She tried to eliminate all refined sugars and processed foods from his diet, a more difficult task because Nick was a picky eater. Two months later, however, she reported that her son was doing very well. His psychologist found him much calmer and his teacher found the improvement "fantastic." Nick's mother also reported that all of his other symptoms, including the skin rash, had disappeared. I had not treated the rash specifically; it had cleared up on its own due to Nick's improved diet and the overall treatment he was following. Nick's hyperactivity only returned when he was sick or strayed from his diet.

DIABETES

Diabetes mellitus is a degenerative disease caused by either lack of insulin or a resistance to insulin, a hormone which is crucial for metabolism of blood sugar (glucose). In a healthy person, the pancreas produces insulin to help metabolize sugar in the blood and maintain blood glucose levels within their normal range. Since diabetics are unable to produce or are resistant to insulin, they cannot move glucose from the bloodstream to the cells and thus cannot maintain a normal glucose level.

There are two major types of diabetes: insulin-dependent juvenile diabetes (Type I), and non-insulin-dependent adult-onset diabetes (Type II).

In Type I diabetes, the body is unable to produce insulin. As a result glucose builds up in the bloodstream and spills over into the urine. The body is "starved" because cells do not get the nourishment—usually provided by glucose—to produce the energy necessary to carry out their normal functions. Symptoms of Type I diabetes include extreme hunger and thirst, along with frequent or excessive urination, often accompanied by weight loss. Type I diabetes usually begins during puberty or adolescence but it can appear in adults if the pancreas is damaged due to injury or disease.

Type II is much more common. About 90% of diabetics are Type II and 80% of them are overweight when diagnosed, which is generally during middle age. Obesity and excess calorie intake create a resistance to insulin—that is, the pancreas continues to produce insulin in response to blood glucose, but the body's cells resist the action of insulin. The combination of obesity and high blood sugar leads to a decrease in the number of insulin receptors, sites to which insulin attaches to initiate conversion of glucose to glycogen or fat for storage. Symptoms of Type II diabetes are the same as symptoms of Type I, with the exception of weight loss.

If poorly controlled, either type of diabetes can lead to heart disease, kidney disease, cancer, hypertension, gangrenous infections, blindness, strokes, and even death.

For information on the **enzymes** for this health condition, see Appendix B.

According to Raymond Peat, Ph.D., an authority on hormonal balancing based in Eugene, Oregon, the conventional view of diabetes as a permanent state is faulty. Diabetes is usually defined by an elevated blood sugar (greater than 140) and glucosuria (elevated sugar in the urine); when glucose reaches a certain level in the blood, it

Type II diabetes can usually be controlled by natural methods, including diet, weight control, enzyme therapy, hormonal balancing, and herbal supplements.

shows up in the urine as well.

Dr. Peat cautions that blood sugar should not be used as the sole indicator of diabetes, since so many factors can raise the level of glucose in the blood (and urine). Among them are fever (such as that occurring during viral infections), a cortisone shot, and even puberty. Young children are often diagnosed with diabetes following the rise in blood sugar after a fever and are placed on insulin. The insulin continues this so-called diabetes, causes insulin dependence, and raises the cortisol (an adrenal hormone) level which exacerbates the problem.

Since elevated cortisol is usually associated with elevated blood sugar, Dr. Peat urges that the levels of cortisol as well as insulin be measured, but many doctors look only at blood sugar. According to Dr. Peat, an actual insulin deficiency (Type I, juvenile diabetes) is rare. The majority of "diabetics" have plenty of insulin and are insulin-resistant, not insulin-deficient, he states.

In addition to excess weight, the two most common causes of insulin resistance are excess (unbalanced) estrogen—estrogen dominance—and excess intake of polyunsaturated fatty acids (PUFAs). The connection between estrogen and insulin-resistance explains why menopausal women have five times more diabetes than men, since estrogen becomes more dominant during menopause, a condition often exacerbated by estrogen replacement therapy.

Most people with high blood sugar have normal insulin and elevated cortisol. The latter is a direct outcome of hypothyroidism (underactive thyroid gland). Thyroid therapy normalizes blood sugar by keeping the cortisol and adrenaline at safe levels. It is imperative to lower cortisol because excess cortisol causes the liver to produce estrogen and excess estrogen desensitizes the skeletal muscles to the action of insulin. Hypothyroidism research pioneer Broda Barnes, M.D., found that although thyroid therapy can increase blood sugar it protects one from the health problems associated with diabetes. (See Appendix A.)

What Causes Diabetes?

A genetic predisposition may be associated with both types of diabetes, but the following are strongly contributing factors:

- Chemical poisoning from substances such as pesticides and certain chemical additives such as alloxan (which is present in bleached white flour and used in commercial wheat products)
  - The use of prednisone (synthetic cortisone)
  - The production of excess cortisol which occurs with hypothyroidism
  - Excess dietary unsaturated oils (liquid at room temperature, SEE QUICK DEFINITION), with the exception of extra virgin olive oil. These include soybean, safflower, sesame, corn, fish, flaxseed, borage, and evening primrose oils. Excess consumption of unsaturated oils suppresses thyroid function which is directly associated with elevated cortisol and insulin-resistant diabetes.[37]
  - Stress, which exacerbates hypothyroidism and suppresses the immune system in general
  - An enzyme-deficient, refined, junk-food diet. In particular, diabetics are deficient in lipase (digests fat) which is required for the metabolism of insulin and for optimum cell permeability, permitting the transport of insulin inside the cell. Insulin metabolism is suppressed in proportion to the amount of undigested fat (triglycerides) in the blood. Lipase deficiency (fat intolerance) leads to the inability to utilize glucose and might also be considered a factor in insulin resistance. If fat can be digested, insulin metabolism can be improved.

For more about the **damaging effects of unsaturated oils**, see Chapter 3: What Causes Enzyme Deficiencies?, pp. 51-54.

Success Story: The Junk-Food Diabetic

Dan, 45, had Type II diabetes and was being treated with oral diabetic drugs. He took these faithfully, but his diet was a diabetic's nightmare, consisting mainly of fast foods and processed foods containing refined sugar. Dan ate few whole foods such as organic fruits, vegetables, meat, or poultry. His urine test revealed the drastic effects of his poor diet: a large amount of urinary glucose, a highly toxic colon, sugar and fat intolerance, severe allergies, and an overly acidic condition with low calcium and low vitamin C.

Even though there are enzyme formulas for each of his conditions, I emphasized to him that popping enzymes without dietary changes was a waste of money. As a prerequisite to enzyme therapy, Dan promised that he would indeed change his diet. Dan said he had no choice—he felt so terrible. Even with this promise, I minimized his treatment, start-

ing with the following formulas:
- Thera-zyme VSCLR: multiple digestive enzyme for fat intolerance
- Thera-zyme SvG: for sugar intolerance
- Thera-zyme Challenge Food Powder: colon cleanse powder which helps reduce colon toxicity and also gets rid of parasites
- Thera-zyme Kdy: for allergy relief
- Thyroid glandular extract: important in all conditions with abnormal blood sugar

Dan changed his diet completely, eliminating fast foods and processed foods. After a month of treatment, his second urine test showed dramatic changes. His colon was no longer toxic and there was no urinary glucose. Dan's doctor told him to stop his oral diabetic drug because his blood sugar was now normal.

Success Story: Getting Off Insulin

Martha was middle-aged and slightly overweight with insulin-dependent diabetes of ten years duration when she consulted Dr. Peat for help in reducing her insulin dosage. He recommended the following program:
- DHEA, 10% in vitamin E oil: 10 mg (three drops) daily for two to three weeks. Caution: DHEA is contraindicated in diabetics who have cancer, since it can convert to estrogen and cause cancerous tumors to grow.
- Thyroid glandular therapy
- Brewer's yeast: up to 4 oz daily for two weeks. This can be added as a paste to chicken broth or another food. Caution: do not take for longer than two weeks, because brewer's yeast is high in phosphorus which, when taken for a prolonged period, can cause loss of calcium.
- A diet high in animal protein: eggs, raw milk/cheese, chicken, and fish. Potatoes are the best vegan source of protein.
- Coconut oil, plus a raw carrot salad daily

In three to four days, Martha had to decrease her insulin dosage. In three weeks, she was off insulin completely.

Prevention and Elimination of Diabetes

Unlike Type I diabetes which generally requires regular insulin injections, Type II diabetes can usually be controlled by natural methods, including diet, weight control, enzyme therapy, hormonal balancing, and herbal supplements. Insulin-dependent diabetics must monitor insulin and glucose levels. In general, physicians consider a fasting plasma glucose level above 140 mg/dl as excessive. The optimum range is actually 85 to 100.

Enzyme Therapy

- Thera-zyme VSCLR: high-lipase multiple digestive enzyme formula
- Thera-zyme SvG: for sugar (sucrose, lactose, and maltose) intolerance
- Thera-zyme Stm: for gastric problems

Thyroid Support

Dr. Barnes discovered that diabetics taking insulin suffered no side effects from the insulin as long as their thyroid gland was functioning optimally.[38] If testing determines that your thyroid function is low, seek the advice of a health professional. If treatment is needed, I recommend a thyroid glandular extract. (See Appendix A.)

Hormonal Balancing

In insulin-dependent diabetics, certain cells in the pancreas, called beta cells, do not function properly to produce insulin. In animal studies in which diabetes was induced by destroying the beta cells of the pancreas, DHEA was found to reverse the damaged beta cells.[39] I am against the use of DHEA in hormonal balancing, however, because if too much is taken, it can convert to estrogen or testosterone. Instead, I recommend pregnenolone powder, which converts to progesterone, and DHEA in the proper amounts according to each body's need. I recommend pregnenolone for all diabetics, young and old alike, at a dosage of 100 mg to 150 mg (about $1/16$ tsp) daily.

As recounted in the case of Martha, Dr. Peat has successfully used DHEA to wean insulin-dependent diabetics from their insulin. However, as cautioned above, DHEA should not be used by someone who has cancer because it can convert to estrogen; research has found that excess estrogen can be carcinogenic.[40]

Dietary Recommendations

Most cases of Type II diabetes can be controlled by diet and many cases of Type I will benefit from proper diet and nutrition as well. A diet of whole, unprocessed foods is recommended for both types. Some diabetics can tolerate whole fresh fruits and some cannot, at least at the beginning of therapy. Each case is individual and, of course, any digestive problems must be remediated with enzyme therapy.

Foods to Avoid

■ Bleached white flour. Not only have the bran and germ been stripped away, but bleached flour also contains a substance from the flour bleach (alloxan) which causes diabetes in animals. Unbleached white flour should also be avoided since it is stripped of essential nutrients.

■ White sugar and all refined sugars, including fructose, corn syrup, and dextrose. Diabetics must be careful about their use of natural sweeteners, including honey, maple syrup, and molasses. Artificial sweeteners should also be avoided. Aspartame is especially bad for insulin-dependent diabetics because it affects blood sugar levels and thus makes controlling them more difficult. According to diabetes specialist H.J. Roberts, M.D., in a study of 58 diabetic patients, "The contributory role of such products in the loss of diabetic control was confirmed by prompt improvement of blood glucose (sugar) levels after abstinence."[41] Dr. Roberts also notes that saccharin has been shown to cause tumors in animals.[42] Both regular and diet sodas, juices with added sugar, and concentrated foods such as dried fruits should all be excluded.

■ Unsaturated oils (those that are liquid at room temperature, with the exception of olive oil). These include soybean, corn, safflower, sesame seed, flaxseed, evening primrose, and fish oils. Also avoid all partially hydrogenated oils such as margarine. In general, the diet must be low in fats, even if they are healthy fats, because of the lipase deficiency associated with diabetes.

EDITOR'S NOTE
The position on unsaturated fats presented here is a controversial one. Many physicians advocate the dietary use and supplementation of essential fatty acids in the form of fish, primrose, borage, and flaxseed oils, among others, in the unsaturated category. There is research to support both positions.

Foods That Help Control Diabetes

■ Complex carbohydrates: potatoes, brown rice, other whole grains. Make sure that grains are whole and preferably organic. Grain-sensitive people should eat heirloom grains such as kamut, spelt, quinoa, and amaranth; heirloom grains are those which have not been hybridized (the wheat found in most wheat products has been for the convenience of modern agribusiness). About 70% of wheat-intolerant people can handle heirloom grains, which are available as whole grains or as flour; they are also used as ingredients in many whole food products such as cereals, breads, and crackers.

■ Dairy: raw, organic milk; raw or at least unprocessed cheese; the least-processed yogurt available. Commercial dairy products, particularly milk, are not recommended.

Key Nutrient Sources for Controlling Diabetes

Certain nutrients are required by the body for the metabolism of glucose, specifically chromium, manganese, zinc, B-complex vitamins (particularly pantothenic acid, or vitamin B5), inositol, and vitamin C. The following are dietary sources of these nutrients (food sources for each are listed in descending order of importance).

- Chromium: brewer's yeast, whole wheat and rye bread, bovine liver, potatoes, green peppers, eggs, chicken, apples, butter, parsnips, and cornmeal (Many diabetics have reported to me that taking small [microgram] amounts of chromium picolinate has helped reduce their insulin dosage. Caution: large amounts of chromium can be toxic.)

- Manganese: pecans, brazil nuts, almonds, barley, rye, buckwheat, split peas, whole wheat, walnuts, spinach, oats, raisins, beet greens, Brussels sprouts, cheese, carrots, broccoli, brown rice, corn, cabbage, peaches, and butter

- Zinc: fresh oysters, ginger root, lamb chops, pecans, split peas, beef liver, egg yolk, whole wheat, rye, oats, lima beans, almonds, walnuts, sardines, chicken, and buckwheat

- B-complex: brewer's yeast, torula yeast, beef and chicken liver, mushrooms, split peas, blue cheese, pecans, eggs, lobster, oats, buckwheat, rye, broccoli, turkey (dark meat), brown rice, whole wheat, red chili peppers, sardines, avocado, chicken (dark meat), and kale

- Inositol: navy beans, barley, whole wheat (wheat germ), brewer's yeast, oats, blackeyed peas, oranges, lima beans, green peas, molasses, split peas, grapefruit, raisins, cantaloupe, brown rice, orange juice, peaches, cabbage, cauliflower, onions, sweet potatoes, watermelon, strawberries, lettuce, tomatoes, eggs, and whole milk

- Vitamin C: acerola, red chili peppers, guavas, red sweet peppers, kale, parsley, collard leaves, turnip greens, green sweet peppers, broccoli, Brussels sprouts, mustard greens, watercress, cauliflower, red cabbage, strawberries, papayas, spinach, oranges, lemons, grapefruit, turnips, mangoes, asparagus, cantaloupe, Swiss chard, green onions, tangerines, and oysters

- Meat and poultry: only organic (free of chemicals, drugs, and hormones) beef, lamb, chicken, or turkey

- Fish: from the least-polluted waters. These are usually white fish—halibut, swordfish, or sole. Salmon contains a high amount of unsaturated fatty acids, so eat it sparingly.

- Fats: coconut oil, butter (preferably raw, organic), and extra virgin olive oil only. Use sparingly, as diabetics are fat intolerant.

- High-fiber foods: fresh whole vegetables, legumes, whole grains, and whole fruits. Dietary fibers (especially oats) lower blood sugar levels, reduce insulin requirements, and decrease the rate of absorption of foods from the intestines into the bloodstream. Get fiber from the whole food itself rather than fiber supplements.

■ Garlic and onions: apparently help lower blood sugar. This action seems to be caused by sulfur-containing compounds, although other ingredients, such as bioflavonoids, may play a role.

■ Nutrients needed to metabolize glucose in the body: see "Key Nutrient Sources for Controlling Diabetes," previous page.

Herbal Remedies

■ Gymnesyl (*Gymnema sylvestre*): Ayurvedic herb used in the treatment of diabetes. It has been shown to reduce the insulin requirement in Type I diabetes, and there is some evidence that it may regenerate or revitalize the cells of the pancreas responsible for producing insulin. Gymnesyl has also shown positive results in Type II diabetes. In fact, some patients were able to discontinue their oral drugs and maintain blood sugar control with gymnesyl alone. In one study of non-insulin-dependent diabetics given gymnesyl along with their oral blood sugar–lowering medication, all patients showed improved blood sugar control, 21 of 22 Type II diabetics were able to reduce their drug dosage considerably, and five subjects were able to maintain blood sugar control with gymnesyl and diet alone.[43] The dose for gymnesyl is 400 mg daily in both Type I and Type II diabetes.

■ *Stevia*: herbal sweetener which helps stabilize blood sugar while not requiring insulin for its metabolism

■ Fenugreek seeds (*Trigonella foenum-graecum*): Defatted fenugreek seed powder given twice daily (50 g) to Type I diabetics resulted in lowered fasting blood sugar and a 54% decrease in 24-hour urinary glucose excretion. In Type II diabetics, the addition of 15 g of powdered fenugreek seed soaked in water significantly reduced postprandial glucose levels.[44]

■ Pterocarpus (*Pterocarpus marsupium*): historically used in India as a treatment for diabetes. It contains a flavonoid called epicatechin which has been shown to prevent and rejuvenate beta cell damage in rats. Epicatechin is also found in green tea (*Camellia sinensis*). Since pterocarpus is not available in the United States, green tea may be a good alternative. Noted health authority Michael T. Murray, N.D., recommends at least two cups of green tea daily.

■ *Huereque*: derived from the root of the huereque cactus which grows in the northwestern Mexican desert. It seems to have a profound effect on lowering blood sugar levels. Daniel Dunphy, P.A., N.D., of the San Francisco Preventive Medical Group, in California, has used this botanical on 15 insulin-dependent patients with adult-onset diabetes. All 15 are now almost or entirely off insulin. Dr.

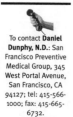

To contact **Daniel Dunphy, N.D.**: San Francisco Preventive Medical Group, 345 West Portal Avenue, San Francisco, CA 94127; tel: 415-566-1000; fax: 415-665-6732.

Dunphy reports that the only drawback to huereque is that, after about six months, its ability to control blood sugar starts to wear off, as if the body has developed a tolerance to it. However, giving the body a month's rest from huereque restores its effectiveness. One option is to switch to nopal (another cactus which reduces blood sugar) for a month, then return to huereque at a lower dose.

Aromatherapy/Essential Oils

Many essential oils have a modulating effect on blood sugar and lead to reduced insulin requirements. Among them are coriander, cypress, dill, eucalyptus, fennel, geranium, ginger, rosemary, and ylang ylang. It is best to choose one or two essential oils to use at a time rather than all of them. Choose based on which odors most appeal to you or how they make you feel. Aromatherapy oils can be used in various ways: put 3-6 drops in bath water; use an aromatherapy diffuser to fill the air with the scent; apply 1-6 drops directly onto the feet (the skin of the feet absorbs oils quickly) or any area of concern; or dilute with massage oil by 15% to 30% and use in massage.[45]

FIBROIDS (UTERINE)

A uterine fibroid is a benign tissue growth, or noncancerous tumor, in the uterus, typically occurring in women over 35. An estimated 25% to 50% of women of childbearing age have fibroids. The fibroid itself is composed of hard, white tissue.

Fibroids (which are also called uterine leiomyomas) lead to an estimated 33% of all gynecological hospital admissions, including surgery (either myomectomy or hysterectomy). They are almost never cancerous and often dissolve spontaneously at menopause. Nevertheless, about 40% of women with large fibroids are infertile; fibroid removal can increase fertility by 60%.

Most women with fibroids have no symptoms at all, but there may be lower abdominal pain, a feeling of pressure in the lower abdomen, and frequent urinination caused by pressure on the bladder, heavy menstrual periods, bleeding between periods, and/or increased menstrual cramps.

What Causes Uterine Fibroids?

Estrogen dominance (an excess of estrogen relative to progesterone) is a primary cause of fibroids. A common source of estrogen dominance is hypothyroidism because an underactive thyroid leads to a progesterone deficiency which throws the hormonal ratio askew.

Success Story: Shrinking a Fibroid Naturally

Roberta, 43, came with several problems, but the most urgent was a melon-sized fibroid in her uterus. Her doctor was giving her Lupron shots to shrink the fibroid to a size that could safely be removed by surgery. In addition to being expensive ($100 per injection), the Lupron made Roberta sick. (Lupron®, a synthetic drug which suppresses both estrogen and progesterone production, has many side effects including some that are common in menopause, such as hot flashes, headaches, emotional lability, decreased libido, and vaginal dryness.)

Roberta also suffered from herpes and had been taking the drug acyclovir for the past ten years. Each time she discontinued it, the herpes came back with a vengeance. Roberta's medical history and physical examination also revealed digestive disturbances and low thyroid function—nearly always present in female health problems. I gave her the following supple-

For information on the **enzymes** for this health condition, see Appendix B.

See *Alternative Medicine Guide to Women's Health 1* (Future Medicine Publishing, 1998; ISBN 1-887299-12-2); to order, call 800-333-HEAL.

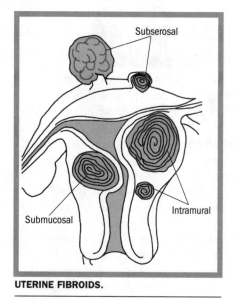

UTERINE FIBROIDS.

ments:

■ Thera-zyme PAN: digestive formula for sugar and gluten intolerance

■ Thera-zyme Rbs: used to control herpes

■ Thyroid glandular extract

■ Natural progesterone (10%) in vitamin E oil

After being on the program for several weeks, Roberta stopped the Lupron shots and the fibroid continued to shrink. A few months later, she had successful surgery. Roberta also weaned herself from the acyclovir while continuing the herpes enzyme formula. As long as she ate a good diet and stayed on her enzymes, she was fine.

Prevention and Elimination of Fibroids

There is no specific enzyme for the treatment of fibroids, but healthy women with no enzyme deficiencies are less prone to forming them. As with other health conditions, testing can determine which enzymes are lacking and the appropriate digestive enzyme formula can then be prescribed. In addition, Thera-zyme TRMA, the immune system formula which is indicated in all forms of tumors, benign or malignant, may be useful. Although TRMA can help shrink a fibroid, it does not address the hormonal imbalance (estrogen dominance) which is the source of the condition.

To correct that imbalance, shrink the fibroid, and prevent a recurrence, natural progesterone (10% in vitamin E oil) can be taken orally and also rubbed on the area of the abdomen over the site of the fibroid. Since hypothyroidism is often a causal factor in estrogen dominance, thyroid glandular extract may be indicated, in combination with the progesterone.

Finally, to prevent further skewing of the progesterone-estrogen ratio, sources of estrogen should be avoided, including birth control pills, estrogenic pesticides (which mimic estrogen in the body), and herbs such as black cohosh, sage, and pennyroyal. (See Appendix A.)

GALLBLADDER DISORDERS

The gallbladder is a small sac-like organ which lies beneath the liver. It stores and concentrates bile produced by the liver. During digestion, the gallbladder contracts and supplies bile to the upper part of the small intestine (the duodenum) to help break down fats. Bile is a water-based solution containing mainly bile salts plus smaller amounts of other substances, including cholesterol. Bile salts have two important functions. First, they have a "detergent function"—that is, they emulsify fats. Second, they facilitate absorption of cholesterol. Without adequate bile salts, up to 40% of the fats consumed are lost in the stool. This can cause a deficiency of nutrient fats and the fat-soluble vitamins (A, D, E, and K).

Ultimately, all cholesterol produced in the liver must be excreted in the bile. Gallstones are formed when cholesterol precipitates (separates from the solution) due to a decrease in bile salts, an increase in the amount of cholesterol in the bile, a decrease in water, or an increased level of acidity in the body. All of these factors must be in balance to keep the highly insoluble cholesterol in solution, so as to avoid the formation of gallstones.

Every year, 20 million Americans have gallstones and more than 300,000 gallbladders are removed due to gallbladder disorders. Although gallstones have been found in fetuses, the average gallstone patient is 40 to 50 years old and the incidence increases with age.

While gallstones are the fifth most prevalent cause of hospitalization in the United States, not everyone with gallbladder problems needs to be hospitalized. Only 20% of people who have gallstones get symptoms—many people have "silent" gallstones which never bother them. It may take as long as eight years for a gallstone to form. Some of the many symptoms of chronic gallstones include belching after meals, pain under the right rib cage or between the shoulder blades, abdominal discomfort or nausea, intolerance of fatty and spicy foods and certain vegetables, clay-colored stools, and headaches.

For information on the **enzymes** for this health condition, see Appendix B.

Symptoms of an acute attack, which needs immediate medical attention, include extreme pain high in the abdomen (especially under the right rib cage) which radiates around to the right shoulder and under the shoulder blade, with possible nausea and vomiting, especially after a heavy, high-fat meal. If the condition persists, the liver, unable to adequately process bilirubin (the pigment in bile) dumps it into the blood, causing jaundice. Although it may save your life, gallbladder removal

If you are having gallbladder symptoms, consult your doctor immediately. Gallbladder disorders need to be taken seriously as they can result in death.

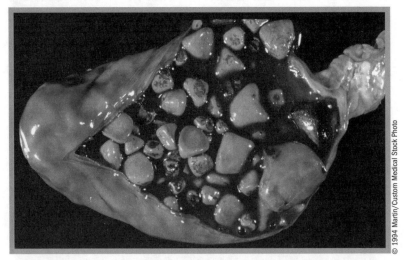

A GALLBLADDER FULL OF STONES. It's estimated that each year some 20 million Americans develop gallstones, making this problem the fifth most prevalent cause of hospitalization. Only 20% of people with gallstones have noticeable symptoms; the remainder have "silent" gallstones which can take up to eight years to form.

© 1994 Martin/Custom Medical Stock Photo

does not correct the underlying problem, which is the liver's inability to convert cholesterol to bile.

What Causes Gallbladder Disorders?

The most common causes of gallstone formation are estrogen dominance, prescription drugs, dietary factors, nutritional deficiencies, and emotional problems.

Estrogen Dominance

Estrogen dominance means estrogen unbalanced by progesterone, an outcome of low thyroid function, consumption of excess amounts of dietary forms of estrogen (yeast and herbal forms of estrogen such as black cohosh, sage, and pennyroyal), and exposure to or ingestion of estrogen mimics or environmental estrogens.

Prescription Drugs

The greatest drug-related cause of gallstones is estrogen, both natural and synthetic, including that found in birth control pills and estrogen replacement therapy, which is probably why six times as many women as men get gallstones. Additionally, cholesterol-lowering drugs, such as Mevacor and clofibrate, increase the risk of gallstones by increasing cholesterol secretion in the bile.[46] In one study of 3,800 people, those taking an anti-cholesterol drug had 22% more bile diseases and a 45% increase in gallstones.[47]

Dietary Factors

The typical American diet of processed foods and heavy consumption of meat, fat, and refined sugars, with few high-fiber foods, has been correlated with increased incidence of gallstones.[48] Refined sugars increase cholesterol synthesis by stimulating insulin secretion. They also increase blood fats (triglycerides) and platelet adhesiveness, or the likelihood that blood cells will adhere to arterial walls. At the same time, refined sugar has none of the B vitamins and trace minerals of the raw sugar cane from which it was derived, while refined fructose contains none of the fiber and nutrients of its mother fruit.

When it comes to fat, it is important to be aware that not all fats are bad for you (if you can digest them) and your body needs a certain amount of the right kinds of fat: the saturated fats such as raw butter and coconut oil, and extra virgin olive oil (a healthy unsaturated fat). Fats to avoid are hydrogenated fats such as vegetable shortening or margarine and all unsaturated oils (liquid at room temperature), including soybean, safflower, flaxseed, sunflower, almond, corn, and fish oils, with the exception of olive oil.

Excessive consumption of unsaturated fats suppresses the thyroid.[49] Since suppressed thyroid function leads to excessive estrogen relative to progesterone and these fats also have properties similar to estrogen, unsaturated fats have a twofold influence associated with gallbladder problems.

Hydrogenated fats contain substances called trans-fatty acids which can inhibit liver enzymes needed to convert cholesterol to bile salts. Thus, margarine and other hydrogenated fats stimulate gallstone formation by inhibiting the conversion of cholesterol to bile.

Nutritional Deficiencies

Refined food diets leave us deficient in many nutrients which are essential to liver and gallbladder health. Deficiencies in either vitamin C or vitamin E have been shown to promote gallstones in test subjects, while control groups eating the same diet with adequate amounts of vitamin C and vitamin E remained free of stones.[50] Vitamin C deficiency has been

EDITOR'S NOTE
The position on unsaturated fats presented here is a controversial one. Many physicians advocate the dietary use and supplementation of essential fatty acids in the form of fish, primrose, borage, and flaxseed oils, among others, in the unsaturated category. There is research to support both positions.

For more about **healthy and unhealthy fats**, see Chapter 3: What Causes Enzyme Deficiencies?, pp. 51-54.

Word of warning: Don't think you can simply take enzymes, herbs, and other supplements to solve your gallbladder condition without adhering to a strict diet.

correlated with increased liver and serum cholesterol, as well as decreased levels of bile acids, making gallstone formation more likely.[51]

Emotional Problems

As with any health condition, there is an emotional component to gallbladder disorders. A person predisposed to gallstones or other gallbladder problems may have a flare-up during an emotional crisis.

Success Story: Gallbladder Relief With Enzymes

The woman in this case is married to a doctor who practices enzyme therapy. In addition, I was already familiar with her medical history when the following events occurred. If not for these two factors, I would not have risked the treatment I used, but would have directed her to the nearest emergency room. I recommend the same to you: if your symptoms resemble hers, immediately consult your doctor or go to the hospital.

Patricia, 45, had been sick intermittently—every two to three weeks—with severe nausea and vomiting for two months. As these bouts of illness progressed, she noticed that her urine was becoming gradually darker—a symptom, along with the nausea and vomiting, of hepatitis. She had suffered from hepatitis in the past and remembered feeling the same malaise. Patricia's husband called me and asked for my opinion. Knowing that Patricia's diet included sugar, synthetic fats, and processed foods, I told him that I suspected gallbladder problems. He did an abdominal exam. Upon palpation, his wife exhibited pain under the right rib cage, an indication of gallbladder trouble.

I advised that Patricia take one Thera-zyme Lvr capsule every 30 minutes to one hour, and told him that if the nausea and vomiting stopped immediately, it was most likely a gallbladder problem. However, if the symptoms persisted, that meant it was an acute, possibly life-threatening attack and she should go straight to the emergency room. As soon as Patricia started the enzyme treatment, her vomiting subsided, her nausea and colic decreased, and she continued to feel better over the next few days.

Patricia then went on a health binge, eliminating fatty foods, junk foods, and sugar from her diet, and adding enzyme-rich raw juices. Subsequent diagnostic tests showed that her liver enzymes were high, but not high enough to indicate hepatitis. An ultrasound revealed the presence of gallstones, confirming the diagnosis.

Success Story: Quick Help for Severe Pain

Another woman in her forties presented with long-standing gallbladder symptoms. She had pain in the upper right abdominal quadrant, directly under the rib cage. It was so severe that she was unable to eat and had lost 20 pounds in the past month. I gave her Thera-zyme Bil, a digestive enzyme for fat intolerance, along with Thera-zyme Lvr, a liver formula. Within hours of taking these enzymes, she felt well enough to eat. She continues to be fine as long as she takes her enzymes, eats a low-fat diet, and avoids certain foods which irritate her gallbladder.

Prevention and Elimination of Gallbladder Disorders

Gallbladder flushes, in which patients consume large amounts of olive oil, have become a popular home remedy in recent years. Howard Loomis, D.C., of Madison, Wisconsin, advises against this procedure, citing it as dangerous, especially for someone who has larger gallstones, because heavy consumption of oil can cause gallbladder contraction. The contractions increase the chances of biliary obstruction—that is, a stone stuck in the bile duct, which requires immediate surgery to prevent death.

Dr. Loomis' enzyme protocol for gallbladder problems (detailed below) is the treatment I recommend if—and only if—you are willing to change your diet. Another word of warning: Don't think you can simply take enzymes, herbs, and other supplements to solve your gallbladder condition without adhering to a strict diet (see Dietary Recommendations below). If you do, you are endangering yourself. There is a point of no return after which gallbladder surgery is necessary to save a life.

Enzyme Therapy

There are two enzyme formulas for gallbladder problems:
- Thera-zyme Bil: multiple digestive enzyme formula for fat intolerance
- Thera-zyme Lvr: liver-gallbladder formula

If the gallbladder problem is mild, I recommend two capsules of Thera-zyme Bil with meals and two capsules of Thera-zyme Lvr after meals. In more serious gallbladder problems, the person will not be able to tolerate two capsules of the Lvr formula and should start with only one capsule after meals. After two weeks, two capsules are normally tolerated. If bilirubin is present in the urine, Dr. Loomis recommends the following protocol:

- Weeks 1 and 2: Take two capsules of Thera-zyme Bil before meals.
- Weeks 3 and 4: Add one capsule of Thera-zyme Lvr after meals to the above program.
- Weeks 5 and 6: Increase to two capsules of Thera-zyme Lvr after meals, still taking Bil.

Taken long enough (the length of time depends upon the severity of the condition), this program will help maintain or decrease the size of gallstones. There is no standard length of time because each case is individual and depends upon the causative factors.

Hormonal Balancing

If testing determines that your thyroid function is low, seek the advice of a health professional. If treatment is needed, I recommend a thyroid glandular extract. Woman should add natural progesterone (10% oral oil or 3% topical cream). (See Appendix A.)

A glandular extract is a purified nutritional and therapeutic product derived from one of several animal glands, including the adrenal, thymus, thyroid, ovaries, testes, pancreas, pineal, and pituitary. It is prescribed by a physician for a person whose corresponding gland is underfunctioning and not producing enough of its own hormone. The various glands are part of the endocrine system which, along with the nervous system, coordinates the functioning of all of the body's systems.

Dietary Recommendations

Researcher J.C. Breneman reports that 100% of his patients found relief of gallbladder symptoms while on an elimination diet of beef, rye, rice, cherries, peaches, apricots, beets, and spinach. The following foods were found to cause symptoms (in descending order of occurrence): eggs, pork, onions, fowl, milk, coffee, citrus, corn, beans, and nuts. Eggs caused gallbladder attacks in 93% of the patients, pork in 64%, and onions in 52%.[52]

To this list of foods to avoid, Dr. Loomis adds cucumbers, radishes, cabbage, chocolate, and tomatoes. Check to see if any of the above foods, especially eggs, give you symptoms of gallbladder stress such as burping or nausea after meals, a pain between the shoulder blades, or clay-colored stools (from lack of bile), among other indications. Increase your intake of vegetables, fruits, and high-fiber foods, especially those containing soluble fiber. Avoid consumption of fatty foods, all fried foods, all commercial oils, margarine and other hydrogenated oils, unsaturated oils with the exception of extra virgin olive oil, all refined sugars, and refined white flour.

A high-fiber diet protects from gallbladder disease by binding cholesterol and bile salts, and decreasing intestinal transit time. A high-fiber diet
can only be achieved with unprocessed, unrefined foods. We need at least
25 grams of fiber daily, with 35 grams being the optimal amount.
Unfortunately, the typical American diet provides only six to eight grams
of fiber daily. In a study in which subjects simply added fiber to their diet,
their blood fats and bile cholesterol decreased significantly.[53]

Fiber is best when it's eaten in the food from which it came rather
than as a supplement. Also, soluble fiber is better than insoluble fiber
in binding cholesterol and intestinal bile salts. All fiber contains soluble parts which are digested by cellulase, and insoluble parts which
cannot be digested. Raw vegetables are good sources of fiber because
they contain the cellulase the body needs to break down the fiber. The
best source is raw carrots; their fiber binds many colon toxins, including those that cause cancer.

Nutritional Supplements

Animals fed a high-fat diet did not develop gallstones as long as vitamin E
intake was adequate. In addition, gallstones, which contain cholesterol and
developed in animals given a vitamin E–deficient diet, dissolved when vitamin E was administered. Vitamin C also appears to be protective, even
in subjects fed a high-cholesterol diet.[54]

Herbal Therapies

Liver support herbs include milk thistle, dandelion, globe artichoke, and
Oregon grape. There are also many herbal remedies, such as Swedish
Bitters, available at health food stores.

Naturopathic Remedies

Naturopaths sometimes use a complex of plant terpenes (essential oils) to
dissolve gallstones. To this remedy is often added lipotropic supplements
(these aid in the transport of fats, which helps to keep fat from accumu-
lating in the liver) such as lecithin.

Homeopathic Remedies

There are many homeopathic remedies for relief of gallbladder symptoms. These include: *Chelidonium* for sharp, quick, stabbing gallbladder pain; *Belladonna* for paroxysms of pain that come and go quickly;
Cina for when the gallbladder pain is worse to the touch and the
liver/gallbladder area is hard to the touch; and *Colocythsis* for pain that
is sharp and relieved by pressure.[55]

GASTROINTESTINAL DISORDERS

Disorders of the gastrointestinal tract are quite common and can lead to improper digestion, malabsorption, and nutritional deficiencies, all of which can contribute to the development of many other diseases. Here I discuss upper digestive tract disorders and intestinal disorders, which include any inflammatory condition of the small or large intestine.

UPPER DIGESTIVE TRACT DISORDERS

Conditions of the upper digestive tract (from the mouth to the stomach) covered here include gastritis, gastric ulcer, and hiatal hernia.

Gastritis

Gastritis is an inflamed gastric mucosa (stomach lining) and the inability to hold acid (HCl or hydrochloric acid) in the stomach, which can produce symptoms ranging from mild to severe, including stomach pain, abdominal tenderness, nausea, and vomiting. Substances such as aspirin and alcohol can exacerbate this condition. Gastritis sometimes precedes gastric (stomach) ulcers.

Gastric Ulcer

Gastric ulcers are open sores or lesions of the stomach lining. Burning or pain in the stomach usually, but not always, occurs with ulcers. An ulcer can result from chronic stress, years of fat intolerance, or severe digestive problems which lead to a faulty pH balance (see below) and a compromised mucosal lining. In addition, the bacteria *Helicobacter pylori* has been linked to inflammation and ulcers in the stomach.[56]

Hiatal Hernia

In this condition, a portion of the cardia (opening of the stomach into the esophagus) bulges through the gap (hiatus) between the diaphragm and the esophagus. Symptoms include regurgitation of stomach contents and esophageal pain or severe burning (heartburn) due to the acidity of these contents; the pain and burning is worse when lying down. Hiatal hernia can lead to an ulcer.

For information on the **enzymes** for this health condition, see Appendix B.

What Causes Upper Digestive Tract Disorders?

Many people think that stomach problems which cause indigestion with burning and sometimes nausea are due to excess stomach acid, and take antacids such as Tums or Rolaids to counteract it. However, according to Howard Loomis, D.C., of Madison, Wisconsin, there is no such thing as excess stomach acid, although inadequate acid production can occur. He points instead to a compromised mucosal lining as the cause. If the mucus-secreting cells lining the stomach are not nourished, they will not secrete adequate mucus and you will develop gastric problems, from mild gastric irritation and hiatal hernia to gastritis and ulcers. The entire gastrointestinal tract is lined with mucus-secreting cells and mucus is needed to protect it from perforation. In order to function, these cells must be nourished by foods digested with enzymes.[57]

The road to hiatal hernia and gastric problems usually starts with fat intolerance and the resulting gallbladder symptoms, such as frequent burping. The burping and the continued eating of fats and other foods that irritate the gallbladder can lead to a hiatal hernia. Literally, the person burps his stomach into his esophagus. Prolonged inattention to this problem—that is, failure to implement enzyme and dietary therapy—can lead to gastritis or an ulcer.

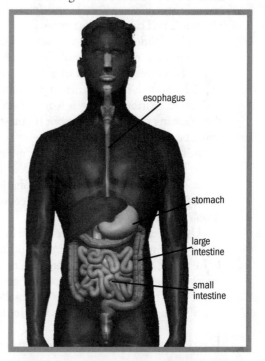

THE GASTROINTESTINAL TRACT. The entire gastrointestinal tract is lined with mucus-secreting cells and mucus is needed to protect it from perforation. In order to function, these cells must be nourished by foods digested with enzymes.

Success Story: Stopping Gastritis and *Helicobacter pylori*

A middle-aged man presented with gastric problems; he had trouble eating because his stomach burned constantly. I immediately gave him Thera-zyme Stm and this relieved the burning, but when he discontinued the enzymes, it returned. I suggested that he might have *Helicobacter pylori*, bacteria common in stomach problems, and recommended that he take Citricidal (grapefruit seed and pulp extract) capsules on a daily basis. Shortly after he added the Citricidal to his enzyme program, his stomach burning disappeared completely.

Success Story: Healing Gastritis and Hiatal Hernia

Joe, 45, had low back pain, nausea and heartburn which were worse in the morning, gallbladder symptoms, and allergies to chemicals and foods (in particular, wheat, sugar, and fat). His urine test indicated poor digestion and assimilation of foods with excess consumption of or intolerance to fat (lipase deficiency) and sugar (disaccharidase deficiency), as well as vitamin C and calcium deficiencies.

Joe's palpation test showed many inflamed areas, especially the epigastrium (area over the pit of the stomach), kidneys, and colon. He described classic symptoms of a hiatal hernia: epigastric pain due to localized gastritis in the herniated portion of the stomach, regurgitation, and severe heartburn that was worse when lying down. I recommended the following enzyme formulas for his most severe problems—epigastric irritation, allergies, and candidiasis:

- Thera-zyme Stm: digestive formula for gastric problems
- Thera-zyme SvG: for sugar intolerance and vitamin C deficiency
- Thera-zyme Kdy: kidney-lymphatic formula.
- Thera-zyme SmI: *acidophilus*-cellulase formula for intestinal problems and candidiasis

Usually, even an ulcer can be healed in about two weeks with Thera-zyme Stm, unless *Helicobacter pylori* or other gastric irritants are present. In Joe's case, his condition worsened on the enzymes. This indicated that the protein in the capsules was causing gastric irritation upon digestion. I suggested he open the capsules and swallow the contents only. After a day of taking the enzymes in this way, his burning pain disappeared.

Prevention and Elimination of Upper Digestive Tract Disorders

The remedy I use for all stomach and upper digestive tract problems is Thera-zyme Stm. This formula helps heal the mucosal lining anywhere in the gastrointestinal tract. Since the cells of the mucosal lining turn over every 14 days, an ulcer or gastritis can be healed in about two weeks, providing all gastric irritants are avoided and proper chiropractic therapy is obtained if needed.

INTESTINAL DISORDERS

Intestinal disorders include all inflammatory conditions of the small or large intestine, such as colitis, diverticulitis (inflammation of the pouches in the intestinal walls), celiac disease (gluten intolerance), irritable bowel syndrome, Crohn's disease (inflammation of the mucosal tissues of the intestines), and chronic (not acute) appendicitis. Some of these conditions are difficult to diagnose and require extensive medical tests. Many people are misdiagnosed. Treating intestinal conditions with enzyme formulas designed for whether the person has diarrhea, constipation, or diarrhea alternating with constipation avoids this problem. These enzyme formulas are discussed in Enzyme Therapy below.

What Causes Intestinal Disorders?

Among the causes of intestinal problems are poor diet, food allergies, viral or bacterial infections, parasites, and stress.

Success Story: Enzyme Therapy Controls Crohn's Disease

Frank, 15, suffered a series of health problems that led to his taking various prescription drugs including prednisone (cortisone) for poison oak, steroids for a bee sting allergy, and penicillin along with other antibiotics for an undiagnosed condition—all within the span of one year. Following this period, he developed a pain in the lower right quadrant of his abdomen and was given Zantac® for his "acid" stomach. A month later, Frank could add diarrhea, night sweats, and a rapid weight loss of 25 pounds to his other symptoms.

A battery of tests, including a colon biopsy, led to a diagnosis of Crohn's disease. The teenager was placed on prednisone and sulfasalazine, the drugs of choice for Crohn's disease. Prednisone is synthetic cortisone which is used for a variety of inflammatory conditions. It does suppress inflammation, but it has serious side effects, including seizures, diabetes and osteoporosis as well as damage to the adrenal glands.[58] Sulfasalazine (Azulfidine®) is recommended as a lifelong treat-

Nausea: Enzyme Therapy for Its Many Causes

Nausea occurs for many reasons, among them indigestion, kidney stress, gallbladder problems, appendicitis, food poisoning, and stomach flu. The following are enzyme therapies for these conditions and thus for nausea.

- Indigestion: Thera-zyme Stm
- Kidney Stress: due to a congested or exhausted lymphatic system which dumps unneutralized toxins back into the blood causing kidney stress; Thera-zyme Kdy
- Gallbladder Problems: Thera-zyme Bil (for fat intolerance and gallbladder problems) to dissolve gallstones and aid in their excretion; Thera-zyme Lvr to relieve gallbladder nausea
- Appendicitis: for chronic cases, protease (Thera-zyme TRMA) and an *acidophilus* formula (Thera-zyme SmI); for acute cases, enzyme therapy combined with surgery

- Food Poisoning: difficult to treat orally because of the nausea and vomiting, but grapefruit seed extract has been reported to inhibit some of the food-borne pathogens such as *Salmonella, E coli*, and *Listeria monocytogenes*

- Stomach Flu: like food poisoning, difficult to treat orally; Thera-zyme Stm, antinausea herbal remedies (ginger root, slippery elm, peppermint), oatmeal tea (cook organic oatmeal, filter the juice, add raw honey to the juice, and drink), or rice tea (same preparation as oatmeal tea); Thera-zymes UrT and Spl can also be helpful

ment for patients with Crohn's disease and colitis. It is high in salicylic acid (aspirin is a compound of this acid) and consequently has the same side effects of taking high doses of aspirin daily, including stomach ulcers and reduced ability of the blood to clot.[59]

Two months later, his doctor concluded that the drugs were not working and recommended surgery. Frank's mother, the owner of a health food store, sent him to me. His urine test indicated that he needed Thera-zyme PAN for a sugar and gluten intolerance, Thera-zyme TRMA for his immune system, and Thera-zyme SmI for small intestine problems. In addition to these three formulas, he was cautioned to avoid wheat and sugar products. Frank was frightened enough by his condition to follow my instructions.

Within three months on this program, Frank had gained 25 pounds. Almost a year later, all of the symptoms of Crohn's disease had disappeared. The disease remains under control as long as Frank stays on a wheat- and sugar-free diet, and continues a maintenance enzyme program.

Success Story: Treating Crohn's Disease With Soil-Based Organisms

Jordan, 20, had a background of good nutrition and no history of bowel problems—no stomach or intestinal flu, or diarrhea. During his freshman year at college, while under much stress and eating a junk-food diet, he suddenly became ill. Jordan's symptoms were extreme and progressed to 12 or more episodes of diarrhea daily, severe stomach pain, abdominal cramps, nausea, fever, chills, and a dramatic weight loss. He consulted a string of physicians and healers, took dozens of toxic drugs, and tried myriad nutritional supplements, but nothing worked.

Jordan was hospitalized several times and, each time, he left the hospital in worse condition with a greater weight loss. At the peak of his illness, his weight had dropped from 180 to 104 pounds, his heart rate raced at 220 beats per minute, and he had as many as 30 bowel movements in 24 hours.

Then Jordan found out about soil-based organisms (SBOs, SEE QUICK DEFINITION), beneficial bacteria in capsule form which help prevent proliferation of intestinal toxins. When Jordan started taking SBOs, he felt worse for the first three weeks. At the end of the first month, he eliminated a black, tar-like material. After that, he experienced surges of energy and his appetite gradually returned. One year after beginning the treatment, he was no longer ill and his weight had climbed back to 180 pounds.[60]

Success Story:
Curing Ulcerative Colitis With Enzyme Therapy

Bernard, 43, was diagnosed with ulcerative colitis. He had the common symptoms of frequent, bloody diarrhea, and severe pain in the lower left abdominal quadrant during attacks. Meat, ice cream, French fries, and gluten-containing foods worsened his condition.

At the start of treatment, Bernard was taking prednisone and Azulfidine, the standard drugs prescribed for his condition. His urinalysis indicated polyuria (excessive urine volume), excessive consumption of fat, vitamin C deficiency, severe sugar intolerance, and low calcium. Further tests indicated the need for a therapeutic formula containing cellulase and probiotics—common in people with yeast infections or parasites. Bernard also had indications of a sluggish thyroid gland; his resting pulse was only 56 beats per minute.

I started him on the following program: a digestive for-

QUICK DEFINITION

Soil-based organisms (SBOs) are beneficial microbes, or probiotics, found in soil. Before chemical farming, the earth was rich in these organisms which naturally destroyed molds, yeast, fungi, and viruses in the soil. Transmitted in the food supply to humans, SBOs perform the same function in the human body, working with the "friendly" bacteria (such as *Lactobacillus acidophilus* and *Bifidobacterium bifidum*) inhabiting the gastrointestinal tract to maintain balance in the intestinal flora and thus ensure a healthy digestive system. Since soil has become depleted of SBOs, the ratio of good to bad bacteria in the intestines has become skewed and a host of health problems, including allergies, candidiasis, hormonal dysfunction, and Crohn's disease, among other gastrointestinal conditions, are the result.

People with a spastic colon are sometimes complex-carbohydrate intolerant and have a tendency to like fats. They respond dramatically to a high-lipase multiple digestive enzyme formula.

mula for sugar intolerance (Thera-zyme PAN), a formula containing B-complex vitamins plus additional disaccharidase enzymes (Thera-zyme Adr), an antioxidant formula for toxins and nasal problems (Thera-zyme Nsl), a cellulase-*acidophilus* formula for yeast infection (Thera-zyme SmI), and the Thera-zyme IrB formula for his irritable bowel condition. He was advised to avoid refined sugars, gluten grains, meat, and junk food.

Three weeks later, Bernard had decreased his prednisone dose gradually, with no recurring episodes of colitis. Retesting showed that he now needed a formula for gastric irritation (Thera-zyme Stm), a normal consequence of taking anti-inflammatory drugs such as prednisone. His resting pulse was still very low (60-64 beats per minute), so I started him on a thyroid glandular extract. Less than two months later, he was no longer taking his drugs and had experienced no recurrence of colitis. Today, three years later, he remains healthy.

Success Story: Multiple Enzymes Stop 20 Years of Diarrhea

Brad, 57, presented with a diagnosis of spastic colon of 20 years duration. His exams showed no evidence of parasites. His symptoms included feeling sick about two hours after eating, with headache, weakness, gas, and abdominal pain. He controlled his diarrhea with four to five doses of Lomotil® daily, but the drug did not control his other digestive symptoms. Brad was milk intolerant; milk consumption led to diarrhea. His diet was typical American fare—overly processed and refined.

Brad's urinalysis revealed an allergy pattern, highly acidic pH, severe vitamin C deficiency, calcium and magnesium deficiency, and a toxic colon. It also showed excess fat and protein consumption, and poor sugar metabolism.

People with a spastic colon are sometimes complex-carbohydrate intolerant and have a tendency to like fats. They respond dramatically to a high-lipase multiple digestive (Thera-zyme VSCLR), so I gave this to Brad along with Thera-zyme SvG for sugar intolerance, vitamin C (Thera-zyme Opt), and Thera-zyme Kdy for his allergies. The herbs in the latter remedy have antiseptic qualities and nutrients that help reduce edema and swollen lymph glands, aid the kidneys in

Iron and the Irritable Bowel

If you suffer from irritable bowel syndrome (IBS), you might want to have your iron levels checked. Too much iron (iron overload or hemochromatosis) supports free radical proliferation, a feature in all inflammatory conditions, and promotes bacterial and yeast infections, often involved in intestinal disorders. Research has correlated excess iron with IBS. While there is not enough data to indicate iron overload as a direct cause, it may be a triggering factor in people who are susceptible to this intestinal problem.[61]

What causes iron overload? One factor is heredity. About one in 200 Americans have genetic hemochromatosis. Diet is another source of excess iron. Processed foods labeled "enriched" are loaded with iron; adding iron to processed foods is a compulsory requirement of the FDA to restore iron lost during processing. Other common sources of iron overload include tap water and iron cookware.[62]

Testing iron status is not automatically part of a standard blood test, so ask your doctor to specifically order it. According to Leslie N. Johnston, D.V.M., author of *Iron Overload = Hemochromatosis = Too Much Iron*, the tests to request are serum iron, total iron binding capacity (TIBC), transferrin, and ferritin. Together, these will provide a reliable analysis of your iron status. Conventional medicine's "normal" range of blood serum iron, transferrin, and ferritin is higher than Dr. Johnston considers healthy. He suggests that serum iron over 100 micromilligrams/liter, transferrin over 25% saturation, and ferritin levels above 50 micromilligrams/liter may indicate iron overload.[63]

If your iron levels are too high, donating blood or undergoing oral chelation therapy (to "bind up" the iron for elimination from the body) may help bring them down. The safest method of oral chelation is sodium succinate capsules; a typical dose is 200-250 mg, twice daily for two weeks twice yearly, depending on blood test results.

For more about **blood iron levels**, see the monograph *Iron Overload = Hemochromatosis = Too Much Iron*, by Leslie N. Johnston. Available from: 4632 North Peoria, Tulsa, OK 74126; tel: 918-425-6209.

cleansing the blood, and reduce the symptoms of allergies (nasal congestion, runny eyes and nose, frontal headache, sometimes nausea, and itching and swelling of the eyes, nose, and throat). In my experience, more people need this enzyme formula than any other single formula.

In less than one month, Brad reported 100% improvement. He was able to stop taking the Lomotil and could eat most foods without any symptoms. A year and a half later, he is still doing fine.

Success Story: Enzymes and Thyroid Supplements End Chronic Diarrhea

Catherine, 41, suffered from obesity (she was 5'3" tall and weighed

230 pounds), hypertension, and severe, chronic diarrhea. She had painful diarrhea attacks six to ten times daily, which she described as "more painful than having a baby." The onset was characterized by a hot flash, weakness, and pain in the colon and rectum. Catherine also suffered from hormonal imbalances following a partial hysterectomy at the age of 26 due to damage from an IUD (intrauterine device, inserted in the uterus to prevent pregnancy). At 40, she went through gallbladder surgery following heavy dieting.

The prescription drugs she was taking included Norvasc® (for hypertension) and Bonine® (for light-headedness and dizziness). Doctors had done many biopsies but could not diagnose the cause of the diarrhea, although they ruled out Crohn's disease. A lactose tolerance test made her very ill. She also reported being intolerant to wheat, pasta, and grains.

Her urinalysis showed a toxic colon, sugar intolerance, very low calcium, excess acidity, and a severe vitamin C deficiency. In addition, her temperature was low (95.5° F) as was her resting pulse (64 beats per minute). This, along with her symptoms of weight gain, insomnia, depression, fatigue, and heart palpitations, indicated hypothyroidism. Her doctor confirmed this and placed Catherine on a natural thyroid glandular extract.

I recommended a low-fat, organic, whole-foods diet, avoiding all refined and synthetic sugars, all gluten foods (wheat, oats, rye, and barley), margarine and other hydrogenated oils, and all commercial polyunsaturated oils. Additionally, I recommended the following enzymes and supplements:

- Thera-zyme PAN: for sugar and wheat intolerance
- Thera-zyme Lvr: for liver/gallbladder problems
- Thera-zyme Opt: vitamin C formula
- Thera-zyme TRMA: protease for soft tissue inflammation, chronic infections (bacterial or viral), the immune system, and certain parasites
- Thera-zyme IrB: for diarrhea and irritable bowel problems

Due to Catherine's menopausal symptoms (night sweats) and low urinary calcium (a precursor to osteoporosis), I recommended thyroid glandular therapy and 10% natural progesterone in vitamin E oil. I also gave her cat's claw, a rain forest herb known for its ability to heal intestinal disorders.

Catherine received her supplements on a Thursday afternoon and took them later in the day. The next morning, they came out intact with her diarrhea—a rare occurrence. Normally, if taken on an empty stomach, the enzymes go from the stomach into the blood within 15 minutes. I recommended that she open the capsules, put the enzymes in water, and drink the solution. She did this and, from the first dose of enzymes, her diarrhea disappeared and has not returned. That was almost two months ago and Catherine is feeling much better and losing weight.

Prevention and Elimination of Intestinal Disorders

Diet is, of course, essential to intestinal health. Along with proper diet, enzyme therapy, herbal remedies, and essential oils can help reverse and prevent intestinal ailments.

Enzyme Therapy

As mentioned previously, since intestinal problems are difficult to diagnose, enzyme therapy treats this type of disorder according to whether diarrhea, constipation, or diarrhea alternating with constipation predominate. The following are the three enzyme formulas to address these conditions:

■ Thera-zyme IrB: for diarrhea, loose stools, multiple bowel movements and bowel movements immediately after eating

■ Thera-zyme LgI: for constipation or infrequent bowel movements, and a hard, dry stool

■ Thera-zyme SmI: for severe constipation with hard, dry stools, alternating constipation and diarrhea, parasites, and yeast infections

Other formulas useful for intestinal disorders include:

■ Multiple digestive formula appropriate to the specific digestive needs, such as Thera-zyme PAN for sugar intolerance, Bil for fat intolerance, and VSCLR for complex-carbohydrate intolerance

■ Thera-zyme Stm: for ulcerative colitis (bloody stool)

■ Thera-zyme Challenge Food Powder: for toxic colon and parasites

■ Thera-zyme TRMA: for soft tissue inflammation, chronic infections (bacterial or viral), the immune system, and certain parasites

Dietary Recommendations

Fiber, present in all whole vegetables, fruits, and grains, is essential for intestinal health. Part of each fiber is soluble and part insoluble, so you need the enzyme cellulase which digests soluble fiber. Since the human body doesn't make cellulase, we must take it in supplemental form or chew raw vegetables well to release the cellulase required to digest the soluble fiber. People who get gas from eating raw vegetables don't chew adequately enough. Some solve the problem by cooking

Part of each fiber is soluble and part insoluble, so you need the enzyme cellulase which digests soluble fiber. Since the human body doesn't make cellulase, we must take it in supplemental form or chew raw vegetables well to release the cellulase required to digest the soluble fiber.

the vegetables, but it's preferable to chew raw food well rather than to cook it because cooking destroys the enzymes. The exception is cruciferous vegetables, such as broccoli, cabbage, and cauliflower, which should be lightly steamed to destroy the thyroid-inhibiting substances they contain in the raw state.[64]

There are three general classes of fiber:

1) Cellulose: a polysaccharide (many carbohydrate units linked together) comprising the main structural material in plant cell walls

2) Noncellulose polysaccharides: includes the noncellulose carbohydrates such as hemicellulose, pectins, gums (such as guar) and mucilages, and algal substances

3) Lignin: the only noncarbohydrate type of fiber; forms the woody part of plants

The various fibers have different functions. The soluble parts of the fiber protect against high cholesterol, while the insoluble parts protect against colorectal cancer. Cereal fiber helps lower cholesterol and balance blood sugar better than the fiber from fruits and vegetables. Pectin, from fruits, binds and eliminates heavy metals, radioisotopes, and other toxins from the gastrointestinal tract. Lignin combines with bile acids to form insoluble compounds, thus preventing the absorption of the bile.

The general recommendation for fiber consumption is approximately 35 grams per day. People in nonindustrial countries who eat totally natural foods consume 24 to 25 grams per day of food fiber. America's favorite foods—meat, fat, refined sugar, and white flour—have little or no fiber. Our standard diet provides a mere six to eight grams per day of food fiber.

Don't confuse fiber as it exists in whole raw foods with fiber supplements, which consist of a gamut of synthetic alternatives including sawdust. To really work, the fiber must not be separated from its mother plant. I am not saying that some of the excellent colon cleanse formulas containing fibers do not help. They are better than nothing when an American low-fiber diet is the standard fare. However, there is no substitute for fiber as it naturally occurs in food. The reported health effects of fiber come from studies on whole food fiber, not fiber supplements which have been extracted from food.

As the colon is the dumping ground for wastes from the gastrointestinal tract, a short colon transit time (the time between ingestion of food and excretion of waste materials) is crucial to eliminate toxins from the body as quickly as possible. Colon transit time is 15 to 18 hours among populations who eat a diet high in raw, high-fiber foods. However, in the United States and other industrialized countries in which a low-fiber diet is common, excretion occurs after two to four days, and up to two weeks among the elderly.

Slow bowel transit time allows certain colon bacteria to convert bile acids into carcinogens. Thus, the standard low-fiber, junk-food diet causes us to convert our own harmless bile acids into carcinogens inside the colon. These carcinogens have been isolated from low-roughage feces but not from high-roughage feces. People who eat high-fiber diets have different bowel bacteria (mainly *Streptococcus* and *Lactobacillus*) which do not convert bile acids into carcinogens. These people pass large amounts of unchanged bile acids in their feces. In particular, raw carrots contain excellent fiber which binds many bowel toxins including carcinogens.

A good rule to follow is "hard in, soft out," meaning raw foods rich in fiber (not softened by cooking) decrease the bowel transit time and produce a high-volume, soft stool with intact bile acids. To make a high-fiber diet work, all refined, synthetic foods must be eliminated. This includes refined sugars, refined flours, white rice, and filtered fruit juices. These should be replaced with enzyme-rich raw foods.

Herbal and Other Natural Remedies

■ Cat's claw (*Uncaria tomentosa*): a Peruvian rain forest herb used for immune system problems and bowel and intestinal disorders, including Crohn's disease, colitis, hemorrhoids, diverticulitis, leaky gut syndrome, and intestinal flora imbalance

■ Chlorophyll perles: fat-soluble chlorophyll extract useful in reducing bowel inflammation. Fat-soluble chlorophyll adheres to the lining of the intestinal wall and retards bacterial growth, removes putrifactive bacteria from the colon, and helps heal the mucosal lining of the gastrointestinal tract. (Chlorophyll closely resembles human blood and is used to cleanse, detoxify, and purify.) I recommend two perles between meals three times daily.

- Grapefruit seed and pulp extract (Citricidal): antiseptic and antimicrobial
- Soil-based organisms: beneficial bacteria for intestinal problems

Aromatherapy/Essential Oils

There are several essential oils useful for chronic diarrhea, particularly nutmeg and orange. If you don't want to buy the oils, try $1/4$ teaspoon of nutmeg in some water once or twice daily. Aromatherapy oils can be used in various ways: put 3-6 drops in bath water; use an aromatherapy diffuser to fill the air with the scent; apply 1-6 drops directly onto the feet (the skin of the feet absorbs oils quickly) or any area of concern; or dilute with massage oil by 15% to 30% and use in massage.[65]

HEADACHES

Headache ranks as the number one health complaint in America. As with many of the health problems discussed in this book, chronic headaches are often a sign of a deeper disorder. While aspirin and painkillers may relieve headache symptoms, the cause must be treated to bring lasting relief.

What Causes Headaches?

Many interrelated factors produce headaches, and most chronic headaches have both structural and physiological causes.

Structural Problems

The most common structural causes of headaches in my experience are subluxations (vertebral misalignments), misaligned coccyx (tailbone), TMJ (temporomandibular joint) problems, and cranial problems.

Atlas Headaches—A headache that arises from a misalignment of the first, second, or third cervical vertebra is commonly called an atlas headache. According to Howard Loomis, D.C., most upper cervical problems are due to some form of head injury, common in sports such as football and from whiplash as a result of an automobile accident. An atlas headache can occur in the back of the head and neck or radiate to the forehead or behind the eyes. In addition to headaches, other problems may develop, such as dizziness, seizures, crib death in an infant (sleeping on the stomach), stroke in an adult, and severe digestive problems.

For information on the **enzymes** for this health condition, see Appendix B.

See *Alternative Medicine Definitive Guide to Headaches* (Future Medicine Publishing, 1997; ISBN 1-887299-03-3); to order, call 800-333-HEAL.

Misaligned Coccyx—A headache can often be traced to a misaligned coccyx (tailbone). According to Ellen Cutler, D.C., a chiropractor and enzyme therapist from Corte Madera, California, when the coccyx is misaligned, the whole nervous system, from the tailbone to the brain, is affected. Symptoms include migraines, sciatica (back and leg pain from a compressed sciatic nerve), low back pain, chronic subluxations, and painful menstruation in women.

Dr. Loomis states that at least 25% of his patients have

To contact **Ellen Cutler, D.C.**: Tamalpais Pain Clinic, Town Center/770 Tamalpais Drive, Suite 203, Corte Madera, CA 94925; tel: 415-924-2273; fax: 415-924-2811.

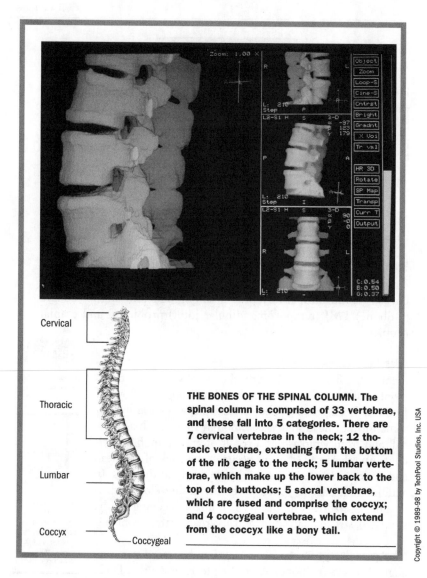

Cervical

Thoracic

Lumbar

Coccyx

Coccygeal

THE BONES OF THE SPINAL COLUMN. The spinal column is comprised of 33 vertebrae, and these fall into 5 categories. There are 7 cervical vertebrae in the neck; 12 thoracic vertebrae, extending from the bottom of the rib cage to the neck; 5 lumbar vertebrae, which make up the lower back to the top of the buttocks; 5 sacral vertebrae, which are fused and comprise the coccyx; and 4 coccygeal vertebrae, which extend from the coccyx like a bony tail.

a misaligned coccyx. He adds that it's easy to detect patients with uncorrected coccyx problems—their condition does not improve despite repeated chiropractic adjustments. He also notes that any severe emotional trauma can lead to a coccyx problem, due to the extreme nervous tension involved. One of the most common emotional causes of coccyx problems is sexual abuse.

The Temporomandibular Joint

TMJ stands for the temporomandibular joint, the joint where the temporal bone, the skull bone that descends in front of each ear, meets the mandible, the bone known as the lower jaw. The TMJ moves every time you chew or talk, making it one of the most active joints in the body. Unlike the ball-and-socket design of most other joints, the TMJ is a sliding joint, distributing the forces of chewing, swallowing, and talking over a wider joint surface which is lined by cartilage for smoother motion. The entire joint is also sheathed with supporting ligaments.

It is the lower jaw that is responsible for the opening and closing mechanism of the jaw. But the TMJ is a unique coupling of two interrelated parts in that movements on one side of the jaw must be coordinated and balanced with movements on the other. These movements are powered by the strong antigravity muscles of the jaw (the masseters and pterygoids), which also allow it to move sideways and up and down.

You can feel the TMJ movement by placing your fingers on the side of your face, just in front of your ears, as you open and close your mouth. Move your fingers up along your hairline and notice how the TMJ extends all the way to your temple.

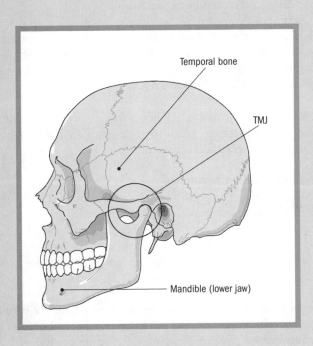

Temporal bone

TMJ

Mandible (lower jaw)

In addition to structural problems, headaches can be caused by a number of physiological imbalances including allergies (resulting from enzyme deficiencies), liver and gallbladder problems, a toxic colon, hormonal problems (hypothyroidism), and in women, estrogen dominance.

TMJ Problems—Although the American Dental Association estimates that 60 million Americans may have TMJ (temporomandibular joint, see p. 151) syndrome with its symptoms of a sore jaw joint, difficulty chewing or talking, and/or headaches, jaw and dental stress as an underlying contributor to headaches is often overlooked by conventional medicine. It is logical that a mouth and jaw under continuous strain affect other parts of the body. Problems such as tooth decay, crooked teeth, impacted wisdom teeth, gum disease, muscle spasm, ill-fitting restorations, and low-grade infections from old fillings all cause stress to the jaw, bringing about muscular and structural compensations.

As the jaw takes on more pressure and pain, it begins to send these sensations to other areas in the skull, which in turn conveys the message to the central nervous system, thereby initiating a complex mechanism which helps to explain the headaches and other chronic symptoms accompanying TMJ syndrome.

Cranial Problems—Cranial (skull) bones may be misaligned due to emotional trauma affecting cranial structure and physical trauma, including the use of forceps during birth.

Physiological Imbalances
In addition to structural problems, headaches can be caused by a number of physiological imbalances including allergies (resulting from enzyme deficiencies), liver and gallbladder problems, a toxic colon, and hormonal (glandular) problems such as hypothyroidism. In women, a common hormonal cause of headaches, including migraines, is estrogen dominance.

Allergy-Induced Headaches—Most people think of allergy symptoms as sneezing, itchy eyes, or dark circles under the eyes, but food allergies produce dozens of other symptoms, including headaches. Whatever you do not digest becomes a poison to the body and the headache will remain until the undigested food (the poison) is eliminated by enzymatic detoxification. Further headaches can be prevented by optimizing digestion with multiple digestive enzymes.

Liver/Gallbladder Headaches—It's common for people with fat intolerance and gallbladder problems to experience headaches. These can be triggered by a meal high in fats or spices and by certain foods, including eggs, pork, onions, poultry, and milk, among others.[66]

Toxic Colon Headaches—A toxic colon, another source of headaches, results from a low-fiber, refined food diet or undigested food which produces a toxin in the colon called indican. Since thyroid hormone has a profound effect on colon health, a toxic colon is almost always associated with an underactive thyroid gland.

The Estrogen Migraine—Hypothyroidism (underactive thyroid gland) leads to estrogen dominance (excess estrogen relative to progesterone) and this, in turn, can lead to migraines and seizures, among many other health problems. Estrogen headaches are common in hypothyroid women, especially those who take birth control pills, use estrogen as a "morning after" pill to prevent conception, or (in menopausal women) use estrogen replacement therapy.

The estrogen migraine is easy to diagnose in premenopausal women because it occurs during ovulation and menses and subsides thereafter. It is often accompanied by vomiting, general malaise, mood swings, and nutritional tendencies such as sugar cravings, excess consumption of chocolate, and other dietary excesses normally controlled except during menses. (See Appendix A.)

See **Allergies**, pp. 65-70. See **Gallbladder Disorders**, pp. 129-135. For more about **indican**, see "A Glossary of 24-Hour Urine Analysis Terms," Chapter 2: Diagnosing Enzyme Deficiencies, p. 40.

Success Story: The Childhood Trauma Behind Chronic Headaches

Beginning when she was three, my daughter Veronica suffered from chronic, severe migraines which were accompanied by vomiting and left her disabled until they passed. These headaches always followed stress, even pleasant stress such as excitement over an upcoming vacation.

At the age of three, Veronica had been molested more than once by the brother of her nanny, but had no recall of her traumatic experience. I never made a connection between the migraines and my daughter's childhood trauma until discussing with Dr. Loomis the importance of correcting a misaligned coccyx. One of the most common emotional causes of coccyx problems is sexual abuse. I immediately took Veronica, then 12, to Dr. Cutler.

Dr. Cutler found that Veronica's coccyx was indeed misaligned and gave her a standard chiropractic adjustment and also applied directional nonforce technique (DNFT) in which gentle touch is exerted along the spine, skull, and pelvis.

As we were driving home from the treatment, my daughter started talking about her childhood experience which, until then, had been completely repressed. She now described each traumatic incident in detail and with complete calm. Although her story was painful to tell, with recall would come a release of the trauma, which apparently had become locked within her coccyx. Seven years have passed since our visit with Dr. Cutler, and my daughter has never had another migraine, though her stresses have been many.

One comment on the coccyx adjustment—during many years of observing clients, I've found that everyone reacts differently when the adjustment is performed. Do not conclude that it hasn't been successful if you do not have the obvious emotional release Veronica had or remember the trauma which contributed to your coccyx misalignment. The adjustment can produce deep benefits that are more subtle.

Success Story: The Headache That 41 Drugs Couldn't Cure

When Lilian, 73, came to the office of Dennis Crawford, D.C., of Folsom, California, she brought a sack containing the 13 drugs she took daily; among them was prednisone which she was taking at a rate of 50 mg a day. Her face was "puffed up like a basketball" and covered with dark purple blotches. These blotches (a side effect of prednisone) were also visible on her arms. She had trouble speaking, seemed confused, and "appeared to be in a stupor," according to Dr. Crawford, a chiropractor who also practices enzyme therapy.

Lilian had been undergoing dental treatment for TMJ (temporomandibular or jaw-joint) problems for six years, when she suddenly developed continuous headaches so severe that they caused vomiting and complete debilitation, and required her to sleep sitting up. Her dentist, concerned that an undiagnosed illness was presenting itself, sent her for extensive medical tests. After $30,000 worth of tests—which included blood chemistries, a brain scan, a biopsy, and an angiogram—she was diagnosed with temporal arteritis, inflammation of the temporal artery which supplies the temporal muscle (closes the

To contact **Dennis Crawford, D.C.**: 10231 Fair Oaks Blvd., Folsom, CA 95268; tel: 916-962-3101.

jaw) and other areas of the face and head, a condition which can lead to blindness or stroke.

In the two years following this diagnosis, 13 different doctors gave Lilian 41 different prescription drugs, including hormones, antibiotics, tranquilizers, and painkillers. However, in Lilian's words, the drugs "only took the edge off" her pain.

Dr. Crawford did a complete chiropractic analysis and treatment, including TMJ and cranial work. Lilian's urine test showed two enzyme deficiencies: cellulase and protease. Cellulase deficiencies often accompany facial nerve pain, Bell's palsy, and other nervous system problems. Protease deficiency is found in TMJ problems and, in fact, in any problem involving soft tissue inflammation, calcium and bone metabolism, protein digestion, and the immune system. Dr. Crawford treated Lilian's cellulase deficiency with Thera-zyme Nsl, an antioxidant formula with vitamin C which helps relieve the inflammation that causes facial pain and paralysis. The prescription for her protease deficiency, Thera-zyme TRMA, also reduces inflammation and generally strengthens the immune system.

Within days after Dr. Crawford's chiropractic treatment and starting enzyme therapy, Lilian's pain went away.

Success Story: No More Tylenol

Another of Dr. Crawford's clients, Joan, 47, had been suffering from daily headaches for nearly two years. She found that by drinking coffee she could get some relief. After that, she took Tylenol®. Since Joan's urinalysis indicated a sugar intolerance, Dr. Crawford recommended Thera-zyme PAN, a digestive enzyme formula for sugar-intolerant people, along with Thera-zyme Adr to support sugar digestion. Joan also suffered from TMJ and was given Thera-zyme IVD, a musculoskeletal support formula.

During his evaluation, Dr. Crawford found Joan's liver was damaged—a common side effect of excessive use of Tylenol. He recommended herbs to detoxify and support the liver. Joan's headaches subsided within a week—the time it took for her to benefit from the liver detoxification program.

Success Story:
Curing Allergy Migraines With Enzymes

Sandra, 10, presented with migraines so severe that they caused loss of vision. Even 250 mg of Naprosyn (an anti-inflammatory drug) did not relieve them. Her parents took her to Dr. Loomis who recognized the classic symptoms of protein and sugar intolerance—protease and disaccharidase deficiencies, respectively. Both of these enzyme deficiencies can cause low blood sugar which, in turn, can result in headaches.

Sandra's symptoms included a craving for sugar and cold liquids, a dislike of meat, and an intolerance of raw foods, dairy, and fats. Palpation and urinalysis indicated the following needs:

- Thera-zyme HCL: for protein, fat, and sugar intolerance
- Thera-zyme Kdy: kidney-lymphatic support for allergies
- Thera-zyme SmI: for colon support
- Thera-zyme TRMA: with protease for the immune system

Dr. Loomis also advised Sandra's mother to remove sugar and junk food from her diet.

The girl's headaches disappeared soon after the therapy began, but before long she complained that the HCL formula gave her a stomachache. Protease can cause stomach distress in patients who challenge their gastric mucosal lining with anti-inflammatory drugs such as Naprosyn. Dr. Loomis switched her to Thera-zyme DGST, a pediatric multiple digestive enzyme formula with less protease than the HCL formula. That solved the problem, but Sandra's headaches returned about four days after she resumed eating sugar.

Prevention and Elimination of Headaches

Since most headaches have both structural and physiological components, they require physical and nutritional therapies, along with recognition of dietary and hormonal imbalances.

Enzyme Therapy

Following is a list of enzymes and supplements used to address all of the causes of headaches listed above:

- Multiple digestive formula appropriate to individual digestive needs
- Thera-zyme Spl: for the spleen and the immune system; helps increase oxygen in the body; good for cranial problems and mild, nagging headaches
- Thera-zyme Sym: for headaches related to upper cervical problems
- Thera-zyme CLM (calm): nervous system support which helps relieve nervous tension in general and nervous/emotional problems associated with a misaligned coccyx in particular
- Thera-zyme IVD: useful for TMJ-related headaches; helps repair broken bones, ligaments, and herniated discs

■ Thera-zyme Kdy: kidney-lymphatic formula for frontal headaches primarily due to allergies

■ Thera-zymes SmI (small intestine), LgI (large intestine), and Challenge Food Powder: help relieve headaches associated with a toxic colon; SmI for constipation, diarrhea, or constipation alternating with diarrhea, yeast overgrowth, and parasites; LgI for constipation; Challenge Food Powder reduces indican, cleanses the colon, and eliminates parasites

Hormonal Balancing

Migraine resulting from estrogen dominance can be cured with thyroid glandular therapy and natural progesterone, in conjunction with a whole-foods diet and enzyme therapy.

Nasal Specifics

One of Dr. Cutler's specialties is cranial work called nasal specifics, pioneered by the late Richard Stober, D.C., a chiropractor influenced by osteopathy. As discussed previously, cranial bones may be misaligned due to both physical and emotional traumas.

Cranial bones articulate around and with the tissues and bones of the nasal passages. In a nasal specific treatment, a finger cot (a small rubber tube that is usually used to cover a finger) is attached to a bulb, then inserted through one nostril and into each of three nasal passages on that side of the skull. The bulb is inflated until the cot expands within the nasal passage. The procedure is then repeated in the three nasal passages accessed through the other nostril. This treatment indirectly "pumps" the pituitary gland, allowing realignment of distortions in cranial bones. The procedure takes only seconds, but it can be highly effective; migraine pain can completely disappear after this treatment, reports Dr. Cutler.

HERPES

Herpes refers to a family of viruses which produce a variety of diseases. The most common types are: herpes simplex virus 1 (HSV-1, cold sores or fever blisters); herpes simplex virus 2 (HSV-2, genital herpes); varicella-zoster virus (VZV, chicken pox in children/shingles in adults); Epstein-Barr virus (EBV, associated with mononucleosis); and cytomegalovirus (CMV, inhabits the salivary glands and is potentially fatal). In common usage, the word herpes indicates herpes simplex. The following discussion is limited to herpes simplex and herpes zoster.

Herpes Simplex
Both facial and genital herpes are caused by the herpes simplex virus. After the first attack, the virus remains dormant in nerve cells. Recurrent attacks start with a burning sensation soon followed by blisters which generally itch and are painful. Within a few days to several weeks they burst, dry up, and disappear. Facial and genital herpes are contagious during outbreaks.

While herpes simplex is annoying, embarrassing, irritating, and painful, it is rarely dangerous, except in two cases: when it infects the eyes or when it attacks newborns. Although herpes infection of the eye is rare—it happens about once in every 500,000 cases—it is serious. If an outbreak occurs near the eyes or on the forehead, do not touch it or rub your eyes, because if it infects the eyes, it could lead to blindness. Seek immediate treatment.

Neonatal herpes can be transmitted from a mother to a newborn infant, often during passage through an infected birth canal (a Caesarean section can protect the infant from transmission). During an infected baby's first month, this is a life-threatening disease because the infant's immune system is not sufficiently developed to fight the virus. Herpes in infants generally attacks the central nervous system and has a 50% to 60% fatality rate. Babies who do survive often suffer from significant brain damage and/or blindness.

For information on the **enzymes** for this health condition, see Appendix B.

Herpes Zoster (Shingles and Chicken Pox)
The common childhood infection called chicken pox is caused by the varicella-zoster virus. During a childhood bout of chicken pox not all of the viral organisms are destroyed. Some lie dormant in sensory (skin) nerves for life. In certain adults, the virus reawakens and causes

shingles, a painful, blistering rash which follows the course of a nerve and appears on different parts of the body, most commonly the forehead and cheeks, abdominal area, buttocks, and groin.

What Causes Herpes?

Recurrent herpes is clearly stress-related. Anxiety is the greatest predictor of a herpes eruption. Other factors that can reactivate the virus are nutrient deficiencies, exposure to the sun, and colds, flu, or other illnesses (especially accompanied by fever).

Nutritional Factors

Although herpes is a virus, its outbreak is often triggered by nutritional factors. The two most important of these are calcium metabolism problems (aggravated by sunlight) and an overly acidic oral pH (SEE QUICK DEFINITION).

Another culprit is deficiencies in fatty acids along with the fat-soluble vitamins A, D, and E, all of which are involved in the transport of calcium into the soft tissues of the body. Vitamin D helps transport calcium from the stomach into the blood. Fatty acids (especially oleic) and lauric acid transport calcium from the blood into the tissues. Even if you get plenty of vitamin D from your diet and exposure to sun, if you have a fatty acid deficiency, the calcium will not be able to get into the tissues from the blood. This leads to sun sensitivity and can cause sun rashes or welts (especially around the belt or clothing lines where there is pressure), as well as itchy skin.

An acidic oral pH is the medium favored by the herpes virus. The optimum oral pH is slightly alkaline, but fluctuations occur and can be aggravated by consuming too many acidic or acid-forming substances such as protein, tomatoes, and ascorbic acid. Normally, saliva buffers and restores the optimum pH before the herpes virus can gain a hold, but if your saliva is already too acidic, eating acidic foods may shift the pH balance long enough to allow the virus to enter.

Success Story: Taming a Boy's Herpes

Michael, 4, had a severe case of facial herpes with painful outbreaks during which much of his face was covered with large scabs. These outbreaks occurred every time he got sick, which was frequently, and each episode lasted two to

The term **pH**, which means "potential hydrogen," represents a scale for the relative acidity or alkalinity of a solution. Acidity is measured as a pH of 0.1 to 6.9, alkalinity is 7.1 to 14, and neutral pH is 7.0. The numbers refer to how many hydrogen atoms are present compared to an ideal or standard solution. Normally, blood is slightly alkaline, at 7.35 to 7.45. The pH of a 24-hour urine sample can range from 5.5 to 7.4. The optimum range is slightly acidic, at 6.3 to 6.7.

Over a one-year period, I treated Michael with several enzyme formulations for sugar and gluten intolerance and to boost his immune system. Gradually, the herpes outbreaks subsided, occurring only when he was run down from an infection, cold, or flu.

three weeks. Michael also had multiple food allergies (gluten, dairy, fruit, and sugars) and elevated liver enzymes (an indicator of hepatitis or inflammation of the liver) from taking antifungal medications, such as nystatin and Flagyl®, for candidiasis.

Over a one-year period, I treated Michael with several enzyme formulations including: Thera-zyme PAN, a multiple digestive formula for sugar and gluten intolerance; Thera-zyme Kdy, for his allergies; and Thera-zyme TRMA to boost his immune system. In addition, I told his mother to give him Thera-zyme MSCLR and Thera-zyme Lvr at the onset of each herpes attack.

Gradually, the outbreaks subsided, occurring only when Michael was run down from an infection, cold, or flu. These attacks were controlled with Thera-zyme MSCLR and Thera-zyme Lvr, and they lasted only three days instead of the painful three weeks he had endured before.

Success Story: The Woman Who Couldn't Kiss Her Boyfriend

When Julie, 38, entered my office, her entire upper lip was swollen and painful. According to Julie, this severe facial herpes episode was brought on by kissing her bearded boyfriend. I would normally be skeptical of contact with a bristly beard being the cause of an outbreak, but Julie was especially sensitive to the virus—an earlier attack had cost her the sight in one eye.

At the onset of symptoms, a herpes attack can usually be warded off by taking a dose of Thera-zyme MSCLR and, when needed, Thera-zyme Lvr. However, Julie was beyond that initial stage, and several days of enzyme therapy were required to deal with the outbreak. Due to her prior history of herpes, I also recommended lomatium, an antiviral herb. With this treatment, Julie's lip healed. From that point on, she was never without her remedies which enabled her to control outbreaks.

Success Story: Reversing Genital Herpes

Bob, 28, had been suffering from genital herpes for two years. His flare-ups occurred every two to three months and were triggered by a combination of sun, stress, and a cold. Episodes were severe, lasting for two weeks and including skin lesions, nausea, fever, muscle cramps, and migraines. His only relief was to soak in the bathtub for long periods. He had been on Zovirax, an antiviral, since the onset of his problem, but it did not resolve it.

I used the following enzymes:

- Thera-zyme PAN: multiple digestive formula for sugar intolerance
- Thera-zyme MSCLR: antihistamine formula to help relieve his herpes inflammation and skin eruption
- Thera-zyme Rbs: to nourish epithelial tissue (skin and the linings of the body's cavities and passageways such as the respiratory tract) and prevent and heal canker or cold sores
- Thera-zyme Lvr: for liver support
- Thera-zyme Kdy: for allergies
- Thera-zyme TRMA: for his immune system and soft-tissue trauma

For Bob's stress-activated herpes, I also added Stress Release, a homeopathic remedy I call the "basket-case" remedy.

On the enzyme program, Bob was able to stop taking Zovirax and, as long as he kept taking his enzymes, he was fine. After four months, he scaled down his enzyme dosage from three doses to one dose daily. Stress brought on an attack, but it was milder, lasting only two days instead of two weeks and the symptoms were greatly decreased. No skin lesions appeared, he just felt "flu-ish" and had a headache. Bob now regulates his dosage of enzymes and knows to increase them during times of sickness or stress.

Prevention and Elimination of Herpes

Preventing a herpes attack is best done through stress reduction and a specific diet. When implemented at the earliest symptoms (a burning sensation or slight itching), enzyme therapy and ointments can help keep an outbreak under control.

Enzyme Therapy

Herpes is one of the acute conditions which has a specific enzyme therapy—based on amylase and herbal formulas. Sometimes only one formula is used and, at other times, several are required, depending on the severity of the case and on clinical judgment.

- Multiple digestive enzyme formula, specific to the individual's needs
  - Thera-zyme MSCLR: natural antihistamine high in amylase
  - Thera-zyme Rbs: for protection and cure of sun-induced cold sores and for sun sensitivity, sun rashes, and sun poisoning
  - Thera-zyme Lvr: for liver problems
  - Thera-zyme TRMA: immune system formula for any kind of infection; also helps relieve anxiety, which is linked to herpes outbreaks
  - Thera-zyme Kdy: for allergies that can lead to herpes

Dietary Recommendations

There are certain dietary restrictions that appear to help inhibit the herpes virus. Studies have shown that the amino acid lysine blocks the growth of the herpes virus, while the amino acid arginine accelerates it. This discovery has led to the use of lysine as an anti-herpes supplement. However, taking large doses of an isolated amino acid on a daily basis can upset your amino acid balance. It is preferable to simply avoid foods high in arginine—especially chocolate, nuts, and seeds—and add foods high in lysine to your diet. Lysine-rich foods include seafood, chicken, turkey, eggs, dairy, brewer's yeast, and green foods such as barley grass, blue-green algae, and spirulina.

Healing Ointments

Over-the-counter ointments can help heal a herpes outbreak. Formulations containing lithium, zinc, and vitamin E are especially effective because they aid in blocking the inflammatory reaction.

INJURIES

Enzymes can be useful not only for relieving pain and inflammation (including after surgery), but as an aid in healing sports injuries and other trauma, including sprains, strains, broken bones, disc problems, tendonitis, injured ligaments, muscle soreness, and bruising.

Success Story:
Enzymes for Healing From a 30-Foot Fall

Ariel, 15, lost her grip while swinging on a rope across a ravine and fell 30 feet. She was unconscious for at least 15 minutes. A mass of cuts and bruises from head to toe, she was taken to the hospital, in too much pain to move. Her face was swollen like a balloon by the time she got there. X rays revealed that the only serious damage was one fractured vertebra which the doctor told her would heal on its own. She was given narcotic painkillers and sent home.

I treated Ariel immediately, giving her the following enzymes five times daily:

■ Thera-zyme TRMA: to reduce the pain, inflammation, swelling, and bruising

■ Thera-zyme MSCLR: to reduce muscle pain, stiffness, and spasms

■ Thera-zyme Kdy: to help her bruised kidneys and the nausea that accompanied the pain

■ Thera-zyme IVD: to help heal the fractured vertebra

On the painkillers the first day at home, Ariel could walk slowly. On the second day, she stopped taking the medication because it made her sick and caused a rash. With only an occasional aspirin along with her many enzymes, she was already able to control the pain. On the third day, when Ariel could sit up long enough to ride in a car, we took her to a chiropractor who began a series of treatments. By the end of the week, Ariel was sitting, standing, and walking with ease. Without these therapies, it would have taken far longer for her to heal from such a serious fall.

Success Story:
Overnight Relief for a Sprained Ankle

While playing basketball, Bruce, 18, came down from a high jump with all of his weight planted on one twisted foot. Disregarding the injury, he played out the game.

For information on the **enzymes** for this health condition, see Appendix B.

Tailoring Enzymes to the Inflammation Type

Each of the main plant enzymes is indicated for relieving a specific type of inflammation due to injury or other trauma:

Protease relieves the type of inflammation that requires ice, and alleviates soft tissue trauma, such as when the skin is cut or broken, either by accident or in surgery. Protease also relieves muscle spasms if they are related to a protease-induced calcium deficiency. Thera-zyme TRMA is the formula with the highest source of protease and also contains minerals to help relieve bruising (hematoma).

Amylase has an antihistamine effect and helps relieve the redness of inflammatory skin conditions. It, along with lipase and fatty acids, relieves many kinds of skin irritation. Amylase is great for athletes because it increases joint mobility and helps relieve sore muscles. Thera-zyme MSCLR is the highest source of amylase.

Lipase relieves cold lymphatic swelling, the kind that requires heat. Lipase can also relieve muscle spasms if they are related to a lipase-induced calcium deficiency. Thera-zyme VSCLR is the highest source of lipase but many other enzyme formulas also contain lipase.

Catalase is an antioxidant enzyme which helps relieve inflammation and the edema of injury. Thera-zyme TRMA is high in catalase. This formula cannot be used by people who have gastric irritation (hiatal hernia, gastritis, or ulcers), but they can substitute Thera-zyme Stm, also high in catalase.

Afterwards, he arrived at my office hopping on one foot, the ankle swollen. I suggested he try natural therapy for a day, then if the ankle hadn't improved, he should get an X ray taken.

I gave Bruce Thera-zyme TRMA for the inflammation and bruising and rubbed the essential oil Pane Away on the site of the injury. The next morning, the swelling was almost gone and Bruce walked without a limp.

Enzyme Therapy for Injuries

The appropriate enzyme formulas or herbal remedies for injuries depend on the type of problem. A few examples follow:

■ Broken Bones: Thera-zyme IVD helps repair broken bones, ligaments, and herniated discs; other indicated formulas may be Thera-zyme Para, a calcium formula, and Thera-zyme TRMA for bruising and pain.

■ Bruises: Thera-zyme TRMA taken immediately after the injury reduces the possibility of bruising and sometimes deters it entirely;

people with gastric problems should take Thera-zyme Thy instead.

■ Disc Problems: A ruptured disc requires protease to reduce inflammation (Thera-zyme TRMA). A herniated disc requires the marshmallow–rose hips formula (Thera-zyme IVD) to help deliver protein to the disc; since water follows protein, the disc gets rehydrated and the pain is relieved.

■ Joint Pain/Arthritis: Before giving supplements for joint pain, I make sure the client is not ingesting NutraSweet™ or low in thyroid function, both of which can cause joint pain, among other symptoms. If these causes are not present, Thera-zyme Mal (for males or menopausal women) or Thera-zyme Fem (for women at any age) can be useful in relieving the pain and swelling of arthritis. Thera-zyme OSTEO may also be helpful as it was developed specifically for arthritis.

■ Muscle Soreness and Strains: Thera-zyme MSCLR helps relieve sore muscles from excessive exercise, and muscle and joint stiffness, especially following rest, as in the morning or after driving or sitting.

■ Tendonitis, Carpal Tunnel, Tennis Elbow: Thera-zyme TRMA is indicated for people without gastric problems; Thera-zyme Thy for those with gastric problems who cannot tolerate protease.

Aromatherapy/Essential Oils

The essential oil blend called Pane Away mentioned previously contains birch, helichrysum, clovebud, and peppermint, all of which act to relieve pain and inflammation. Pane Away can be applied (3-6 drops, once or twice daily) directly on the injured area unless it is an open wound. In the case of open wound, apply the oil on the feet (if the open wound is not located there) or near the wound, but not directly on it.

INSOMNIA

Over 50 million Americans suffer from sleep disorders, including insomnia, excessive drowsiness, and restless movement during sleep. Here we discuss insomnia which consists of difficulty falling asleep, staying asleep, or both.

What Causes Insomnia?

Billions of dollars are spent each year on sleeping pills and tranquilizers—in spite of their severe side effects. If you cannot sleep, there is a reason and it is probably nutritional, emotional, hormonal, or perhaps a bit of each. For example, you might have a protease deficiency, one of the symptoms of which is anxiety. If you feel overly anxious, it is difficult to fall asleep. Worry about not sleeping increases your anxiety until you are caught up in a vicious cycle of insomnia.

An underactive thyroid gland is a common cause of insomnia. Unfortunately, this easily remedied imbalance often goes undetected.

Success Story: Reversing Insomnia

Roger, 43, suffered from depression and insomnia. In addition, every time he did fall asleep, his legs would cramp and wake him up, causing him to pace the floor through the night. Several doctors had diagnosed him as having "restless leg syndrome," but none could help him. Roger even spent time in a sleep clinic, but to no avail.

His urinalysis showed sugar intolerance and malabsorption, along with an extreme calcium deficiency. In addition, his thyroid gland was underactive. Since depression and insomnia are major complaints of hypothyroid adults, I advised Roger to take a natural thyroid glandular extract. I also gave him Thera-zyme PAN, a multiple digestive enzyme formula for sugar intolerance. The calcium deficiency explained Roger's "restless legs," since people who lack sufficient calcium often develop nocturnal leg cramps or a nighttime cough. For this, I gave Roger Thera-zyme Para, an enzyme formula containing calcium lactate.

The first symptom that subsided (in less than a week) was his leg cramping. A fast response was expected since his body could quickly digest and absorb the badly needed calcium. Roger's underactive thyroid and the resulting depression and insomnia took longer to correct but, within several months, he was sleeping through the night and his depression had lifted.

For information on the **enzymes** for this health condition, see Appendix B.

Insomnia Checklist:
What Enzymes Will Help You Sleep?

Below is a list of symptoms followed by a suggested enzyme therapy or other treatment. Find the symptom that best describes your sleeping problems. If several apply to you, discuss an appropriate treatment with an enzyme therapist.

■ You are anxious, a worrier, and you sigh a lot; your anxiety increases when you go to bed: Thera-zyme TRMA (Caution: TRMA is not advised for people with gastric problems)

■ You have trouble falling asleep due to nervousness or severe emotional stress: Thera-zyme CLM

■ You fall asleep early, but cannot stay asleep; you sometimes have nightmares or bad dreams: You may have a problem digesting sugar. Try avoiding refined sugars and take Thera-zyme Adr to help sugar intolerance.

■ You can't fall asleep because your mind races and you can't stop thinking: This also may be due to problems with sugar digestion. Avoid all refined sugars and take Thera zyme SvG to help you relax.

■ Your legs cramp or are restless; you cough during the night: You may be calcium deficient; take Thera-zyme Para.

■ You are so restless that you toss and turn all night: You may have trouble relaxing your muscles. This is often accompanied by sore muscles after exercise or stiffness after rest, especially in the morning or after driving or sitting. Take Thera-zyme MSCLR for muscle soreness.

■ You have trouble staying asleep, are restless, grind your teeth, and have itching around your rectum or groin: You may have parasites. There are several formulas to get rid of them, including Thera-zyme Challenge Food Powder, Sml, and TRMA, along with grapefruit seed extract. The appropriate therapy will depend upon your specific symptoms.

■ You can't sleep because you are in pain due to an injury: Almost any injury can cause insomnia. If you suffer from pain due to an injury, seek qualified chiropractic or other care. Enzymes can help relieve pain that prevents sleep: Thera-zym Sym (for headaches related to upper cervical problems); IVD (for TMJ-related pain); TRMA (for pain of injury or chemotherapy); Stm (for stomach pain); and OSTEO (for arthritic pain).

■ Men: Your sleep is interrupted by frequent nighttime urination: Prostate problems can be the cause of frequent urination. Other symptoms include a feeling of incomplete bowel evacuation, loss of libido or pain with intercourse, pain in the groin, or pain down the front of the legs. Thera-zyme Mal and natural thyroid therapy is indicated.

■ Women: You are frequently awakened by hot flashes: Hot flashes indicate the need for hormonal balancing. Thera-zyme Fem, natural progesterone in vitamin E oil, and thyroid therapy is indicated.

Success Story: Too Stressed to Sleep

Sarah, 55, a regular client of mine, had previously suffered from a lung infection each winter. Since starting an enzyme therapy and thyroid support program, Sarah had been doing quite well and had come far in strengthening her immune system. Now, however, she was facing a stressful situation in her life and that brought on a new problem: she couldn't sleep. "I toss and turn all night, and I'm a nervous wreck," she complained. To make matters worse, she was often awakened by nightmares.

To be sure that she was taking adequate thyroid glandular extract, I reminded Sarah to check her temperature upon rising in the morning and again at noon. This was especially important at the time, because the need for thyroid hormone increases not only during periods of sickness and stress, but also during the winter season. I recommended the following enzyme formulas:

- Thera-zyme MSCLR: to help relax her muscles
- Thera-zyme CLM: enzyme formula containing tranquilizing herbs
- Thera-zyme Adr: for sugar intolerance; helps relieve insomnia, nightmares, and panic attacks

Sarah's insomnia and nightmares ceased. Her stress was reduced by the formulas she took and—since she was able to sleep again—her immune system held up. Sarah was able to make it through the winter without succumbing to a seasonal lung infection.

Prevention and Elimination of Insomnia

Insomnia can be successfully treated without toxic drugs. In addition to enzyme therapy, you may need to change your diet or have your thyroid tested.

Enzyme Therapy

The following enzyme-herbal formulas can break the insomnia cycle and help you get a good night's sleep:

- Thera-zyme Para: for hyperirritability, insomnia or restless legs during sleep, and night cough
- Thera-zyme MSCLR: muscle-relaxing formula for insomnia due to restlessness
- Thera-zyme CLM: containing tranquilizing herbs; for unresolved emotional problems, restlessness, nervousness, insomnia, and nightmares
- Thera-zyme Adr: for sugar intolerance and troubled sleep or

nightmares; useful during times of high stress since the sucrase/B-vit-amin combination helps transport sugar to the brain—a major requirement for relaxation

■ Thera-zyme SvG: for people who cannot relax, become serene, or meditate, those with the "racing mind syndrome"

■ Thera-zyme TRMA: for anxiety-ridden people who sigh a lot

KIDNEY STONES

Kidney stones are accumulations of mineral salts which can lodge anywhere along the course of the urinary tract. There are three types of stones: calcium oxalate, calcium phosphate, and uric acid. Calcium oxalate stones are the most common (80% of all cases).

The predominant symptom of kidney stones is sudden severe back pain which may come and go and often radiates from the back across the abdomen and into the genital area or inner thighs. This pain may be associated with nausea, vomiting, abdominal bloating, blood in the urine, pain on urination, and sometimes chills and fever. Kidney stones in the urinary tract are extremely painful and, if untreated, can be life threatening. In the United States, seven to ten of every 1,000 hospital admissions are due to kidney stones.

What Causes Kidney Stones?

A tendency toward kidney stone formation may be genetically influenced—if one parent is a stone-former there is an increased risk in the children. Other factors include diet, nutrient deficiencies, and cadmium toxicity.

Dietary Factors

Eating refined carbohydrates, including sugar, seems to be a major factor in the formation of stones. Sugar consumption stimulates the pancreas to release insulin, which in turn stimulates increased calcium excretion through the urine. When unbalanced by adequate calcium, consuming high-phosphorus foods and beverages, such as meat and soft drinks, also leads to increased calcium loss via the urine. Thus, the all-American fare of refined carbohydrates, meat, and soft drinks is a prescription for kidney stones.

Avoiding foods high in oxalic acid (the compound in oxalates, mineral salts forming the majority of kidney stones) is a common recommendation. These foods include beets, carrots, celery, cucumbers, grapefruit, kale, parsley, peanuts, rhubarb, spinach, and sweet pota-

For information on the **enzymes** for this health condition, see Appendix B.

toes. However, recent findings suggest that such foods are not responsible for kidney stone formation. In fact, consuming oxalic acid from food increases urinary oxalates by a relatively small amount. One study showed that only 16.3% of 392 stone-formers were found to have excess urinary oxalates.[67]

I emphasize this because so many nutritious foods happen to be high in oxalic acid. Rather than eliminating them from your diet, correct your nutritional imbalances by cutting out refined sugars and avoiding all other refined foods. Instead, eat an organic, whole-foods diet, with adequate protein (from fish, organic meat or poultry, organic eggs, raw or fermented milk products), organic fruits and their juices, and organic vegetables and salads.

Nutritional Deficiencies

Magnesium helps in the dissolving of oxalates in the urine, allowing them to be excreted before stones are formed. Vitamin B6 is essential for the normal metabolism of oxalic acid. Deficiencies of either vitamin B6 or magnesium will increase kidney stone risk—and anyone who subsists on processed foods is most likely deficient in both.

Both vitamin A deficiency and vitamin C deficiency may promote kidney stone formation. Smokers are nearly always deficient in vitamin C—each cigarette destroys as much vitamin C as there is in one orange. Also, people who are sick or under stress are usually deficient in vitamin C. However, as discussed with other health conditions, taking supplements without changing the diet is not the way to address nutrient deficiencies. The lacking vitamins should be obtained from food sources.

Cadmium Toxicity

Cadmium is a trace metal which can damage the kidneys, and exposure is associated with increased risk of kidney stones.[68] Cigarette smokers have abnormally high levels of cadmium in their blood and thus run a higher risk of forming stones. Joggers should avoid running along highways because they risk inhaling cadmium from automobile exhaust. In addition to cigarette smoke and automobile pollution, cadmium can be found in drinking water, fertilizers, fungicides, pesticides, refined grains, coffee, tea, and soft drinks. Certain metalworkers, such as coppersmiths, are chronically exposed to cadmium.

Success Story: Preventing Recurrent Kidney Stones

Alice, 55, was desperate to avoid another round in a long history of painful kidney stone episodes, two of which required hospitalization.

Her urinalysis and palpation revealed that she was both sugar and fat intolerant. She also showed a severe allergy pattern. Of particular interest was her urinary sediment which showed high oxalates—an indication of fat intolerance and a high consumption of coffee, tea, or

Alice, 55, was desperate to avoid another round in a long history of painful kidney stone episodes, two of which required hospitalization. Her urinalysis and palpation revealed that she was both sugar and fat intolerant. She also showed a severe allergy pattern.

cola. Alice ate a lot of high-fat and refined foods (white flour, sugar, rice, pasta) and drank an excessive number of cola beverages.

I advised her to change her diet, to avoid excessive fats and cut out refined foods and colas altogether. I also recommended the following enzyme formulas:

- Thera-zyme HCL: digestive formula for fat and sugar intolerance
- Thera-zyme UrT: for kidney stones and all urinary tract problems; this formula must be taken with at least 4-6 oz of water
- Thera-zyme Kdy: for allergies, which can sometimes lead to kidney pain

Alice changed her diet according to my instructions and took her enzymes faithfully. In the five years since, she has not had another episode of kidney stones. Although she no longer needs the urinary tract formula, Alice keeps it handy, just in case she feels a twinge of pain.

Success Story:
She Didn't Know She Had Kidney Stones

Iris, 80, suffered from fatigue, insomnia, osteoporosis, the inability to gain weight, and one symptom she could not adequately describe—diffuse pains near her bladder. With further questioning, I discovered that she had several urinary tract symptoms, including urgency to urinate while passing only small amounts at each voiding (which kept her awake at night) and frequent burning with urination (cystitis). Her health history also indicated long-standing low thyroid function and the resulting need for progesterone. A urinalysis revealed severe sugar intolerance, vitamin C and calcium deficiencies, kidney-lymphatic stress (indicating allergies), plus traces of hemoglobin (pigment in red blood cells) in her urine (hematuria).

I gave Iris the following:

- Thera-zyme PAN: for sugar intolerance and environmental sensitivities
- Thera-zyme Kdy: for her multiple allergies
- Thera-zyme Opt: containing a food source of vitamin C

- Thera-zyme Para: containing calcium
- Thera-zyme UrT: for kidney stones and all urinary tract problems

I also recommended a thyroid glandular extract to boost her immune system, improve her appetite, and help her sleep. Finally, I added 10% natural progesterone in vitamin E to help reverse the osteoporosis, which was advanced in this frail woman, and as a further aid to her immune system.

I told Iris that if the blood in her urine did not disappear within two weeks, she most likely had a kidney stone, regardless of test results. Two weeks passed and the hematuria did not abate, nor did her other symptoms. Iris remained on the Thera-zyme UrT until both the blood in her urine and the other urinary tract symptoms disappeared.

After several months, not only did the hematuria disappear, but Iris no longer had the frequent urge to urinate and began passing more normal amounts of urine—which allowed her to sleep through the night. The burning sensation during urination was also gone and she even began to gain weight. It has been several years since I treated Iris and she has had no further urinary or kidney problems.

Prevention and Elimination of Kidney Stones

Both the urine and the blood have an optimum pH (SEE QUICK DEFINITION) range, and keeping pH levels within these ranges will help prevent the formation of kidney stones. The blood creates its own acid-base balance from the acidity and alkalinity provided from the digestion of food along with the proper ratios of water, carbon dioxide, and oxygen. Everybody drinks water and breathes, but not everybody eats raw, unrefined foods, high in food enzymes. Food enzyme therapy can correct the pH balance of the body, thus preventing kidney stones.

In addition to enzyme therapy, I also carefully monitor the client's diet and suggest nutritional supplements as appropriate.

The term **pH**, which means "potential hydrogen," represents a scale for the relative acidity or alkalinity of a solution. Acidity is measured as a pH of 0.1 to 6.9, alkalinity is 7.1 to 14, and neutral pH is 7.0. The numbers refer to how many hydrogen atoms are present compared to an ideal or standard solution. Normally, blood is slightly alkaline, at 7.35 to 7.45. The pH of a 24-hour urine sample can range from 5.5 to 7.0. The optimum range is slightly acidic, at 6.3 to 6.7.

Enzyme Therapy

I conduct specific tests to determine which of the following formulas are necessary, but often it is a combination of the three. In people with urinary tract conditions with a trace of blood in the urine, these formulas will aid in healing and the blood should disappear.

- Multiple digestive formula for the individual's needs
- Thera-zyme UrT: contains food sources of the nutritional deficiencies often found in kidney stone–formers—vitamins A and C. If the stone is small, the pain from kidney stones is sometimes eliminated overnight by using this formula. In severe cases requiring medical attention, Thera-zyme UrT is still indicated to prevent recurrence.
- Thera-zyme TRMA: a formula for the immune system; added when there is a urinary tract or kidney infection
- Thera-zyme Kdy: for when the kidneys appear sore and stressed (when the urinalysis shows low volume or low specific gravity)

Enzyme formulas to treat nutritional deficiencies often found in kidney stone–formers include:

- Thera-zyme Adr: B vitamins
- Thera-zyme CLM: magnesium
- Thera-zyme Opt: vitamin C
- Thera-zyme Nsl: antioxidant/vitamin C formula

Nutritional Supplements (Dietary Sources)

- Magnesium: found in kelp, whole grains, yeast, nuts, coconut meat, and fruit (whole or juices)
- Vitamin B6: found in brewer's yeast, wheat germ, fish and beef, brown rice, bananas, avocados, egg yolks, kale, spinach, potatoes, and popcorn

MENOPAUSAL SYMPTOMS

Women usually experience menopause at some point between the ages of 45 and 55 (the average age is 52), when their monthly menstrual cycle becomes irregular and then stops. In addition to hot flashes, accompanying symptoms may include water retention, weight gain, memory loss, irritability, depression, thinning of the vaginal walls, decreased libido, and arthritis. Women who undergo a hysterectomy (surgical menopause through removal of the uterus and/or ovaries) may experience the same symptoms as with natural menopause.

Causes of Menopausal Symptoms

Contrary to what most women are told, the unpleasant symptoms of menopause are not from an estrogen deficiency, but are rather the result of years of damaging effects on the pituitary gland from estrogen dominance, that is, excess estrogen in relation to progesterone. When the first menses is missed, the estrogen level has usually not decreased but progesterone has been decreasing, sometimes for years. It is the lack of adequate progesterone that stops menses in both young and older women alike. The lack of progesterone may also bring about increased loss of calcium from bones, making them brittle and more likely to break—a condition known as osteoporosis.

Along with the decrease of progesterone production, causes of estrogen dominance include an underactive thyroid gland (hypothyroidism) and the ingestion of estrogens—from estrogen drugs (as in hormone replacement therapy or birth control pills), environmental estrogens, or phytoestrogens (plant-derived estrogens such as black cohosh).

In many women, the declining levels of progesterone which occur with aging (after about age 35) are accelerated by hypothyroidism, since the production of progesterone from cholesterol is dependent on adequate thyroid function (plus vitamin A and certain enzymes). Estrogen replacement therapy (ERT; also called hormone replacement therapy, or HRT) will actually worsen the situation. In fact, it is difficult to remediate the condition without adequate thyroid therapy, even if progesterone is used.

For information on the **enzymes** for this health condition, see Appendix B.

Common complaints are night sweats or hot flashes and a pounding heart. Hot flashes are associated with estrogen

Hot flashes and other menopausal symptoms can be controlled by the correct use of natural progesterone and thyroid glandular extract plus enzyme therapy and a diet of whole foods.

dominance and low blood sugar, leading to increased surges of adrenaline followed by cortisol (both adrenal gland hormones). Hot flashes usually increase at night, because darkness exacerbates stress, causes blood sugar to fall, adrenaline and cortisol to rise, and lowers calcium levels. Hot flashes decrease during the day as the blood sugar rises. This situation is worse during the winter because of the reduced hours of sunlight.

Success Story: Ending 15 Years of Menopausal Symptoms

For Rachel, 49, it had been 15 years since she had undergone a hysterectomy, but she still felt like she was going through menopause. She had hot flashes and trouble sleeping, couldn't lose weight, and suffered from arthritis. In addition to her menopausal and arthritic symptoms, Rachel had severe allergies and trouble breathing through her nose. "I feel like I'm going downhill and there's nothing I can do

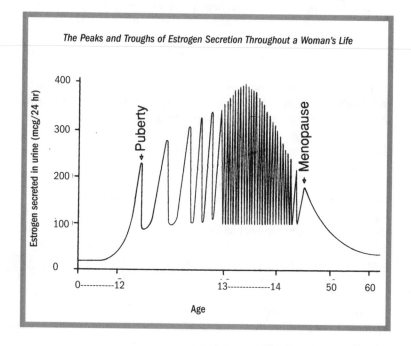

The Peaks and Troughs of Estrogen Secretion Throughout a Woman's Life

about it," Rachel concluded.

Her palpation test and urinalysis revealed that she was both sugar and fat intolerant, had kidney-lymphatic stress, low thyroid function (probably of long duration), and calcium and vitamin C deficiencies.

Rachel's diet was low in protein, fruit, and salt—the main dietary requirements for optimum thyroid function. In addition, she often ate soy-based foods, including tofu and protein drinks containing soy (soy is a thyroid inhibitor).

I advised Rachel to increase her daily protein intake with fish and organic food sources including poultry and potatoes. I also told Rachel that if she could keep her blood sugar up, she would sleep better and have fewer hot flashes. The fastest way I know of to increase blood sugar is to drink a glass of orange juice mixed with a bit of organic sea salt (up to ¼ tsp). I told her to drink this as often as necessary.

I then started Rachel on the following enzyme formulas:

■ Thera-zyme HCL: multiple digestive formula for both fat and sugar intolerance

■ Thera-zyme Para: to help her sleep

■ Thera-zyme Nsl: antioxidant/vitamin C formula for her nasal problems

■ Thera-zyme Kdy: allergy formula

■ Thera-zyme OSTEO: for arthritis

For Rachel's menopausal symptoms, I recommended a natural thyroid glandular extract to help optimize her thyroid function, along with 10% oral natural progesterone in vitamin E.

Rachel changed her diet, while conscientiously taking her enzymes, thyroid hormone, and progesterone each day. Her persistence paid off, but it was a slow over the course of about six months. As the weeks went by, she noticed a change in her energy level and moods; her hot flashes became less frequent; and her allergies became tolerable and she began to breathe through her nose. Her sleep improved, she started losing weight, and her joints stopped aching. Finally, Rachel said that she felt like herself again.

Success Story: Hot Flash Relief

Jean, 48, suffered from hot flashes as well as allergies. Her urinalysis showed that she had severe digestive problems (fat and protein intolerance), low calcium, a vitamin C deficiency, plus kidney-lymphatic stress. In addition, her thyroid was underactive.

Jean had been on estrogen replacement therapy for several years and her diet contained large amounts of thyroid inhibitors, including unsaturated fatty acids, raw cruciferous vegetables (cabbage, cauli-flower, broccoli; lightly steaming them destroys the thyroid inhibiting substances they contain), and tap water (containing fluoride and many other thyroid inhibitors).[69] Soy also figured prominently in Jean's diet; some evidence indicates that soy products may affect the thyroid.[70] In addition, Jean also engaged in extensive endurance exercise which further depletes thyroid function (reversible when the exercise is reduced).

I explained to Jean that to relieve her symptoms she needed to increase the protein, fruit, and salt in her diet, eliminate dietary thyroid inhibitors, and decrease her endurance exercise to walking briskly rather than running. I recommended the following enzyme supplements:

- Thera-zyme Bil: multiple digestive formula for fat and protein intolerance
- Thera-zyme Para: an enzymatic calcium formula
- Thera-zyme Kdy: for her allergies

More specifically for Jean's hot flashes, I recommended a natural thyroid glandular extract to help improve her thyroid function, along with 10% progesterone.

It took Jean over a year to completely recover, due to the many years of poor diet combined with the ERT. In fact, that therapy had led to a severe estrogen dominance which required large doses of progesterone to correct (three drops, five times daily). In addition, Jean's strenuous exercise regimen caused her to need higher than usual doses of thyroid hormone.

Gradually, her hot flashes became less intense and less frequent, her sleep improved, and her energy level rose. Now Jean is on a maintenance program of the multiple digestive enzyme formula, Thera-zyme Bil, a thyroid glandular extract, and a small daily dose (three drops) of natural progesterone—and she no longer complains of hot flashes.

Prevention and Elimination of Menopausal Symptoms

Hot flashes and other menopausal symptoms can be controlled by the correct use of natural progesterone and thyroid glandular extract plus a diet of whole foods and enzyme therapy. Progesterone decreases hot flashes by opposing estrogen. As noted above, thyroid hormone is needed for the manufacture of progesterone.

Enzyme Therapy

Many women benefit from taking extra protease and/or lipase enzymes which are often deficient during menopause. Calcium is carried in the blood partly as an ionic (salt) and partly as protein-bound calcium. Protease, the enzyme that digests protein, supplies both the required digested protein for protein-bound calcium and adequate acidity required for the ionic or salt form. Lipase is required to carry calcium across the intestinal wall and for the production of female hormones. A deficiency in either of these enzymes could contribute to osteoporosis. The multiple digestive enzyme formula required depends on each individual's digestive problems, for example:

- Thera-zyme Bil: for fat and protein intolerance
- Thera-zyme HCL: for fat, sugar and protein intolerance
- Thera-zyme VSCLR: highest in lipase; for women who are fiber intolerant and eat excessive amounts of fat (these women may have trouble losing weight, be diabetic, or have high blood fats)
- Thera-zyme Stm: containing no protease; for women with gastric problems

Other enzyme formulas are used as needed. For instance, Thera-zyme OSTEO is indicated in women who develop arthritic symptoms during menopause, and Thera-zyme Fem or Mal can be used for all of the symptoms of menopause, including hot flashes and arthritic symptoms.

Hormonal Balancing

Progesterone will balance the excessive estrogen which leads to menopausal symptoms. I recommend 10% oral natural progesterone in vitamin E oil.

Thyroid Support

I suggest a natural thyroid glandular extract to improve thyroid function. If you are hypothyroid, also increase your salt, fruit, and protein intake. To avoid hot flashes, try eating a salty snack right before going to bed. Also, a small carbohydrate snack such as fruit, fruit juice, or crackers will help keep blood sugar up and cortisol down as the night progresses. (See Appendix A.)

Factors to Consider Before Using Estrogen Replacement Therapy

In the United States, an estimated 15% to 18% of postmenopausal women (about three million) currently take estrogen. Numerous articles and advertisements in the mainstream media testify to estrogen's usefulness in preventing hot flashes, and in protecting women from osteoporosis and heart disease. They even imply that estrogen has youth-restoring properties. In these same articles, the risks—cancer, gallbladder disease, and blood clots—are underplayed. Yet hundreds of medical studies describe the many dangerous side effects of estrogen when unopposed by adequate progesterone and thyroid hormones.

Even the words "estrogen replacement therapy" are misleading, since HRT usually "replaces" much more estrogen than a woman normally produces. At the peak of fertility, most women produce 30 to 40 micrograms of estrogen daily—the usual HRT dosage is *15 times* that amount. Even so-called "low-dose HRT" is a 100% replacement dose of 30 micrograms daily.

Promoters of HRT imply that, all of a sudden, at menopause, a woman simply ceases to make estrogen, rendering her a helpless target for emotional problems, hot flashes, and osteoporosis. On the contrary, although estrogen production does decrease, it is the decrease in progesterone during menopause and the resulting lowered ratio of progesterone to estrogen that is responsible for the aging effects of menopause, including osteoporosis.[71] Women can secrete a significant amount of estrogen after menopause or even after a total hysterectomy (in which the ovaries have been removed) because estrogen is made by most body cells, especially damaged fat cells. Breast cells normally do not make estrogen unless they become cancerous and then they, too, make estrogen.

I do not believe that any woman needs to take additional estrogen because, along with that produced in your body, you ingest it through phytoestrogens (plant-derived estrogen) in your diet and through exposure to or ingestion of pesticides, which mimic estrogen in the body. However, if you do choose ERT, you should take natural (not synthetic) progesterone along with it to afford some measure of protection from estrogen's carcinogenic effects.

Even though the side effects of HRT include weight gain, leg cramps, dark spots on the skin, migraines, increased tendency to gallbladder disease, and increased risk of endometrial and breast cancer, many women choose HRT because of its supposed beneficial effects. However, even the reputed benefits of HRT should be looked at more closely.

■ Does estrogen prevent hot flashes?

Estrogen does diminish hot flashes, but in an unnatural manner. Metabolized into a form which promotes the actions of adrenaline, it increases excitation in the brain, tones and speeds up all body processes, including the nervous system, and tightens blood vessels. Research has shown that estrogen can block the liver's ability to eliminate adrenaline; a similar effect has been observed in the brain's enzyme systems, which accounts for estrogen's amphetamine-like or cocaine-like action in the brain.[72]

In a typical hot flash, there is first an adrenaline surge. This triggers a cortisol surge for the purpose of raising blood sugar. There is then an adrenal relaxation stage—as the adrenals relax, a hot flash occurs. Estrogen works by keeping adrenaline up so there is never any adrenaline letdown.

■ Is estrogen cardioprotective?

Women are told that HRT can prevent heart disease, but excess estrogen is actually bad for the heart. Researchers have found that estrogen used for more than a few months after menopause can elevate the incidence of vascular disease. In a study of 1,234 postmenopausal women, 50 to 83 years old, no benefits from estrogen use were observed. Disadvantages of postmenopausal estrogen use included premature vascular disease and stroke, breast pathology, increased clotting, and increased risk of developing tumors, including cancerous ones.[73]

■ Does estrogen prevent Alzheimer's disease?

On the contrary, one of estrogen's toxic effects is to cause calcium to deposit in soft tissues. Most people are aware of the association of Alzheimer's disease with poisoning from heavy metals, such as aluminum and mercury, but calcium deposits have also been found at the site of damaged areas in the brain.[74]

■ Does estrogen prevent osteoporosis?

Rather than preventing osteoporosis, estrogen dominance is a causal factor in this destructive bone disease.[75] Progesterone, on the other hand, prevents and cures osteoporosis even in elderly women. In addition, natural (not synthetic) thyroid glandular extract promotes both bone formation and resorption (the breaking down of old bone material so new bone can take its place). Both are necessary for healthy bones.

MENTAL DISORDERS

A number of my clients have been diagnosed with mental disorders by psychologists or psychiatrists after their general physicians were unable to find anything physically wrong with them. Many were placed on drugs. Some were even told to try electroshock therapy. This is unfortunate, as a number of these supposed mental and emotional conditions have their roots in physical causes which can be remedied without toxic drugs.

What Causes Mental Disorders?

Abnormal brain chemistry leading to mental illness is often a direct result of abnormal body chemistry due to nutritional problems and/or hormonal imbalances. These include sugar intolerance (the inability to digest disaccharides into simple sugars), protease deficiency (difficulty digesting protein), and hypothyroidism (an underactive thyroid gland).

Sugar Intolerance

Sugar intolerance can lead to emotional and mental problems as well as physical. Mental and emotional symptoms and conditions caused by sugar intolerance include: insomnia or nightmares, panic attacks, depression, mood swings, irritable, aggressive, or violent behavior, bipolar and schizophrenic disorders, autism, and attention deficit disorder (ADD). The worst symptoms arise in people who are sugar intolerant, B-vitamin deficient, and have hypothyroidism which causes low blood sugar (glucose).

Glucose, formed in the body from the digestion of sugars, protein, and carbohydrates plus the B-complex vitamins, is a major requirement of brain nutrition. There are three primary factors that prevent glucose from arriving in the brain. First, the body is unable to digest sugar. Second, the body cannot adequately digest protein (46% of digested protein is eventually converted to sugar). Third, there is a deficiency of B vitamins, which are required to transport sugar into the brain.

For information on the **enzymes** for this health condition, see Appendix B.

Most Americans are sugar intolerant to some degree, either because they eat too much of it or because they do not produce enough disaccharidases (the sugar-digesting enzymes: lactase, sucrase, and maltase) in the small intestine. Most people eat too much sugar, far exceeding the capacity of the digestive system to make disaccharidases to process it. In addition, refined white sugar (sucrose), white flour, and white rice are devoid of B vitamins, so even if you can digest the sugar or the starch (flour and rice), you still cannot transport it into the brain.

Protease Deficiency

People who are deficient in protease cannot digest protein. Even those who become vegetarians still have trouble digesting plant protein. Protease deficiency leads to a buildup of excess alkaline reserves (an alkaline pH, SEE QUICK DEFINITION) because there is not enough digested protein to supply the necessary acidity. Symptoms of an overly alkaline system are anxiety and frequent sighing. Since protease-deficient people have excess alkaline reserves in the blood, it is difficult for their bloodstream to carry calcium—another factor which leads to anxiety.

The term **pH**, which means "potential hydrogen," represents a scale for the relative acidity or alkalinity of a solution. Acidity is measured as a pH of 0.1 to 6.9, alkalinity is 7.1 to 14, and neutral pH is 7.0. The numbers refer to how many hydrogen atoms are present compared to an ideal or standard solution. Normally, blood is slightly alkaline, at 7.45. The pH of a 24-hour urine sample can range from 5.5 to 7.4. The optimum range is slightly acidic, at 6.3 to 6.7.

Hypothyroidism

Hypothyroidism appears to be closely linked to depression and symptoms of mental illness. Since it leads to digestive problems and low blood sugar, low thyroid function, and sugar intolerance have overlapping symptoms. (See Appendix A.)

Success Story: To the Bottom and Back

Victoria, a vice president of an international bank, was well-read, articulate, and creative with a lively sense of humor. In her mid-40s, she became increasingly confused, disoriented, and depressed. She deteriorated emotionally, mentally, and physically: over the course of two years, she developed breast cancer, became arthritic, and gained over 100 pounds.

Victoria was subsequently diagnosed with bipolar disorder (manic depression), panic disorder, and obsessive personality disorder. Her psychiatrist prescribed a wide range of psychiatric drugs—including Prozac®, Paxil®, BuSpar®, Depakote®, Zoloft®, lithium, Xanax®, Tegretol®, Moban®, Wellbutrin®, Effexor®, and imipramine—none of which improved her condition. Rather, they caused multiple side effects including nausea, vomiting, loss of bowel control, and her extreme weight gain.

At this point, Victoria's doctor referred her to me for an evalu-

Most Americans are sugar intolerant to some degree, either because they eat too much of it or because they do not produce enough disaccharidases (the sugar-digesting enzymes: lactase, sucrase, and maltase) in the small intestine.

ation of her nutritional needs. He was open to the idea that some of her mental problems were caused by inadequate nutrition and hormonal imbalance.

Victoria, now 50, was taking imipramine, Xanax, and Tegretol in relatively high doses. Her temperature was only 95° F (I had never seen one so low), but it spiked to 104° F after she took imipramine—of great concern, given reports of sudden death (especially in children and adolescents) after ingestion of the drug. Victoria's diet consisted of junk foods, sweets, soft drinks, and coffee. She appeared almost catatonic and could barely climb onto the therapy table because of her large size and severe arthritis. Although I talked to her extensively, I could not tell whether she heard or understood what I said.

After a urinalysis and palpation test, I recommended the following enzyme therapy:

■ Thera-zyme PAN: for sugar intolerance to help alleviate her mood swings, insomnia, and depression

■ Thera-zyme Adr: sugar-digesting formula for her panic attacks and depression

■ Thera-zyme TRMA: containing protease to strengthen her immune system and help relieve inflammation and anxiety

■ Thera-zyme Kdy: lymphatic drainage formula to relieve low-back (kidney) pain, nausea, frontal headaches, and allergies

I also gave Victoria a thyroid glandular extract for her underactive thyroid and 10% oral natural progesterone.

Within a few weeks, there was a gradual but profound change in her behavior. She started to lose weight. Her speech was faster and more articulate with normal emotional expression, and she revealed a sense of humor. Both TRMA and natural progesterone are antitumor agents, and they worked for Victoria—to date, she is still cancer free.

Victoria still has her ups and downs—depending on whether she is taking her enzymes or not—but she has improved enough to become a student at a local college and begin living her life again.

Success Story: Mental Illness or Sugar Intolerance?

Tony, 16, came to see me after having been released from a psychiatric hospital following a second suicide attempt. He had been diagnosed with cerebral palsy and manic depression. He complained of anger, anxiety, nightmares, and hearing voices.

Tony was agitated, had involuntary body movements (characteristic of cerebral palsy, but also a side effect of antipsychotic drugs), and his whole face was swollen and puffy—side effects from the drugs he had been given to control his behavior. These included trazodone, an antidepressant that causes drowsiness, for his insomnia; lithium, for manic depression; Paxil, an antidepressant similar to Prozac; Navane®, a psychotropic prescribed to control his auditory hallucinations; and Cogentin®, intended to offset the many side effects of the other drugs. The medications did not seem to be helping him; in fact, their adverse reactions were adding to his suffering.

Tony's urinalysis was relatively normal, revealing only low calcium and poor kidney concentration which caused kidney pain. I suspected that the many he drugs he was taking were having a masking effect. Further testing revealed multiple enzyme deficiencies, respiratory problems, a toxic colon (high indican), and, most important, extreme sugar intolerance.

I recommended the following enzyme formulas:

■ Thera-zyme Bil: multiple digestive enzyme formula for fat intolerance

■ Thera-zyme Adr: for sugar intolerance, with symptoms including nightmares, anger, mood swings, and depression

■ Thera-zyme Rsp: for his respiratory problems

■ Thera-zyme Kdy: to relieve his kidney pain

■ Thera-zyme TRMA: to help relieve anxiety and detoxify the drugs in his system

Tony had a sluggish thyroid function, common in people diagnosed with mental or emotional problems, so I gave him a thyroid glandular extract. For his toxic colon, I added a colon cleanse powder (Thera-zyme Challenge Food Powder). In just a few days, Tony showed noticeable improvement: his edema (the puffy, swollen appearance of his face) disappeared and his insomnia and depression lessened. Under a psychiatrist's supervision, his mother began decreasing Tony's medications. He continued to improve, and is currently off all of his drugs. The involuntary movements ceased when he stopping taking the drugs.

When her doctor prescribed Prozac, her depression lifted and her bulimia improved, but neither completely disappeared. Terry hated taking the drug, but could not do without it. When she stopped taking Prozac for more than ten days, her depression would return.

Success Story: Lithium Blues

Jane, 22, had been taking lithium since the age of 15, when she had been diagnosed as having a bipolar disorder. Her initial doses were so high that they caused her to vomit daily for several years. Even though the dosage was gradually reduced over the years, Jane felt like a prisoner to the drug and wanted to be free of it. She eventually found a doctor who believed she had been misdiagnosed and offered to help her stop the lithium by cutting her dosage in half each week. At this point, she came to see me for additional support. Even though she desperately wanted to stop taking the drug, Jane was afraid that she would be unable to control her emotions without it.

Jane had multiple health problems, including frequent kidney and bladder infections, cystic acne, stomach discomfort, chronic constipation alternating with diarrhea, chronic intestinal pain, premenstrual syndrome (PMS), and migraines. A urinalysis, along with her health history, indicated that she was sugar intolerant.

I recommended Thera-zyme PAN for Jane's sugar intolerance, along with other enzyme-herbal remedies to help correct her nutritional deficiencies. These included Thera-zyme UrT and TRMA for her bladder and kidney infections, respectively; SmI, for her constipation and intestinal discomfort; and Lvr to help detoxify the effects of lithium. In addition, I supported her low thyroid function with a thyroid glandular extract and gave her 10% oral natural progesterone to help her PMS.

While following this therapy, Jane was able to cut down on lithium, under her doctor's supervision, and was completely off the drug within a month. She continues to improve both physically and emotionally.

Success Story: Trading Prozac for Enzymes

Terry, 26, had a history of depression, bulimia (an eating disorder which involves vomiting up food to keep from gaining weight), and frequent flu, colds, and sinus infections indicating a suppressed immune system. When her doctor prescribed Prozac, her depression lifted and her bulimia improved, but neither completely disappeared. Terry hated taking the drug, but could not do without it. When she stopped taking Prozac for more than ten days, her depression would return.

Her urinalysis and physical exam indicated poor sugar metabolism, a toxic colon (high indican), kidney congestion, and inflammation requiring protease. She also exhibited many signs of hypothyroidism, including low temperature (96.4° F) and low resting pulse (only 54 beats per minute), along with her depression and suppressed immune system. I sent Terry to a doctor who confirmed hypothyroidism and placed her on a natural thyroid glandular extract. In addition to the thyroid glandular, I added oral natural progesterone; one of its many health benefits is that it helps reduce anxiety.

I also recommended the following enzyme formulations to help alleviate her digestive problems:

- Thera-zyme PAN: for sugar and/or gluten intolerance
- Thera-zyme Kdy: to help the kidneys cleanse the blood and to aid lymphatic drainage
- Thera-zyme TRMA: to heal her immune system and alleviate anxiety
- Thera-zyme Challenge Food Powder: a colon detoxification program

Three weeks later, Terry's resting pulse had increased to 59 beats per minute and her oral temperature to 97.4° F. She reported no depression whatsoever and had not needed Prozac during those three weeks—a record for her. In addition, her bulimia almost entirely disappeared over the next month. Her diet, digestion, and thyroid function continued to improve. Today, three years later, she is free of depression and bulimia.

Prevention and Elimination of Mental Disorders

Anxiety, insomnia, panic disorder, depression, and other symptoms and conditions of the Prozac epidemic can safely be alleviated by enzymes and other natural remedies. In addition to the following enzyme and thyroid therapy, I recommend that people suffering from anxiety drink naturally carbonated mineral water. The carbon dioxide in carbonated water helps supply extra oxygen to the brain, restore acid-alkaline balance, and calm the person down by relaxing nerves and muscles.[76]

Enzyme Therapy

There are four enzyme formulas for sugar intolerance; some people need only one, some need several.

■ Thera-zyme HCL: multiple digestive formula for sugar, fat, and protein intolerance; I add PAN if gluten intolerance is also present

■ Thera-zyme PAN: multiple digestive formula for sugar and gluten intolerance

■ Thera-zyme Adr: high in sucrase plus B vitamins for symptoms which include dizziness when bending over, seizures, panic attacks, depression, insomnia, nightmares, stress, and low blood pressure

■ Thera-zyme SvG: containing disaccharidases, amylase, and food sources of vitamins A, E, and C and tryptophan, the amino acid precursor to the neurotransmitter (SEE QUICK DEFINITION) serotonin, a mood elevator; relieves other sugar intolerance symptoms including a frequent sore or irritated throat, speech impediments such as stuttering or stammering, loss of voice (laryngitis), poor memory, and the inability to relax, become serene, or meditate

Other enzymes may be indicated to ease anxiety and nervousness:

■ Thera-zyme TRMA: primary immune system formula which helps relieve anxiety; people who take Xanax are candidates for this formula

■ Thera-zyme CLM: calming for nervous, emotionally distraught people; helps relieve insomnia

Thyroid Support

If testing determines that your thyroid function is low, seek the advice of a health professional. If treatment is needed, I recommend a thyroid glandular extract. Certain herbs, such as the Ayurvedic herbs *Coleus forskohlii* and *Gugulipid*, also have a stimulating effect on thyroid function.

Hormonal Balancing

I recommend oral natural progesterone to women who are

hypothyroid. To both men and women, I sometimes give pregnenolone, a primary anti-aging steroid with healing effects. (See Appendix A.)

OSTEOPOROSIS

Osteoporosis literally means "porous bones." Bone is living tissue that renews itself every two to seven years through a process of bone resorption (bone loss, breaking down of old bone material to make way for new bone) and new bone formation. Bone loss without adequate rebuilding of bone produces osteoporosis which, if allowed to progress, makes the bones brittle and subject to fracture.

What Causes Osteoporosis?

Osteoporosis is caused by hormonal imbalance, hypothyroidism (underactive thyroid gland), enzyme and other nutritional deficiencies, and bone calcium loss and calcium malabsorption due to dietary

factors. Other factors that induce bone loss are exposure to heavy metals, especially aluminum (in baking powder, cookware, and antacids) and cadmium (in cigarette smoke), conditions such as hyperparathyroidism (too much parathyroid hormone), malabsorption and colon problems, the inability to convert vitamin D to its hor-

For information on the **enzymes** for this health condition, see Appendix B.

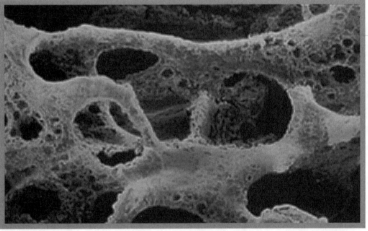

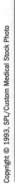
Copyright © 1993, SPL/Custom Medical Stock Photo

OSTEOPOROTIC BONE. Osteoporosis is generally regarded as a metabolic bone disorder. The rate of bone loss (resorption) speeds up while the rate of making new bone tissue slows down. Levels of calcium and phosphate salts decline so that the bones (osteo) become porous, brittle, and susceptible to fracture for lack of new bone tissue to replace the old tissue that has been removed.

monal form due to low magnesium or inadequate HCl, lactose intolerance, low phosphorus levels (which leads to the deposit of calcium in soft tissue), excess phosphorus (which leads to the loss of calcium from hard tissue), too much or too little exercise, and stress.

Hormonal Imbalance and Hypothyroidism

A proper hormonal balance is essential in preventing and reversing osteoporosis. Adequate progesterone is of particular importance because this hormone is necessary for building new bone. The thyroid gland fills several vital functions regarding bone health. Thyroid hormone promotes both bone resorption and new bone formation, and is needed for the manufacture of progesterone from cholesterol. Thus, hypothyroidism has a serious detrimental effect on the bones.

Environmental estrogens and estrogen replacement therapy contribute to estrogen dominance (excess estrogen in relation to progesterone) which, without the adequate balance of progesterone's bone-building function, promotes bone loss.

Dietary Factors in Calcium
Bone Loss and Malabsorption

Loss of calcium from bones leads to the thin, porous bones of osteoporosis. However, lack of dietary calcium is not the source of the increase in incidence of osteoporosis. In addition to the causal factors discussed above, the standard American fare of refined, processed foods, high-phosphorus soft drinks, and high protein, sugar, and salt consumption is the dietary culprit. Other dietary practices that increase the likelihood of calcium excretion and bone loss include excess intake of sugar, coffee, and alcohol.

The effect of a nutrient-depleted diet is twofold. Without proper nutrients, the body cannot absorb the calcium ingested in food or supplement form and is forced to draw it out of the bones to remedy the deficit. Further, inadequate nutrition fails to supply the body with the range of nutrients needed for bone rebuilding. Thus, poor diet both contributes to bone loss and prevents bone formation.

The high-phosphorus content of red meat (and high-phosphorus soft drinks such as colas) contributes to bone loss. Consuming large amounts of phosphorus can raise the levels in the blood, skewing the normal calcium to phosphorus ratio. This causes the parathyroid glands (endocrine glands close to the thyroid), which help regulate calcium and phosphorus metabolism, to pull calcium from the

For more on the effects of **estrogen replacement therapy**, see Menopausal Symptoms.

Environmental estrogens and estrogen replacement therapy contribute to estrogen dominance (excess estrogen in relation to progesterone) which, without the adequate balance of progesterone's bone-building function, promotes bone loss.

bones to supplement blood calcium levels.[77] Most of the body's calcium is (or should be) in the bones and teeth, with some in the tissues and blood. The small percentage in the blood is essential to the function of vitamin D and the parathyroid hormones (and to the blood-clotting mechanism and muscle and nerve function), therefore it is also vital to bone health as well as calcium metabolism.

Along with these factors, the proper metabolism of calcium depends on adequate digestion of protein, sufficient hydrochloric acid (HCl) for digestion, proper blood pH (SEE QUICK DEFINITION) levels, the proper ratios of both phosphorus and magnesium to calcium, and the presence of many nutrients. These nutrients include appropriate levels of vitamin D (which the body must be able to convert to its hormonal form), vitamins A, C, E, and K, and minerals such as boron, sodium, zinc, copper, silicon, and strontium. Adequate fatty acids and the proper hormonal balance are also required.

Ultraviolet light from the sun is important in calcium metabolism, too. It converts skin oil to vitamin D, which transports calcium from the stomach into the blood. Certain fatty acids, especially oleic acid (present in milk, butter, and extra virgin olive oil), are vital in the transport of calcium from the blood to tissue. If you have vitamin D, but not enough essential fatty acids to provide transport, your blood calcium level will increase at the expense of your tissue calcium level. If your skin itches or you get hives, welts, or cold and canker sores when exposed to the sun, you may have tissue calcium starvation due to an essential fatty acid deficiency.

Sometimes calcium is deposited in soft tissue rather than in the bones where it is needed. There are several causes for this. One important factor is the pH of the blood, which is normally in the narrow, slightly alkaline pH range of 7.35 to 7.45. To maintain this range, the blood must keep an adequate level of acidity in the form of hydrogen ions and chloride ions, plus just the right amount of alkalinity in the form of bicarbonate ions. To accomplish this, it is important to ensure optimum digestion of foods either by eating lots of raw foods and/or by taking a multiple digestive enzyme supplement with meals. For example, inadequate digestion of protein, lowers your pH (makes it more acidic) and your body will not be able to properly utilize calcium.

Common over-the-counter supplements also upset the pH balance, leading to digestive disturbances which in turn result in further calcium metabolism problems. For instance, calcium carbonate supplements, such as Tums, exert an alkaline influence on the blood and cause calcium to precipitate in the urine, the stool, and, in the worst case scenario, in the soft tissues. When the blood is too alkaline, adequate HCl is not available for digestion in the stomach.[78]

The natural way to raise acid to an optimum level is to digest protein with protease, which supplies the necessary hydrogen ions, and to increase chlorides with lipase. Chloride and other minerals are carried in the blood by lipase, so if you are low in lipase, you will not be able to maintain an adequate chloride level.

On the other hand, acidifying supplements such as betaine HCl, used by people who think it will help with digestion, cause excess acid reserves in the blood. This has far-reaching digestive consequences because pancreatic enzymes are activated in the duodenum (upper end of the small intestines, beginning at the connection to the stomach) only at an alkaline pH. Once again, be careful of random supplementation, as it can throw off your body chemistry, compounding the problems you thought you were treating.

Likewise, don't make the mistake of thinking you can get all of the nutrients required for bone health in pill form. If simply taking vitamin and calcium supplements prevented bone loss, osteoporosis would not be so widespread in the United States today. Many people are calcium deficient even though they take calcium supplements. These people cannot absorb or utilize the calcium supplements for any combination of the reasons discussed above.

Success Story:
Reversing Osteoporosis In a 25-Year-Old Runner

Pam, 25, was a dedicated runner; she ran at least ten miles daily, and participated in several marathon races yearly. Although she looked like she was at the peak of health, Pam had not menstruated for six months (a common occurrence in women who diet or exercise to the extreme). When she consulted her doctor, one of the tests he performed was for bone mineral density (BMD). It revealed that Pam had

Reversing Osteoporosis With Progesterone

According to John R. Lee, M.D., of Sebastopol, California, some women begin losing bone mass in their mid-thirties, at the rate of 1% to 1.5% each year. Many of them have lost 25% to 30% of their bone mass by the time they reach menopause. This loss increases for three to five years at menopause, then once again levels off to 1% to 1.5% yearly. It is not uncommon to see 50% bone loss in a 65-year-old woman. In women with such frail bones, even a slight misstep can lead to a fractured hip which, for many, begins a rapid decline; 20% of women who fracture their hips die within a year.

Dr. Lee has found, however, that taking natural progesterone results in progressive increase in bone mineral density and clinical improvement in patients, including fracture prevention. Progesterone supplementation can benefit women of all ages; Dr. Lee reports reversal of osteoporosis in women over 70.[79]

osteoporosis with more than 15% bone loss—an amount one would expect to find in a woman twice her age.

Pam came to me in hopes of reversing the bone loss. A urine analysis revealed sugar intolerance, low calcium, and low vitamin C. Pam's health history indicated a diet high in starches and low in protein. Her thyroid proved to be severely underactive, which meant she was likely to be low in progesterone, a critical female hormone in the prevention and cure of osteoporosis.

First of all, I cautioned Pam about her diet: no more quick sugar fixes or "carbohydrate loading" before her daily exercise. I then told her that if she was serious about stopping the bone loss, she would simply have to cut down on the exercise—otherwise the supplements I was giving her would be a waste of money.

Pam promised to make the changes and I started her on the following program:

■ Thera-zyme PAN: digestive formula for her sugar intolerance
■ Thera-zyme Para: enzymatic-calcium formula
■ Thera-zyme Opt: enzymatic-vitamin C formula
■ Thyroid glandular extract
■ Natural progesterone in vitamin E oil

In addition to this treatment, Pam stopped running ten miles daily and walked vigorously instead. She increased her protein and fruit intake, while eliminating all refined sugars and junk food. She began to feel better and within six seeks her menses returned. I advised her to wait a year before getting another BMD test. Twelve months later, the test showed that, not only had the osteoporosis halted, but Pam had gained back about 50% of her bone loss. In another year, the bone loss was entirely reversed.

Pam still enjoys daily exercise and has taken up skiing. She continues to protect her bone health with a whole-foods diet, natural thyroid glandular, and natural progesterone.

Prevention and Reversal of Osteoporosis

While proper diet is essential in the prevention of osteoporosis, enzyme therapy is often necessary for proper food digestion so that calcium can be efficiently metabolized. In addition, hormonal balancing—in particular, progesterone supplementation—can not only prevent, but also reverse osteoporosis.

Enzyme Therapy

Many women subject to osteoporosis benefit from taking extra protease and/or lipase enzymes. Protease, the enzyme that digests protein, is required to carry calcium in the blood. Without proper digestion of protein, both protein-bound and ionic calcium levels in the blood will not be adequate. Lipase is required to carry calcium across the intestinal wall and for the production of female hormones. Thus a deficiency in either of these enzymes could contribute to osteoporosis.

Which multiple digestive formula is needed is determined by urinalysis and palpation. The following are useful formulas, which contain lipase and protease, among other enzymes:

■ Thera-zyme Bil: for fat and protein intolerance and gallbladder problems

■ Thera-zyme HCL: for fat and sugar intolerance and to aid in the digestion of protein (Note: this formula does not contain hydrochloric acid but, by providing lipase, helps the body produce it)

■ Thera-zyme PAN: emphasizes sugar intolerance and also contains protease and lipase, but in lower amounts than Bil or HCL

■ Thera-zyme VSCLR: high-lipase formula especially for people who have weight problems, diabetes, high blood fats, or hypertension

■ Thera-zyme Para: a pH-balanced enzyme and calcium formula for calcium deficiency

See *Alternative Medicine Guide to Women's Health 2* (Future Medicine Publishing, 1998; ISBN 1-887299-30-0); to order, call 800-333-HEAL.

Hormonal Balancing

In men and women alike, optimum thyroid health is necessary in order to stimulate bone resorption and formation and to manufacture adequate progesterone from cholesterol to maintain the correct level of this hormone. As was the case with Pam, supplementation with natural progesterone and a thyroid glandular extract can actually reverse the bone loss of osteoporosis and prevent further loss by promoting bone formation.

Dietary Recommendations

Whole, unprocessed, organic foods contain all the minerals, vitamins, and other nutrients you need to build bones. For full benefit, remember the following guidelines:

■ Eat a variety of whole foods including green, leafy vegetables, root vegetables, whole grains, whole fruits, raw milk and cheese, fish, and organic poultry and beef.

■ Eat adequate protein, salt, and fruit to stimulate thyroid function.

■ Eliminate processed foods from your diet, especially white sugar, white flour, white rice, and margarine. Avoid excessive intake of coffee, alcohol, and carbonated soft drinks.

PARASITES

A parasite is any organism that lives in or on a host organism, in this case, the human body. Of the dozens of specific parasites that affect our health, the major groupings include microscopic Protozoa, roundworms, pinworms, hookworms (Nematoda), tapeworms (Cestoda), and flukes (Trematoda).

Parasites tend to reside in the intestines, but they can also migrate to the blood, lymph, heart, liver, gallbladder, pancreas, spleen, eyes, and brain. The numerous symptoms and health conditions they produce include: constipation, diarrhea, gas, bloating, irritable bowel syndrome, joint and muscle aches, allergies, anemia, skin problems, sleep disturbances, chronic fatigue, and gradual immune dysfunction.

What Causes Parasitic Infections?

Parasites are most often transmitted through contaminated drinking water, uncooked or undercooked meat or fish, unwashed vegetables, close contact with household pets, and contact with fecal matter.

Success Story: The Seven-Inch Worm

Cindy, 27, came to me with mild stomach problems. Upon testing, I found that she needed Thera-zyme Stm, a multiple digestive enzyme formula that nourishes the tissues of the stomach. A palpation test also revealed a need for Thera-zyme SmI, although Cindy said she had none of the usual symptoms, such as a yeast infection or diarrhea, associated with the need for it.

I suspected either a yeast problem or a parasite, and gave Cindy the Thera-zyme Stm and SmI to take home. Three days later, she reported that I had been correct about the parasite, that she had passed a seven-inch worm. After that, her stomach problems were resolved.

Success Story: A Seven-Year Itch

Ted, 44, had suffered from bowel irritation, severe anal itching, and rectal bleeding for seven years. In addition, he had developed skin rashes on his wrists, ankles, and thighs. These symptoms were continually present, but were exacerbated by certain foods. Ted also reported getting so tired after eating that he fell asleep (another sign of food aller-

For information on the **enzymes** for this health condition, see Appendix B.

How to Avoid Parasites

There are several precautions which will help you avoid parasites:

Food

- Do not eat raw beef; it can be loaded with tapeworms and other parasites (not to mention *E. coli* bacteria).
- Do not eat raw fish, including in sushi; you are almost certain to get worms if you eat raw fish.
- Wash hands after handling raw meat or fish (including shrimp); don't put your hands near your mouth without washing them first.
- Use separate cutting boards for meat and vegetables; spores from meat can seep into the board and contaminate vegetables or anything else you put on the board.
- Wash utensils thoroughly after cutting meat.
- Wash vegetables and fruit thoroughly, particularly salad items, as they often harbor parasites. Wash in water to which you have added grapefruit seed extract (a few drops) or household bleach (1 tsp of the bleach per gallon of water). Soak for 15-20 minutes, then soak in fresh water for 20 minutes before refrigerating.

Pets

- Do not sleep near your pets; they harbor worms and other parasites.
- De-worm your pets regularly and keep their sleeping areas clean.
- Do not let pets lick your face.
- Do not let pets eat off your dishes.
- Do not walk barefoot around animals.

General

- Do not drink from streams and rivers.
- When traveling, don't drink the water.
- Always wash your hands after using the toilet.
- Wash your hands after working in the garden; the soil can be contaminated with spores and parasites.

gies). To care for his allergies, I placed Ted on Thera-zyme Kdy and Thera-zyme Bil, a multiple digestive enzyme for fat and protein intolerance. The severe anal itching and his health history made me suspect that, in addition to allergies, Ted also had large parasites (worms), so I gave him Thera-zyme TRMA, a formula for eliminating worms which would also boost his immune system.

Ted followed this program for two weeks, then one day suddenly had loose stools, which was unusual for him. He observed long, wormlike strands in his stool. All of his symptoms subsided and he felt dramatically better for the first time in seven years.

Success Story:
Flushing Out Parasites With Enzymes

The parents of Tonya, 10, brought her to me with a number of complaints. Testing revealed severe digestive and nutritional problems, including serious allergies, a toxic colon (high indican), and a calcium deficiency. I recommended Thera-zyme Bil for her fat intolerance, Thera-zyme Kdy for her allergies, and Thera-zyme Challenge Food Powder for her toxic colon and suspected parasites.

After several weeks of enzyme treatment, my suspicions of an infestation of worms were confirmed. Tonya's parents called with the news that their daughter had excreted worms. Over the next month, with good dietary changes and continued enzyme therapy, Tonya's digestive problems and allergies became minimal and only returned when she neglected to take her enzymes or ate junk food.

Prevention and Elimination of Parasites

Both enzyme therapy and nutritional supplements can be helpful in preventing and getting rid of parasitic infection.

Enzyme Therapy

In addition to a multiple digestive enzyme formula, appropriate to individual digestive needs, there are three formulas to treat parasitic infection. The patient's symptoms and the results of palpation determine which should be used.

■ Thera-zyme SmI: a probiotic or friendly bacteria formula high in cellulase. When my testing indicates the need for SmI, the patient may have candidiasis, parasites, a toxic colon, or a combination.

■ Thera-zyme TRMA: high in protease, this formula is recommended for larger worms

■ Thera-zyme Challenge Food Powder: for people who have symptoms of parasites such as itchiness around the rectum and groin and restless sleep with grinding of teeth

Nutritional Supplements

■ Grapefruit seed and pulp extract (Citricidal): nontoxic antimicrobial with the advantage that very few people are allergic to it; can be effective against *Candida albicans*, *Giardia lambia*, and other parasites, fungi, and bacteria

■ Soil-based organisms (SEE QUICK DEFINITION): an intestinal formula of beneficial bacteria from soil which help prevent proliferation of intestinal toxins

QUICK DEFINITION

Soil-based organisms (SBOs) are beneficial microbes, or probiotics, found in soil. Before chemical farming, the earth was rich in these organisms which naturally destroyed molds, yeast, fungi, and viruses in the soil. Transmitted in the food supply to humans, SBOs perform the same function in the human body, working with the "friendly" bacteria (such as *Lactobacillus acidophilus* and *Bifidobacterium bifidum*) inhabiting the gastrointestinal tract to maintain balance in the intestinal flora and thus ensure a healthy digestive system. Since soil has become depleted of SBOs, the ratio of good to bad bacteria in the intestines has become skewed and a host of health problems, including allergies, candidiasis, hormonal dysfunction, and Crohn's disease among other gastrointestinal conditions, are the result.

PREMENSTRUAL SYNDROME (PMS)

Premenstrual syndrome (PMS) is a condition that affects at least 60% of women. For the majority, symptoms begin a few days before the onset of their menstrual period, but some women suffer for two weeks out of every month. PMS symptoms range from mild to severe, but generally include cramping, abdominal discomfort, kidney (low-back) pain, sore breasts, irritability, mood swings, depression, frustration, crying spells, migraines, nausea, and sometimes vomiting. More severe symptoms associated with PMS include cyclic seizures (seizures that occur during menses and ovulation as a result of estrogen surges).

What Causes Premenstrual Syndrome?

A primary cause of PMS is hormonal imbalance, but poor diet, enzyme deficiencies, and kidney-lymphatic stress are also factors.

■ Hormonal Imbalance: As discussed in numerous other health conditions in this book, low thyroid function (hypothyroidism) leads to estrogen dominance (an excess of estrogen relative to progesterone) because the thyroid is involved in producing progesterone from cholesterol.

■ Enzyme Deficiencies: Adequate protease and lipase, both of which are required for normal calcium metabolism, are important in preventing PMS symptoms. In addition, protease digests the protein needed to convert the thyroid hormone to its active form, and lipase is necessary for the synthesis of progesterone and for digestion of foods containing fat-soluble vitamins, such as A, D, and E, which are crucial in the entire process of hormonal production.

For information on the **enzymes** for this health condition, see Appendix B.

See *Alternative Medicine Guide to Women's Health 1* (Future Medicine Publishing, 1998; ISBN 1-887299-12-2); to order, call 800-333-HEAL.

■ Kidney-Lymphatic Stress: Before and during their periods, women with kidney-lymphatic stress, what I call "kidney or back PMS," may have low-back pain, nausea, vomiting, and frontal headaches.

Success Story: Low Thyroid Plus Too Much Exercise Caused PMS

Liz, 45, a dedicated marathon runner, presented with serious PMS problems along with heavy menstrual bleeding. Her PMS symptoms included severe cramps, sore breasts, fatigue, and mood swings. The moodiness was so severe that her husband jokingly offered to stay in a motel during her monthly episodes.

I suspected that Liz's problems were exacerbated by her level of endurance exercise, which can create a transient hypothyroidism and lower progesterone. In fact, Liz noticed a decline in her general health after participating in the New York Marathon. She felt more fatigued than ever, and her PMS symptoms got worse. A visit to her gynecologist did nothing to reassure her. The doctor suggested pain pills, birth control pills, or, if nothing else worked, a hysterectomy. Liz declined.

At that point, she consulted me. Her urinalysis indicated severe malabsorption, sugar intolerance, allergies, and a vitamin C deficiency.

I recommended the following program:

- Thera-zyme PAN: for sugar intolerance
- Thera-zyme Opt: for her vitamin C deficiency
- Thera-zyme Kdy: for allergies
- Thera-zyme Fem: a PMS formula
- Natural thyroid glandular extract
- 10% natural progesterone in vitamin E oil

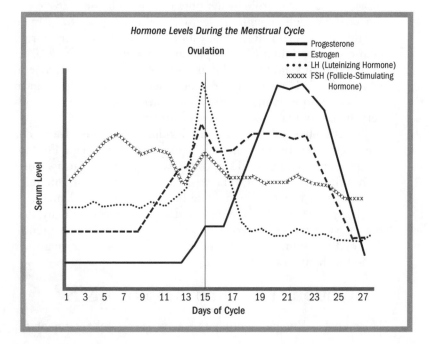

Hormone Levels During the Menstrual Cycle

Ovulation

Progesterone
Estrogen
LH (Luteinizing Hormone)
FSH (Follicle-Stimulating Hormone)

Serum Level

Days of Cycle

PMS symptoms can be relieved by hormonal balancing with thyroid therapy and adequate natural progesterone. Sometimes a 3% progesterone cream can relieve pain and irritability, but more often a stronger 10% oral progesterone is needed.

Within one week, Liz's energy came back. She no longer felt the need for an afternoon nap, but had an even flow of energy throughout the day, rarely experiencing lows. Her PMS gradually improved. By the second month of treatment, her mood swings, sore breasts, and heavy bleeding ceased, and "my husband stopped joking about going to a motel," Liz reported. It took a bit longer to get rid of the cramps, so she increased her dosage of the PMS formula and relieved the pain by rubbing progesterone cream wherever it hurt. "Even my digestive problems have improved," she announced.

Success Story: Relieving Cramps With Enzymes

Tracy, 15, had PMS, along with severe menstrual cramps, headaches, and general malaise during her menses. She had been placed on natural thyroid by her physician, but I found that she was not taking a high enough dosage. I encouraged Tracy to increase her thyroid supplement gradually until her oral temperature during menses was optimum (98° F upon arising and 98.6° F to 99.0° F during the day) and to take a daily dose of natural progesterone in vitamin E oil. I recommended that Tracy increase the protein in her diet because, as mentioned above, protein is required to convert the thyroid hormone to its active form.

Tracy's physical exam indicated kidney-lymphatic stress. For this, I gave her Thera-zyme Kdy along with Thera-zyme Fem for her menstrual cramps. (Taking these two enzyme formulas, along with progesterone, can relieve cramps in about 20 minutes.) Finally, Tracy needed Thera-zyme Para, a calcium supplement.

Tracy took the progesterone and thyroid hormone daily, and the enzymes only during menstruation. After only one month, Tracy's PMS symptoms were relieved and she sailed through her period without a twinge of pain.

Prevention and Elimination of PMS

Hormonal balancing is often the most successful treatment for

PMS symptoms, but a proper diet and enzyme therapy can also be instrumental.

Hormonal Balancing

PMS symptoms can be relieved by hormonal balancing with thyroid therapy and adequate natural progesterone. Sometimes a 3% progesterone cream can relieve pain and irritability, but more often a stronger 10% oral progesterone is needed. The dosage is dependent on the severity of the symptoms.

Enzyme Therapy

The following enzyme formulas can be helpful for PMS and menstrual problems:

■ A multiple digestive enzyme formula to address individual digestive needs

■ Thera-zyme Fem: helps relieve the symptoms of estrogen dominance, including irritability, mood swings, depression, edema, and/or pelvic pain

■ Thera-zyme Para: calcium formula taken from mid-cycle to menses, since calcium levels start falling at ovulation and bottom out at the end of each menses

■ Thera-zyme Kdy: lymphatic drainage remedy which helps the kidneys cleanse the blood; for premenstrual and menstrual nausea and vomiting

Dietary Recommendations

I always encourage PMS sufferers to increase their protein intake to optimize thyroid function, as stated earlier. This is especially important for vegetarians, since they tend to eat a limited amount of protein while consuming excess unsaturated fats, which further suppress thyroid function.[80]

To help relieve PMS symptoms and menstrual cramps, women should be sure they eat a whole foods diet, especially foods containing calcium and magnesium. Organic fruit juices are good sources of both.

PROSTATE ENLARGEMENT

The chestnut-sized prostate gland is the part of the male genitourinary tract in which problems are most likely to occur. One of the most common disorders is benign prostatic hypertrophy (BPH) or enlargement of the prostate.

After age 55, up to 60% of men suffer from the effects of BPH. Each year, over 300,000 of these men have surgery at an annual cost of more than $1 billion. Prostate enlargement can lead to bladder and kidney infections, and eventual bladder obstruction resulting in retention of urine in the blood, kidney damage, and sexual disability.

Early symptoms of BPH include progressive urgency to urinate, frequent nocturnal urination, difficulty urinating (with reduced force or dribbling), pain in the lower back or around the groin, a feeling of incomplete bowel evacuation, and painful intercourse.

What Causes Prostate Enlargement?

Like all chronic degenerative diseases, disorders of the prostate originate in part from a diet of processed foods devoid of the nutrients required for health. The trace mineral zinc is particularly vital, as it is found in higher concentrations in the prostate than in any other organ in the body. According to Michael B. Schachter, M.D., author of *The Natural Way to a Healthy Prostate*, zinc is the single most important prostate nutrient.[81] Other factors that contribute to prostate problems are excess alcohol intake and exposure to or ingestion of environmental estrogens.

For information on the **enzymes** for this health condition, see Appendix B.

Do not assume that you have BPH—the symptoms of BPH and prostate cancer are similar. If you have any of the symptoms associated with BPH, consult your physician.

A study by Camille Mallouh, M.D., Chief of Urology at New York's Metropolitan Hospital, found that men with BPH had 80% higher serum cholesterol levels than those without prostate problems.[82] Although this may be attributed to a high-fat diet, an underactive thyroid could also be a factor. Since hypothyroidism is associated with high cholesterol, I suspect that men with BPH, as well as prostate cancer, may have a higher incidence of hypothyroidism than men with healthy prostates.

Many researchers believe that the growth of prostate tissue resulting in BPH is associated with the conversion of testosterone to its more active form, dihydrotestosterone (DHT). They argue that the accumulation of DHT is responsible for excessive cellular growth and tumor formation in the prostate. However, according to Raymond Peat, Ph.D., it is excess estrogen rather than DHT that causes prostate enlargement. Dr. Peat suggests that, just as female health problems arise as the ratio of progesterone to estrogen decreases, male health problems arise as the ratio of androgens (the "male" hormones such as testosterone) to estrogen decreases. Studies show that not only estrogen but also hormones stimulated by estrogen encourage cell division and, thus, can contribute to BPH.[83]

Success Story: An Enzyme Cure for BPH

Tom, 28, might seem like an unusual choice for an example of benign prostatic hypertrophy, which usually occurs in men over 50. However, while I've successfully treated older men for the condition, I find Tom's case especially interesting *because* of his age. It's a reminder that many conditions are not limited to specific age groups.

Even though he seemed too young for it, Tom's symptoms all pointed toward BPH. He had pain in his groin that shot down through his legs. He felt unable to completely empty his bowels. He was up every two hours throughout the night because of the need to urinate. Intercourse had become painful.

His urine analysis showed kidney-lymphatic stress, low calcium, a toxic colon (high indican), and the presence of leukocytes (white blood cells). The sediment test which pinpoints digestive problems revealed both fat and sugar intolerance.

A palpation exam indicated urinary tract and prostate problems and confirmed the kidney-lymphatic stress. Tom's temperature (less than 97.5° F) and resting pulse (under 75 beats per minute) were both low, suggesting an underactive thyroid.

I started Tom on the following formulas, many of them containing the herbs saw palmetto, pygeum, and hydrangea, which are known for their role in reducing prostatic swelling:

■ Thera-zyme HCL: multiple digestive formula for fat and sugar intolerance

■ Thera-zyme UrT: urinary tract formula which relieves frequent or painful urination, urgency to urinate with passing small amounts, and cystitis (inflammation of

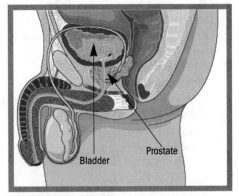

THE PROSTATE GLAND.

Bladder

Prostate

Disorders of the prostate originate in part from a diet of processed foods devoid of nutrients. The trace mineral zinc is particularly vital, as it is found in higher concentrations in the prostate than in any other organ in the body.

the urethra)

- Thera-zyme Kdy: kidney-lymphatic stress formula; also relieves edema
- Thera-zyme Mal: anti-inflammatory prostate formula containing enzymes and herbs which relieve prostatic swelling

I also recommended thyroid glandular extract to help stimulate Tom's low thyroid function.

After one month of treatment, all of Tom's symptoms were alleviated. The frequent trips to the bathroom at night, groin pain, pain upon intercourse, and the feeling of incomplete bowel evacuation had all disappeared. Tom continues to take his digestive formula and thyroid glandular extract, and every six months he has another urine test, just to ensure he stays out of prostate trouble.

Prevention and Elimination of BPH

There is no single program that fits everyone, but I have observed that most men who have enlarged prostates need natural products such as saw palmetto to reduce the swelling and prevent recurrence of the problem.

Thyroid Support

If a sluggish thyroid gland is indicated, I suggest thyroid glandular therapy to improve thyroid function, strengthen the immune system, and help relieve the edema associated with prostate enlargement. (See Appendix A.)

Hormonal Balancing

I recommend that BPH sufferers take pregnenolone powder. This hormone is a precursor to progesterone, so supplementing with pregnenolone is a safe way to raise progesterone levels which will act to reduce the swelling and inflammation of BPH. (See Appendix A.)

Enzyme Therapy

Several enzyme formulas to treat an enlarged prostate are listed below;

the appropriate ones will differ for each person:
- Multiple digestive enzyme formula specific to individual needs
- Thera-zyme Mal: anti-inflammatory, to relieve prostatic swelling
- Thera-zyme UrT: urinary tract formula to relieve frequent or painful urination, urgency to urinate with passing small amounts, and cystitis
- Thera-zyme Kdy: helps drain the lymphatic system and reduce swelling, and aids the kidneys in cleansing the blood
- Thera-zyme TRMA: antioxidant to block free-radical activity, which is involved in all inflammatory conditions and pathologies

Nutritional Supplements

As mentioned earlier, zinc is essential to prevent and reverse prostate disorders. The following are good sources of zinc:
- Pumpkin seeds: they also contain traces of progesterone-like phytosterols required by a healthy prostate
- Bee pollen: used by Europeans since the early 1960s to treat both BPH and prostate infections, bee pollen contains zinc and magnesium, both of particular importance to prostate health

Herbal Remedies

Research has shown that the following herbs can be effective in the treatment of an enlarged prostate:
- Saw palmetto (*Serenoa repens*): From the berry of a palm tree, saw palmetto extract has been shown to reduce prostate enlargement as well as conventional medications such as Proscar, without the side effects.[84] Saw palmetto is among the herbs in the Thera-zyme Mal formula.
- *Pygeum africanum*: Derived from an African evergreen tree, *Pygeum* contains substances called phytosterols which help reduce inflammation. BPH patients show elevated levels of prostaglandins, hormone-like fatty acids involved in inflammatory processes, which drop significantly with the use of *Pygeum*.[85]
- Horsetail (*Equisetum arvense*): An astringent for the genitourinary system, horsetail is used for both inflammation and enlargement of the prostate. Some herbalists combine horsetail with hydrangea to treat prostate problems. The Thera-zyme UrT formula contains both of these herbs.
- Hydrangea (*Hydrangea arborescens*): A diuretic (increases urine flow), this herb is used to treat an inflamed or enlarged prostate, urinary infections, and kidney stones.

SEIZURES

Seizures or convulsions can be defined as a variety of nonvoluntary contractions (single or in series) of the voluntary muscles, due to sudden uncontrolled changes in the electrical activity of the brain. Symptoms occur in varying degrees, from mild—with only slight muscle twitches and tingling—to violent, jerking whole-body movements. More severe seizures are sometimes associated with intense feelings of fear, hallucinations, and/or a lapse of consciousness. Seizures with loss of consciousness are called grand mal seizures.

What Causes Seizures?

The most common causes of seizures that I have observed in my clinical practice are estrogen dominance, excess intake of unsaturated fatty acids, and the use of aspartame (NutraSweet™), monosodium glutamate (MSG), and other "excitatory" amino acids. Other causes include fluoride toxicity, blood sugar problems, nutritional deficiencies, structural problems, and, in infants, a sharp rise in body temperature.

Estrogen Dominance

An excess of estrogen in relation to progresterone, a condition known as estrogen dominance, can cause seizures.[86] Ideally, women should have five to ten times more progesterone than estrogen.[87] The lower the ratio of progesterone to estrogen, the higher the risk of seizures, especially during menses when there is a surge of estrogen.

The primary sources of excess estrogen are an underactive thyroid (hypothyroidism), birth control pills, estrogen replacement therapy (ERT), excessive intake of phytoestrogens (plant-derived estrogens), and exposure to or ingestion of pesticides (environmental estrogens.)

For information on the **enzymes** for this health condition, see Appendix B.

All forms of estrogen are toxic to the body if not adequately balanced by progesterone.[88] Women with estrogen dominance are more prone to estrogen toxicity conditions such as cyclic seizures, migraines, hypoglycemia (low blood sugar), and fluid retention. Women in this category are much more likely to be vulnerable to aspartame-related migraines and seizures as well. (See Appendix A.)

Seizures can be due to brain tumors or other brain dysfunction. These should be medically ruled out before pursuing alternative treatment.

Excess Intake of Unsaturated Fatty Acids

Just as estrogen's toxic effects have to do with the ratio of progesterone to estrogen, the toxicity of unsaturated fatty acids depends on their ratio to saturated fats (coconut oil and raw butter). Unsaturated fats are all oils liquid at room temperature with the exception of extra virgin olive oil; these include soybean, safflower, sesame, corn, evening primrose, canola, flaxseed, and fish oils.[89] Excess consumption of these oils can be a contributing factor in seizures.[90]

EDITOR'S NOTE
The position on unsaturated fats presented here is a controversial one. Many physicians advocate the dietary use and supplementation of essential fatty acids in the form of fish, primrose, borage, and flaxseed oils, among others, in the unsaturated category. There is research to support both positions.

Aspartame and Excitatory Amino Acids

Substances containing aspartate, such as aspartame (NutraSweet), or glutamates, such as monosodium glutamate (MSG)—as well as minerals chelated with aspartate or glutamate—can freely enter the brain and reportedly cause toxic effects, including seizures in susceptible people. The amount of these substances ingested does not determine whether they will induce a seizure or not; a small amount can trigger a seizure in some people, while others can consume excessive amounts and be unaffected.

Aspartic acid (aspartate) and glutamic acid (L-glutamine or glutamate) are among the "excitatory" amino acids, which must be naturally balanced with the inhibitory, or calming, amino acids such as alanine, glycine, taurine, and GABA. Excitatory amino acids are naturally released during the digestion of whole-food proteins, but the release happens slowly and consequently the brain is not flooded with them. However, when they are consumed in isolated or concentrated forms, as in Nutrasweet or MSG, the brain receives a mega-dose of them all at once and problems may ensue.[91]

Aspartic and glutamic acids have similar chemical structures and show comparable toxicity in animal studies. Research has shown that excess glutamate and aspartate can flood the excitatory receptors on the external surface of nerve cells and excite them to death.[92]

Factors that may lower the threshold to seizures among those who consume aspartate and glutamate include:[93]

■ Exaggerated low blood sugar caused by consumption of diet drinks

■ Depletion of the neurotransmitter norepinephrine in aspartame-induced insomnia, which has been found in animal studies to provoke seizures

■ Excess caffeine and sodium found in some diet drinks

■ Excess fluid intake resulting from the intense thirst induced by aspartame

■ Excess phenylalanine (an essential amino acid) which handicaps

Seizures occur in 15% of people sensitive to aspartame, most of whom suffered their first convulsions after consuming a diet product. A single dose of aspartame can trigger a seizure in susceptible patients. Children who have unexplained seizures should be questioned regarding their ingestion of aspartame and glutamates.

the nutritional flow of other amino acids to the brain and can lead to a lowered seizure threshold in certain individuals

Seizures occur in 15% of people sensitive to aspartame, most of whom suffered their first convulsions after consuming a diet product. No other underlying cause could be found in most of these patients, despite extensive tests such as CT (computerized tomography, formerly CAT) scan, MRI (magnetic resonance imaging), EEG (electroencephalogram), and even an angiogram of the cerebral blood vessels. Aspartame-caused seizures disappear or dramatically decrease when aspartame is avoided, even without antiepileptic drugs.[94]

A single dose of aspartame can trigger a seizure in susceptible patients. Consider the following gruesome examples: a nursing infant convulsed when his mother drank a diet soda. A woman with epilepsy convulsed within minutes of chewing a piece of sugar-free gum sweetened with aspartame. A 16-year-old female with previously unexplained seizures experienced a seizure in a clinical experiment after eating one serving of chocolate pudding sweetened with aspartame. A 31-year-old nurse had a grand mal seizure within hours of drinking two liters of an aspartame-sweetened drink.[95]

Children who have unexplained seizures should be questioned regarding their ingestion of aspartame and glutamates. If such substances can be eliminated from their diets, the need for antiepileptic drugs may also be eliminated or at least reduced.

If you are a health-conscious person, you probably already shun products containing aspartame. However, you may not be aware that some vitamin and mineral supplements, even those found in health food stores, contain aspartate or glutamate as chelating agents. If calcium glutamate or calcium aspartate appear on the list of ingredients, it is best to avoid that product.

Fluoride Toxicity

Fluoride poisons at least 100 enzymes.[96] It accomplishes this by binding to sites on the enzyme which prevents the coenzyme (a vitamin or mineral) from activating the enzyme. In addition to its seizure-inducing effects, fluoride can cause cancer, osteoporosis, and other aging diseases. As with aspartame, the toxic effects of fluoride are not dose-related and, in fact, have been observed at levels below those commonly found in most fluoridated city water supplies.[97]

Fluoride decreases calcium in the blood by combining with it to form an insoluble compound called calcium fluoride. At the same time, the parathyroid glands (endocrine glands close to the thyroid) are extremely sensitive to fluoride. Continuous doses cause the parathyroid glands to become overactive, one of the effects of which is calcium depletion which can result in seizures.[98]

Blood Sugar Problems

Glucose deficiency may be a universal cause of seizures. I have had many clients with seizure disorders resulting from both sugar intolerance and hypothyroidism leading to low blood sugar and brain starvation of glucose. Seizures related to blood sugar problems occur more frequently at night, often during sleep, when adrenaline rises and causes a surge of cortisol—the body's effort to raise blood sugar.

Nutritional Deficiencies

Deficiencies in certain nutrients are implicated in seizures. These include the B vitamins, especially folic acid and vitamin B6, and the minerals magnesium, calcium, manganese, and zinc.

Sudden Increase in Body Temperature in Young Children

Most parents are told to give their babies aspirin or Tylenol to lower fevers, because high fevers cause seizures. The late Robert Mendelsohn, M.D., author of *How to Raise a Healthy Child...In Spite of Your Doctor*, disagreed. He argued that it is the sudden, rapid rise in body temperature that can cause a seizure, not the fever itself. However, he noted, "By the time you become aware of the child's temperature, the probability is that this rapid rise has already occurred, and unless the child has already convulsed, the danger period has passed."[99]

Fortunately, convulsive fevers are rare, and seldom serious. Yet, to prevent future seizures, many doctors prescribe long-term therapy with phenobarbital or other antiepileptic drugs—in spite of their terrible side effects.

Do You Have a Neck Problem? A Simple Test Can Tell You

Howard Loomis, D.C., of Madison, Wisconsin, developed the following test to determine if you have an upper cervical (neck) problem:

Lie on your back on a table with your arms crossed on your chest. Raise both legs simultaneously, keeping your knees straight. Then lower your legs. If you can't do this, whether you are nine or ninety, you have a problem.

Next, have a partner stand behind you, place his or her hands on top of your head (not face), and push your head horizontally towards your feet, keeping your head on the table. This compresses the spinal column.

After this procedure, raise your legs again. If it is more difficult to raise them, you have an upper cervical problem. If this is the case, a chiropractic adjustment can help. When it has been successful, you should be able to raise your legs without difficulty both times in the above test. The enzyme formula Thera-zyme Sym can aid your body in maintaining the adjustment.

Structural Problems

Misalignments in the first three cervical (neck) vertebrae can cause seizures. Nearly all head injuries cause upper cervical problems. Thera-zyme Sym is the enzyme formula for this, but chiropractic treatment is also indicated.

Success Story: Solving the Holiday Seizures

Melissa, 6, was brought to me by her distraught mother. The girl was bright and seemed healthy, but the family doctor had recently diagnosed her as having epilepsy and announced there was no cure—her child could look forward to a lifetime of using antiepileptic drugs. Melissa's mother refused to give her the drugs.

In the process of getting Melissa's complete history, I learned that the seizures occurred during "special" times of the year: Christmas, Easter, her birthday, and other festive periods when children are more likely to indulge in sweets. Melissa's mother recalled one seizure that followed a breakfast of pancakes with syrup. I suspected sugar intolerance and advised her mother to eliminate all refined sugar (white sugar, fructose, and corn syrup) and synthetic sweeteners from Melissa's diet and have her eat only whole, unprocessed food. In addition, I gave her Thera-zyme PAN, a digestive enzyme formula for sugar-intolerant people. Her mother followed my suggestions, paying close attention to holiday treats. Melissa's seizures then disappeared, never to return.

Success Story: Zapping Junk-Food Seizures

Zach, 10, was taking antiepileptic medication when his mother brought him to me. He was subject to seizures brought on by eating sugar or by playing video games with rapidly blinking lights. Zach's diet was typical junk-food fare: high in refined white sugar and artificial sweeteners, including products containing aspartame.

In addition to the obvious need to change his diet, my tests revealed the need for the digestive enzyme formulas Thera-zyme PAN and Thera-zyme Adr for his sugar intolerance. Taking digestive enzymes and eating properly eliminated Zach's seizures. Relapses occurred only when he reverted to his junk-food mode and did not take his enzymes.

Success Story:
Ending Six Years of Grand Mal Seizures

James, 47, had suffered from grand mal seizures for six years. They usually happened when he was sleeping and were followed by intense headaches, nausea, disorientation, and incontinence. James reported feeling dizzy and disoriented even without recent seizures, and he felt his behavior was erratic.

Urinalysis and palpation indicated that he was hypothyroid plus severely sugar intolerant (unable to digest disaccharides such as sucrose, lactose, and maltose into simple sugars such as glucose, fructose, and others). Both conditions lead to low blood sugar and therefore low brain glucose which worsens during a long period of no food, as in sleep. With the brain starved of its main energy supply, the result can be seizures.

To help James, I first suggested that he eliminate from his diet all refined sugars and synthetic sweeteners, most notably NutraSweet. Next I gave him a natural thyroid glandular extract for his hypothyroid condition, Thera-zyme PAN for sugar and wheat intolerance, and Thera-zyme Adr to help his body digest sucrose and transport the resulting glucose into the brain.

Once he was on the enzyme program, James' seizures stopped completely, only returning temporarily if he ate excessive amounts of fruit or bread. This positive outcome is a confirmation of the alternative medicine view that, when given the proper nutrition and the correct enzymes to ensure digestion, absorption, and assimilation, the body can heal itself, even of a severe disorder such as grand mal seizures.

The treatment to be implemented for seizures depends on the underlying cause. Proper diet and enzyme therapy are necessary to prevent and eliminate seizures due to sugar intolerance, while progesterone supplementation is recommended for those due to estrogen dominance.

Success Story: Cutting Out Fluoride Stops Seizures

Freddy, 8, began having chronic seizures when his family moved to a new state. His urine test and physical exam revealed mild digestive problems, but I didn't think them serious enough to induce seizures. Further testing ruled out structural problems. The fact that Freddy had recently moved from one state to another made me suspect an environmental factor. I asked about the family's source of drinking water and was not surprised to find that they were now drinking fluoridated tap water. In addition, Freddy used fluoridated toothpaste and received regular dental fluoride treatments.

I recommended minor dietary changes, gave the boy Thera-zyme DGST, a multiple digestive formula for mild digestive problems. I advised his mother to eliminate all of Freddy's fluoride intake. His mother was more than happy to comply. She bought a reverse osmosis water filter (a two-step system which filters not only heavy metals and minerals, but also microbes), got rid of the fluoride toothpaste, and requested that their dentist stop fluoride treatments. Once this program was under way, Freddy's seizures stopped and never came back.

Another boy, Tod, 12, lived in a town where the water supply was fluoridated. He developed seizures of increasing severity but remained conscious during the episodes, a feature not usually observed in severe epilepsy. A neurosurgeon performed a number of tests as well as exploratory neurosurgery, but found no reasons for the seizures. When fluoridated water was eliminated from his diet, Tod had no further attacks.

These stories are not uncommon. Many people who develop fluoride-toxicity symptoms while living in cities with fluoridated water become symptom free when they move to cities without fluoridated water.

Success Story: Adjusting an Atlas and a Diet

When Sam, 23, first came to see me, he was so lethargic that he fell asleep on the examining table. The severe seizures from which he suffered required him to take several antiepileptic drugs to keep them in check. However, the drugs were so strong that Sam was in a constantly drowsy state. Understandably, he wanted to get off the drugs, but avoid having more seizures.

Sam's tests indicated low thyroid function, sugar intolerance, and low calcium. His diet—a standard fast-food regimen high in refined sugars—didn't help. He also had a problem with his atlas (first cervical vertebra). As mentioned earlier, a misalignment in the first three cervical vertebrae can cause seizures.

First of all, I told Sam that he would have to change his diet. In his fatigued state, he was reluctant to take on the "work" of shopping for and preparing whole foods, but the alternative—living an isolated, inactive life due to drug-induced lethargy—was worse. He promised to try.

For enzymes, I gave him Thera-zymes PAN and Adr to improve sugar digestion and aid in the transport of glucose into the brain, Thera-zyme Para for his low calcium, and Thera-zyme Sym because of his atlas problem. For his hypothyroidism, I gave him a thyroid glandular extract.

Sam then went to a chiropractor and had his atlas adjusted. When his structural problem was taken care of, his diet altered, and the enzyme therapy in place, his seizures stopped. However, it took a long time of gradually reducing the dosages (under the guidance of his physician) before Sam was completely off the powerful prescription drugs.

Prevention and Elimination of Seizures

The treatment to be implemented for seizures, of course, depends on the underlying cause. Proper diet and enzyme therapy are necessary to prevent and eliminate seizures due to sugar intolerance, while progesterone supplementation is recommended for those due to estrogen dominance. However, aspartame, a leading cause of seizures, should be avoided by everyone. For structural problems, mainly atlas misalignment, I recommend chiropractic adjustments.

Enzyme Therapy

Once again, the correct enzyme formula depends on what is causing the seizures. The following are formulas I use often:

- A multiple digestive formula according to the individual's specific needs; this always includes a formula for sugar intolerance, either Thera-zyme PAN or, in people who are both fat and sugar intolerant, Thera-zyme HCL

- Thera-zyme Adr: indicated for seizure disorders in people who are sugar intolerant
- Thera-zyme Sym: indicated in people who have upper cervical problems (C1, C2, and C3)

Hormonal Balancing

Natural progesterone (10% in vitamin E oil) can stop a seizure regardless of its cause. It is especially useful in estrogen-induced seizures (cyclic seizures during ovulation and menses), but it works for other seizures as well.

Thyroid glandular therapy, by normalizing blood and brain glucose, is instrumental in eliminating seizures in those whose thyroid gland is sluggish. When blood sugar is normal, there is no adrenaline surge with its attendant surge in cortisol, the mechanism behind seizures in hypothyroid people. (See Appendix A.)

Dietary Recommendations

All sugar-intolerant people, especially those suffering from seizures, should avoid all refined sugars (white sugar, corn syrup, fructose, commercial honey) and all synthetic sugars, especially NutraSweet. Even organic whole sugars such as sucanat (whole sugar cane) and raw honey can be problematic. The source of dietary sugar should be organic whole fruits and fruit juices.

Blood sugar can be maintained at night by eating a salty snack, drinking fruit juice, or eating a light protein snack just before bed. Stevia, an herbal sweetener, is also useful for stabilizing blood sugar.

Nutritional Supplements

To avoid seizures, it is important to get sufficient B vitamins, especially folic acid and vitamin B6, as well as the minerals magnesium, calcium, manganese, and zinc. I am against the use of chelated colloidal minerals because they may contain toxins such as aluminum, arsenic, and iron.[100] I recommend getting all of your minerals from whole organic foods. Good sources, especially for calcium and magnesium, are organic fruits and juices.

SKIN PROBLEMS

Enzyme therapy and hormonal balancing are especially valuable for treating the common skin disorders acne and psoriasis.

ACNE

Acne is an inflammatory condition of the skin's hair follicles which results in blemishes such as whiteheads, blackheads, pimples, and cysts. While sweat glands detoxify the body by excreting waste through sweat pores, sebaceous glands secrete an oil (sebum) through the hair follicles. Sebum helps keep the skin moist, but as aging occurs, the oil secretion slows down, causing dryness and loss of elasticity.

During puberty, testosterone—a major male hormone also present in females—stimulates secretion of sebum. In acne-prone individuals, excess oil accumulates in hair follicles and feeds the always-present bacteria. As the oil breaks down into fatty acids, the dead cells lining the follicles stick together, clogging the pores and causing blemishes. Sebaceous cysts can also develop as small swellings on the face, scalp, or back. These subcutaneous nodules of sebum often become chronically infected.

What Causes Acne?

Factors contributing to acne are heredity, hormonal imbalances, poor diet, and emotional problems. Heredity is not covered here because, although you may be predisposed to acne, you can avoid it by taking the steps discussed in this section.

Hormonal Imbalance

Raymond Peat, Ph.D., of Eugene, Oregon, believes that acne is causally related to low thyroid function, low progesterone, and vitamin A deficiency. When thyroid hormone and/or vitamin A are deficient, the body cannot convert cholesterol into the hormone progesterone. Likewise, without sufficient cholesterol, conversion cannot occur. By inhibiting both estrogen and testosterone, progesterone helps prevent and cure acne.

For information on the **enzymes** for this health condition, see Appendix B.

217

If you lack the necessary enzymes, food particles pass as undigested clusters into the blood. The body's immune system identifies these strange particles as foreign matter called antigens and creates an antibody as a defense. The result is an allergic reaction, which can produce acne.

Dietary Factors

Certain people have trouble digesting specific foods, which leads to food intolerance or allergies. Normally, enzymes break foods apart into their individual nutrients which then pass into the blood. But if you lack the necessary enzymes, food particles pass as undigested clusters into the blood. The body's immune system identifies these strange particles as foreign matter called antigens and creates an antibody as a defense. The result is an allergic reaction, which can produce acne.

Processed foods are another cause of acne, and include all junk foods, refined foods (white flour, white sugar, and other refined sugars), processed meats (deli foods), unsaturated fats, margarine and other fake foods, and commercial meat, poultry, and dairy products which contain chemicals and hormones. Sometimes, simply treating any food allergies and avoiding junk or processed foods will prevent acne. However, if you have hormonal problems, changing your diet will not be sufficient to heal the acne.

Emotional Problems

The role of emotions in creating a health condition should never be overlooked. Emotional problems suppress the immune system and reduce thyroid function, both effects contributing to acne. Addressing problems and working to resolve them need to be an integral part of any therapeutic program.

Success Story: Painful Cystic Acne Relieved

The day Claire, 18, walked into my office, her face was inflamed and covered with large cysts and scabs. It hurt so much, she couldn't touch it. She had suffered from this acne for five months along with other symptoms which she explained as follows: "I don't feel like myself. I'm spacey, lightheaded, and tired all the time. I'm so moody that I've lost a lot of my friends. I'm really self-conscious and depressed." Despite the fact that she ate a vegan diet with no animal or dairy products, in her own words she felt "horrible."

At the age of 13, Claire had suffered from mild acne and started antibiotic treatment, including tetracycline and related medications (Minocin® and minocycline), Augmentin®, and amoxicillin, which she continued for four years. At 14, she began what extended to three years of oral contraceptives for ovarian cysts—an ill-advised prescription given that the estrogen in birth control pills can actually *cause* ovarian cysts,[101] not to mention that synthetic progesterone (progestin) is carcinogenic and inhibits the body's production of progesterone.

Then Claire received a shot of Depo-Provera® (a progestin, normally prescribed as a contraceptive) for the cysts. The reported side effects of Depo-Provera are numerous and include irregular menstrual bleeding, headache, abdominal cramps, nausea, depression, insomnia, pelvic pain, and acne. After the injection, Claire gradually developed severe cystic acne. Although she was desperate, she was afraid to take yet another suggested drug because of its widely reported toxic side effects.

Although the breakout on her face was her major complaint, Claire had other health problems and frequently got sick with flu, colds, and bronchitis, indicating a weakened immune system. She still had painful cysts in one ovary and her periods were irregular. She suffered from constipation and nausea that was so constant it was difficult for her to eat. Social engagements caused her great anxiety because she was self-conscious about her acne.

Claire's urine analysis showed extreme sugar intolerance, which fit with her sugar cravings. Her urine analysis also revealed a severe vitamin C deficiency, low calcium, a salt deficiency, and severe allergies. Other testing showed a sluggish thyroid gland, adrenal gland insufficiency, candidiasis (an overgrowth of the yeast-like fungus *Candida albicans*), and liver and spleen problems (related to the many drugs she had been taking and a suppressed immune system). Claire's history revealed a series of traumas, including rape, physical abuse by her father, and anorexia. In fact, she had moved away from her family to start a healthier life on her own.

Claire had serious structural problems including a misaligned atlas (the vertebra supporting the skull) due to an injury, and a misaligned coccyx (tailbone) which frequently occurs in women who have been sexually abused. One leg was two inches shorter than the other which produced abdominal muscle cramps. These problems were healed by chiropractic therapy over a period of time.

See **Candidiasis**, pp. 94-96. For more about chiropractic treatment of a misaligned coccyx, see "Success Story: The Childhood Trauma Behind Chronic Headaches," Headaches, pp. 153-154.

My first effort was to work on Claire's immune system, clear the yeast infection, relieve the nausea and allergies, improve her diet and digestion, and help balance her hormonal system. For these problems I gave her the following supplements:

- Thera-zyme PAN: for sugar intolerance
- Thera-zyme Adr: for severe sugar intolerance and mood swings
- Thera-zyme Nsl: for vitamin C deficiency and nasal problems
- Thera-zyme Skn: for acne
- Thera-zyme Kdy: for allergies, nausea, and hypoglycemia
- Thera-zyme TRMA: for the immune system and to relieve anxiety
- Thyroid glandular extract
- Natural progesterone (10%) in vitamin E oil

In addition, Claire used many healing topical creams to help relieve the inflammation on her face. These included:

- Natural progesterone (3% cream): relieves pain and helps heal cysts and scars
- Alpha hydroxy acid: helps shrink the pores and slough off dead skin
- Zinc: an important mineral for skin health
- French green clay: helps draw out toxins and pus from infections

Dietary changes were an essential component in Claire's healing. Her vegan diet, devoid of protein, along with her inadequate salt and fruit intake, would not promote her healing because these foods are necessary to maintain good thyroid function. I strongly recommended that she start eating protein daily. She grudgingly obliged, beginning with raw cheeses, potatoes, and occasionally fish. I also told her to eliminate: all thyroid-inhibiting food such as raw cruciferous vegetables (cauliflower, broccoli, cabbage, and Brussels sprouts) which should only be eaten steamed (cooking kills the thyroid-inhibiting substances); all unsaturated oils (canola, safflower, soybean, flax); fluoridated water and toothpaste; and foods with pesticide residues (which are estrogenic and therefore suppress thyroid secretion).[102] I advised her to eliminate soy products as well because there is some evidence that soy also may affect thyroid function.[103]

A month after beginning treatment, Claire came down with a respiratory flu from which it took her a month to recover. I gave her Thera-zyme Rsp to help relieve her relentless cough, in addition to TRMA for the infection. Over the next year, Claire's immune system improved and, with it, her acne, although flare-ups would occur with periods of bad diet and high stress. Gradually, the cysts began to shrink. Her forehead was the first to clear.

Claire came in often to update her program. I used other enzymes as her body indicated; a round of Thera-zyme Lvr to cleanse her liver and Thera-zyme Spl to aid in healing her spleen and supporting her immune system.

It has now been almost two years. Her acne has disappeared and her immune system has healed, except for allergies.

Success Story: Candidiasis Treatment Clears Up Acne

Marion, 43, walked into my office and rattled off a long list of health problems, including: food allergies, especially to sugar, frequent bladder infections, premenstrual syndrome (PMS), hot flashes, candidiasis, and acne. The acne, though not severe, was her major complaint, since she was concerned about her looks. "I used to have a beautiful complexion, and look at me now!" Marion pointed to several cysts and added that her doctor wanted to excise the one on her nose.

Her diet was fairly healthy, consisting mainly of meals at high-quality restaurants which served pasta, fish, salads, gourmet soups, steamed vegetables, and potatoes or rice.

A urinalysis indicated sugar intolerance, low calcium, excess acidity, and kidney-lymphatic stress leading to allergies. Further testing confirmed a *Candida albicans* yeast overgrowth and also indicated a urinary tract inflammation. Marion's thyroid test indicated low thyroid function which is why, even with her relatively good diet, she still had acne. It was obvious that she needed thyroid and progesterone therapy in addition to a multiple digestive enzyme formula, an allergy formula, and a remedy for candidiasis.

During the treatment, I discovered that the formula for Marion's candidiasis had a profound effect on her acne. Thera-zyme SmI contains both cellulase, which digests pathogenic yeast, and probiotics (friendly bacteria, SEE QUICK DEFINITION) essential for colon health. Almost overnight, her acne started to clear, which I attribute to the probiotics. Marion's cysts took longer to disappear, but they did so as her thyroid function improved and she took adequate progesterone to balance her estrogen level.

> **QUICK DEFINITION**
>
> **Friendly bacteria,** or probiotics, refer to beneficial microbes inhabiting the human gastrointestinal tract where they are essential for proper nutrient assimilation. The human body contains an estimated several trillion beneficial bacteria comprising over 400 species, all necessary for health. Among the more well known of these are *Lactobacillus acidophilus* and *Bifidobacterium bifidum*. Overly acidic bodily conditions, chronic constipation or diarrhea, dietary imbalances, consumption of highly processed foods, and the excessive use of antibiotics and hormonal drugs can interfere with probiotic function and even reduce the number of these microbes, setting up conditions for illness.

For her urinary tract (bladder) problem, I gave her Thera-zyme UrT, a special formula for inflammation of the bladder (cystitis). During periods of infection, I gave her Thera-zyme TRMA, which has a healing effect on all soft tissue including skin. Later, I suspected that the cause of her frequent bladder infections was the use of spermacidal foams as birth control. My suspicions proved correct—when she eliminated them, her bladder problems ceased.

Success Story:
The Importance of Getting Enough Protein

When Stephen, 15, came into my office to be treated for acne, his complexion looked clear, but upon closer examination, scattered acne eruptions were apparent. He was taking adequate amounts of enzymes, as well as thyroid supplements, and was eating fairly well. However, his protein intake was minimal and I recommended that he increase it.

Stephen started eating organic eggs, raw cheese, raw milk and yogurt, more potatoes, and some fish. In less than two weeks, his acne disappeared. This is because adequate protein is required for good thyroid function and for the conversion, in the liver, of the inactive form of thyroid hormone (T4) to the active form (T3). As mentioned above, low thyroid function is a causative factor in skin problems.

Acne Prevention and
Elimination Program

The following therapies are useful in avoiding and eliminating acne.

Enzyme Therapy

With the help of a professional enzyme therapist, find out what multiple digestive enzyme formula you need to facilitate digestion. This will vary according to the specific enzyme and dietary deficiencies of the individual.

For acne cases, I often recommend the following:

■ Thera-zyme Skn: for the liver, intestines and kidney; specifically addresses skin problems such as psoriasis, eczema, and acne

■ Thera-zyme Kdy: kidney-lymphatic formula which helps relieve many symptoms, particularly allergies

■ Thera-zyme TRMA: primary immune system formula, for any kind of infection and for soft tissue trauma which is always present in skin problems; also relieves anxiety

■ Thera-zyme Adr: for severe sugar intolerance and related mental and emotional problems including mood swings

■ Thera-zyme Nsl: antioxidant/vitamin C formula; since free radical pathology accompanies all diseases, useful for any inflammatory condition, especially in people who have a vitamin C deficiency

Thyroid Support and Progesterone Therapy

Thyroid and progesterone therapy are essential in the healing of acne if your thyroid gland is sluggish and/or you have other hormonal imbalances. As explained above, thyroid hormone deficiency can lead to a low level of progesterone, and progesterone is important in both preventing and healing acne. For people with an underactive thyroid, I recommend a thyroid glandular extract. (See Appendix A.)

In studies conducted by Dr. Peat, both males and females consistently reported that the use of natural progesterone in either oral (10% in vitamin E oil) or topical (3% cream) form at the first sign of a pimple stopped its development; it also prevented outbreaks, or resulted in relatively clear skin within a few days.[104] Women can use the progesterone liberally—either the cream or the oil. For men, I recommend the cream; be careful to apply only a tiny dab to each pimple. A word of caution: while progesterone therapy is effective for men as well as women, men should be careful not to inhibit their testosterone to the extent that they lose their facial hair or libido, although this condition reverses within a few days of stopping the treatment.

Dietary Recommendations

Avoid synthetic and processed foods, including all refined sugars and grains. There are many nutrients important in preventing skin problems. To supply these, an organic, whole-foods diet is preferable to taking megadoses of synthetic vitamins and minerals. Such a diet will provide adequate amounts of minerals (including zinc), folic acid, the entire vitamin B complex (including biotin), and the fat-soluble vitamins such as A and E, all of which are important in skin health.

Cultured milk products, including yogurt, as well as sauerkraut and other fermented vegetables are abundant with friendly bowel bacteria. These friendly bacteria are essential in maintaining the healthy functioning of the intestinal tract. They are also involved in the production of enzymes such as protease, lipase, and lactase, along with B vitamins, and they produce their own antibiotic substances which can kill at least 27 types of pathogenic bacteria. They thus aid healing of skin diseases, including acne.

For healthy thyroid function, eat thyroid-friendly foods and avoid thyroid-inhibiting foods. The friendly foods include all organic animal protein (beef, lamb, eggs, raw and cultured dairy products), fish, especially halibut and other white fish, and coconut oil. As mentioned in Claire's case, inhibitors include all unsaturated oils with the excep-

For healthy thyroid function, eat thyroid-friendly foods and avoid thyroid-inhibiting foods. The friendly foods include all organic animal protein (beef, lamb, eggs, raw and cultured dairy products), fish, especially halibut and other white fish, and coconut oil.

tion of extra virgin olive oil, cruciferous vegetables, and, according to some research, soy products. Fluoride and toxins such as mercury in dental fillings can also affect thyroid function.[105]

As discussed earlier, if you have trouble digesting specific foods, this may be due to food allergies. With the help of an enzyme therapist, find out what foods you are allergic to and minimize your consumption of them.

Acne Creams and Oils

Products containing the following ingredients are the most effective in treating acne:

■ Natural progesterone: oral 10% progesterone in vitamin E oil and 3% topical cream; relieves pain and helps heal cysts and scars; the vitamin E in the oil is an added benefit for the skin

■ Alpha hydroxy acid: a component in many skin creams; helps shrink the pores and slough dead skin

■ Zinc: important mineral for skin healing; certain skin enzymes require zinc to become activated

■ French green clay: a special clay that helps draw out toxins and pus from infections

■ Salicylic acid: an anti-inflammatory component in skin creams; the active ingredient in aspirin

■ Retinyl palmitate: pure vitamin A, *not* Retin-A. Although vitamin A is needed for progesterone production, I do not recommend internal use of vitamin A. Instead, eat foods containing vitamin A; all whole foods contain this important vitamin. I only recommend retinyl palmitate, a pure form of vitamin A, which can be applied directly to the skin. Unfortunately, most acne sufferers use synthetic forms of vitamin A, including Retin-A (topical) and Accutane (oral). According to the *Physicians' Desk Reference*, Accutane is known to cause birth defects and has been associated with a number of severe reactions, including inflammatory bowel disease, decreased night vision, corneal opacities, and clinical hepatitis.

PSORIASIS

Psoriasis is characterized by excessive cell replication. In the affected areas, cells reproduce at 1,000 times the normal rate, exceeding even the rate in skin cancer. Normal skin regenerates itself approximately every 28 days. In psoriasis patients, this process occurs every three to four days. As the skin produces new cells at this alarming rate, the surface area becomes red and inflamed, and can rise to three times its normal thickness.

There are a number of forms of psoriasis, but all involve scaly red patches of various shapes. The patches appear on the scalp, knees, elbows, buttocks, and sites of repeated trauma, but there are cases in which the entire body surface is involved. Usually, psoriasis begins with a small, scaly spot that does not heal. As time goes on, the original spot gets worse and others appear. Psoriasis may affect the nails as well.

Psoriasis is the fourth most common skin disease in the United States, after acne, warts, and eczema. In 50% of people with psoriasis, there is a family history of the condition. Psoriasis sufferers also have a higher than average rate of rheumatoid arthritis. About one person in 20 with psoriasis has some form of arthritis, and about one person in 20 with arthritis has psoriasis. .

Psoriasis manifests at any age; peak onset usually occurs between the ages of 15 and 35, but it may begin as early as age three and as late as 55. It strikes regardless of sex or skin color, but the incidence among darker-skinned people appears to be less than among lighter-skinned people.

What Causes Psoriasis?

The cause of psoriasis has not been determined, but the factors associated with it include food allergies, metabolic problems, liver and colon problems, hypothyroidism, and stress. Psoriasis is also classified as a psychosomatic illness and has long been treated with psychotherapy.

As with many health conditions, diet also appears to play a role. Germany had a high incidence of psoriasis prior to World War II. During the war, the disease nearly disappeared when certain foods, notably sugar, were in short supply. After the war, as the economy recovered and the food supply returned to prewar standards, psoriasis came back.

The cause of psoriasis has not been determined, but the factors associated with it include food allergies, metabolic problems, liver and colon problems, hypothyroidism, and stress.

According to researcher Helmut Christ, M.D., "Psoriasis is not a skin disorder, strictly speaking, but is instead an inherited metabolic disturbance which is triggered by environmental or stressful conditions, like faults in the diet, flu-like conditions, the administration of penicillin, death of a family member, surgery, etc."[106]

Specific metabolic factors which have been linked to psoriasis are an imbalance in substances called cyclic AMP and cyclic GMP, abnormal fatty acid metabolism, elevated levels of homocysteine in the blood, abnormal fumaric acid metabolism, hypothyroidism, and abnormal elimination of toxins. Structural problems and nutritional factors can also contribute.

Decreased Cyclic AMP in Relation to Cyclic GMP

There are two substances in the body that work in concert to create the production of new cells and normal cell growth and maturation. These substances are called cyclic GMP and cyclic AMP. Cyclic GMP is associated with the production of new cells. Cyclic AMP is associated with cell growth and maturation. In a healthy person, the two substances are in balance with each other. In a person with psoriasis, there is excessive cyclic GMP (cell production) in relation to cyclic AMP (cell maturation) at the sites in the body where psoriasis occurs.

A major factor in the decrease of cyclic AMP levels is undigested protein, a result of protease deficiency. Factors that increase the levels of cyclic GMP include candidiasis, intestinal bacterial toxins, certain antibodies present in people with allergies, and leukotrienes, substances involved in inflammation.

For more on **homocysteine**, see Cardiovascular Disease, pp. 102-103.

Therapies which work to reestablish the balance of cyclic AMP and GMP are therefore helpful in reversing psoriasis. *Coleus forskohlii*, an Ayurvedic herb, can help increase cyclic AMP levels. Substances that work to decrease levels of cyclic GMP include antioxidants, such as vitamins A, E, and C, zinc, and selenium, and antioxidant enzymes such as catalase, which is included in many Thera-zyme formulas.

Abnormal Fatty Acid Metabolism

Recent findings show abnormally high levels of arachidonic acid—an end product of unsaturated fat metabolism which has inflammatory properties—in areas of the body affected by psoriasis.[107]

Elevated Blood Levels of Homocysteine

Homocysteine is a by-product of amino acid metabolism. Blood levels of this by-product have been found to be abnormally high in patients with severe cases of psoriasis. These elevated levels of homocysteine may be related to the excessive growth of cells. A study of 323 psoriasis patients showed increased incidence of cardiovascular disease compared to matched controls, especially in those with other predisposing factors. The elevated homocysteine exhibited by psoriasis sufferers may be the reason, as research has linked it to cardiovascular disease.[108]

Abnormal Fumaric Acid Metabolism

Helmut Christ, M.D., reports that the metabolism of fumaric acid—a substance necessary in the energy production mechanisms of the body—may be defective in psoriasis patients. In healthy individuals, fumaric acid is formed in skin exposed to sunlight. Psoriasis patients cannot produce enough fumaric acid and need longer than normal exposure to the sun to produce it. This is why they frequently notice an improvement in their skin during the summer months. Treatment with an ethyl ester of fumaric acid (a compound of ethyl alcohol and fumaric acid) can help remedy this abnormality.[109]

Hypothyroidism

Low thyroid function (hypothyroidism) is associated with many skin

---

The Psoriasis-Eczema Connection

John Pagano, D.C., has found that psoriasis and eczema are related not only in cause but in treatment. He reports that three out of four cases of eczema cleared up with the same therapy he used for psoriasis. The major differences in treatments for the two conditions include different topical creams and spinal adjustments. The most important chiropractic adjustments for psoriasis (in descending order of importance) are the sixth, seventh and ninth thoracic (midback) vertebrae, whereas for eczema, the third, fourth, sixth, and ninth thoracic vertebrae are more often implicated. Both involve the third cervical (neck) vertebra and all of the lumbar (lower back) vertebrae, especially the fourth.

While the type of topical cream varies according to which skin ailment you have, olive oil is recommended for both. Also, sunlight normally helps psoriasis but is usually harmful to eczema.[110]

problems, including psoriasis, eczema, and acne. When the thyroid operates at a reduced level, prolactin (a hormone secreted by the pituitary gland which is responsible for milk production among other functions) levels rise. Excess prolactin is associated with psoriasis because prolactin increases cell division and the production of skin oils. Sunlight decreases prolactin formation, whereas darkness and stress increase it. This may be another connection between exposure to sunlight and the alleviation of psoriasis.

Normalizing thyroid function can cure or at least partially relieve psoriasis. In my practice, I have never seen a client with psoriasis who had normal thyroid function.

Abnormal Elimination of Toxins

Another factor in psoriasis may be the abnormal elimination of toxins. According to John Pagano, D.C., researcher and author of *Healing Psoriasis*, "Psoriasis is the external manifestation of the body's attempt to eliminate internal toxins that have accumulated in the lymphatics and bloodstream by seeping through the intestinal walls."[111] The body's elimination systems, primarily the liver and the kidneys, then try to filter out these toxins. When the liver is overloaded, toxins are eliminated through the skin. In time, as toxins accumulate, psoriasis begins.

Dr. Pagano's treatment is based upon a dietary cleansing program for the colon, the kidneys, and the liver, along with chiropractic therapy. In addition, he often recommends colonics during the cleansing program.

Structural Problems

Dr. Pagano describes physical structural problems—vertebral subluxations (disc misalignments)—correlated with psoriasis. Subluxations in the mid-thoracic (midback) section of the spinal cord from the fourth to the ninth thoracic vertebrae can affect the functioning of the liver or upset normal stomach activity during digestion, according to Dr. Pagano. In addition, subluxations of the third cervical (neck) and the fourth lumbar (lower back) vertebrae disturb lymph centers and their neural and circulatory connections. For this reason, I strongly recommend chiropractic care for psoriasis.

Nutritional Factors

Any undigested food can precipitate problems, but psoriasis is aggravated by certain foods in particular. These include undigested proteins, undigested vegetables from the nightshade family (eggplant, tomatoes, and peppers), refined sugar, pork, and alcohol. Bacteria can convert partially digested proteins into toxic substances called polyamines, which contribute to excessive cell proliferation and psoriasis.

Prevention and Elimination of Psoriasis

For prevention of psoriasis, proper nutrition is essential and enzyme therapy is often needed. To treat an outbreak, I recommend enzyme formulas, herbal remedies, and topical creams.

Dietary Recommendations

While there are variations on dietary recommendations in the treatment of psoriasis, all alternative medicine practitioners agree that a diet of whole, unprocessed foods and no refined or synthetic foods is central. Some experts advocate a vegetarian diet while others believe that organic meat, aside from pork, is acceptable. Sugar and alcohol— with the exception of red wine—are known to aggravate psoriasis. As some people with psoriasis also have arthritis, the nightshade family of foods, which exacerbates arthritis, is on the questionable list.

Enzyme Therapy

As with other health conditions, the enzymes used for psoriasis depend upon individual digestive needs and symptoms. Some people require more protease and others more lipase or cellulase; some are sugar intolerant. I have never noticed a pattern, except that all have hypothyroidism.

Thera-zyme Skn, formulated for psoriasis, eczema, and acne, contains the herb fumitory (see Herbal Remedies, below) and other herbs

The enzymes used for psoriasis depend upon individual digestive needs and symptoms. Some people require more protease and others more lipase or cellulase; some are sugar intolerant. I have never noticed a pattern, except that all have hypothyroidism.

important in healing the skin, including burdock root, Oregon grape root, and figwort.

Herbal Remedies

The following is a list of herbs that are useful in the treatment of psoriasis.[112] Consult a qualified health-care practitioner to determine which are best suited to your particular case.

■ Fumaric acid and its herbal source, fumitory (*Fumaria officinalis*): the ethyl ester of fumaric acid is available in oral capsule form (Psorex) and as a cream (Psoractin). For the cream, follow the directions on the label. The recommended oral dosage is one to three capsules daily, taken with tea, water, or milk.[113] As fumaric acid is metabolically highly active, you should start with a little and build the dosage slowly. Too much can lead to a drop in blood sugar, but this is reportedly rare. There are two signs that you have reached the right dosage. The first, of course, is a slow improvement in the condition. The second is that you will experience a warm feeling and a tingling of the skin and the shoulder and neck region about 15 to 30 minutes after taking the capsule. This indicates that the fumaric acid is working. As long as you feel the warming sensation and lesions are slowly healing, there is no need to increase the dosage.

■ *Coleus forskohlii:* Ayurvedic herb with two healing properties that make it valuable in combating skin problems. First, it helps promote normal cell division, which is not only helpful in controlling psoriasis and eczema, but has also been used in cancer patients to help fight metastasis. Second, *forskohlii* has a stimulating effect on thyroid hormone production. The majority of psoriasis patients have a sluggish thyroid, so *forskohlii* provides an additional healing benefit.

■ Burdock root (*Arctium lappa*): used to cleanse and detoxify the blood and the liver. It is a common remedy for skin conditions such as psoriasis, eczema, and dandruff. For skin problems, burdock is often combined with yellowdock, red clover, or cleavers. Combined with nettles and figwort, burdock is used to treat childhood eczema and nervous eczema.

■ Milk thistle (*Silybum marianum*): contains silymarin, a substance which supports healthy liver function and proper cell proliferation. Thera-zyme Lvr contains milk thistle.

■ Cleavers (*Galium aparine*): antineoplastic (working against the growth of abnormal tissue) and anti-inflammatory; helps drain the lymphatic system. In the treatment of psoriasis it is best combined with yellowdock and burdock.

■ Red clover (*Trifolium pratense*): useful for a range of skin conditions, including psoriasis, especially when combined with yellowdock and nettles. It can be effective for children with skin problems, particularly childhood eczema.

■ Oregon grape root (*Mahonia aquifolium*): cleanses the liver, blood, and spleen, stimulates liver activity and secretion of bile, and strengthens a weak liver. It is not recommended for those with an overactive liver caused by overeating or eating too much rich food.

■ Saffron (*Crocus sativus*): American yellow saffron is often substituted for the Spanish variety and is better for psoriasis. Saffron acts on the stomach and intestines and alleviates skin problems caused by malfunction in the digestive tract. Chamomile may be used as an alternative to saffron.

■ Slippery elm (*Ulmus rubra*): the inner bark is an anti-inflammatory for gastrointestinal irritation and helps heal the mucosal

Success Story: An Unusual Case of Hives

Hugh, 55, came to see me with no particular complaints. He said he wanted to improve his lifestyle and remain healthy. Since his wife had come to me before him, his diet had already been improved. His urine test showed a pattern of fat and sugar intolerance and a vitamin C deficiency, but was otherwise normal. I sent him home with Thera-zyme Bil for fat intolerance, Thera-zyme SvG for sugar intolerance, and a vitamin C formula (Thera-zyme Opt). A month later Hugh called me complaining about hive-like sores which had appeared on his lower back and hands, progressively worsening until they were open and oozing.

I told Hugh that this was probably due to the enzymes digesting toxins which he could not eliminate through normal channels—the urine and feces. I asked him if he had been exposed to any environmental toxins. At first he said no, but with further questioning he admitted to spraying pesticides on his lawn every two weeks without a mask or gloves—and he had just done some spraying. He also told me that his water came from a well on his property.

I told him to come immediately for another test. The second urinalysis and palpation test showed a need for Thera-zyme MSCLR to relieve the hives, a kidney-lymphatic formula for allergies (Thera-zyme Kdy), and a formula to help cleanse the blood and treat soft tissue trauma (Thera-zyme TRMA). Needless to say, Hugh stopped using pesticides. In several days, his wounds began healing and they have not returned.

lining of the entire digestive tract. Due to a worldwide demand for slippery elm, the fine powdered inner bark is in short supply and the coarser outer bark has been substituted, but it lacks the inner bark's healing power.

Topical Remedies

■ Psoractin: in addition to fumaric acid, this cream contains salicylic acid, a common ingredient in anti-inflammatory creams, and allantoin for wound healing. It is easily applied and leaves no stain on the clothing.

■ Licorice root (*Glycyrrhiza glabra*): contains a compound which, when applied to the skin, has a similar effect to cortisone (blocking the formation of inflammatory compounds) without the toxic side effects. Alticort is one brand of cream that contains licorice root.

■ Tea tree oil (*Melaleuca alternifolia*): used to relieve skin and mucous membrane problems including: psoriasis, eczema, and dermatitis; dandruff; poison oak, ivy, and sumac; cradle cap; herpes simplex and canker sores; gingivitis (bleeding gums); fungal infections such as athlete's foot; and severe sunburn. In addition, it has antiseptic, antibacterial, and germicidal properties.

■ Other essential oils: in addition to tea tree oil, essential oils of lavender, bergamot, helichrysum, and thyme can also be helpful in relieving psoriasis.

WEIGHT PROBLEMS

Excess weight has become an American epidemic—59% of adults in the U.S. fall into the category of clinical obesity. In 1990 alone, about 300,000 people died as the result of excess weight, and the health care costs associated with the diabetes, heart disease, high blood pressure, and gallstones it produces were estimated at over $45 billion. In that same year, Americans spent an estimated $33 billion on weight-loss services and products.[114]

Commercial weight-loss products not only often do not work, but may create other problems for those who use them. High-protein diet drinks should be avoided because they are not whole organic protein and are often made with isolated amino acids, which can result in an imbalance in other amino acids. In addition, they are often laced with processed sugars or, worse, artificial sweeteners, and contain synthetic vitamins and minerals. Some of these drinks also contain caffeine or herbal forms of caffeine, such as *ma huang* or ephedra. Anyone can lose weight by reducing caloric intake and hyping themselves up with stimulants, but it is not a healthy approach to the problem and is likely a short-term solution at best.

Over-the-counter diet pills, such as phenylethylamine, should also be avoided. Diet pills work by tricking the brain into thinking you aren't hungry, but what happens when you stop taking them? A return to normal—generally unhealthy—eating patterns, including overeating and bingeing. It's better to eat organic, whole foods, and digest them properly with the help of enzymes if necessary. A person with normal digestion who eats a natural diet is rarely overweight.

What Causes Weight Problems?

In addition to an underactive thyroid gland, which slows metabolism and can therefore lead to weight gain, the following dietary, physiological, and environmental factors are also commonly implicated in weight problems.

■ An excess-starch diet: Most fattening food is starch and people who eat excessive amounts are prone to gain weight. By starch, I mean bread, pasta, rice, and beans. A healthy diet should include thyroid-stimulating foods, such as adequate protein, sea salt, fruit, and coconut oil, in addition to organic vegetables.

For information on the **enzymes** for this health condition, see Appendix B.

Supplying food enzymes to predigest food in the stomach tends to normalize weight—providing that people eat consciously and not out of habit. When taking food enzymes, fat people tend to lose weight and thin people tend to gain weight.

■ Poor digestion: I have observed that supplying Thera-zyme food enzymes to predigest food in the stomach tends to normalize weight—providing that people eat consciously and not out of habit. When taking food enzymes, fat people tend to lose weight and thin people tend to gain weight. The fat person will eat less because he or she is satisfied with less food. The thin person will be able to digest food, get more nourishment, feel better, and have an increased appetite.

■ The obesity-enzyme connection: Lipoprotein lipase (LPL) is an enzyme produced by the body. Its function is to transport fat from the blood into storage in fat cells. The higher the LPL level, the more predisposed you are to store fat. Your inherent LPL level is partly determined by your heredity. That's why if your parents are obese, you probably have higher LPL levels than the children of thin parents, thus predisposing you to store more fat. Dieting will worsen this situation because a low-calorie diet makes LPL more efficient at storing fat.

According to a study published in the *New England Journal of Medicine*, this enzyme also causes dieters to regain the weight they lost during the diet. Even going for hours without food can trigger LPL and, the longer you fast, the more active LPL becomes. This activity level remains high even after you return to your original eating habits. The best way to outsmart LPL is to snack frequently, every four hours, and to eat when you are first hungry, rather than waiting until you are ravenous and then eating a huge meal. Eating small amounts frequently helps keep the blood sugar up and prevents the body from shifting into the fasting mode, which activates LPL.[115]

See **Allergies**, pp. 65-70, **Candidiasis**, pp. 94-96, and **Parasites**, pp. 197-199.

■ Allergies: Edema resulting from the ingestion of allergens or from exposure to environmental allergens can cause weight gain. For example, I know of a young man who lost weight just by eliminating wheat—to which he was allergic— from his diet. Nothing else was altered. In another case, a woman gained ten pounds when she bought a down jacket to which she was allergic. Without following a diet, when she gave away the jacket, the weight disappeared. In general, whatever a person is allergic to, whether it's feathers or fat, can cause weight gain.

■ Hypoglycemia (low blood sugar): This is caused not only by the inability to digest sugar (sucrose, lactose, and maltose) but also protein, because 56% of digested protein is converted to glucose (blood sugar) as needed by the body. People in this category can be either fat or thin, depending on how much of what they eat is digested.

■ Candidiasis and parasites: An overgrowth of the yeast *Candida albicans* and parasitic conditions can cause bloating and weight gain.

■ Enzyme poisons (inhibitors): These include heavy metals (lead, cadmium, mercury), pesticides, synthetic substances such as margarine, and many common chemicals used by industry, agriculture, and consumers. Enzyme poisons can interrupt important metabolic processes in the body, some of which control fat burning and appetite.

Success Story: Losing 80 Pounds Without Dieting

Pauline, 73, came to me for help with her digestion and her weight problem. Barely 5' tall, she weighed 250 pounds and had a noticeable goiter. She also had severe gastric problems for which she gulped as many as 35 Tums daily. A gourmet cook, her diet was a healthy one, although she loved rich desserts. My program for her was simple: a multiple digestive formula for ulcers and other gastric problems (Thera-zyme Stm) and a thyroid glandular extract. Her weight decreased so dramatically that her friends couldn't believe it when she smugly denied having changed her diet. They thought she had sneaked off to a "fat farm" and starved herself. In less than a year, Pauline's goiter and 80 pounds had disappeared.

Success Story:
Chemical Poisoning Behind Weight Gain

Penelope, 38, had a history of being overweight and had undergone a hysterectomy at the age of 24, but, according to her, felt well otherwise. However, she developed life-threatening health problems after she was exposed to chemicals in the workplace. Here is Penelope's account of what occurred:

"Around December 25, I started a new job. There was extensive painting and varnishing of floors going on while I worked 10-hour days for eight weeks. By December 29th, I started to feel sick and developed severe hives. After eight weeks, I had the following symptoms: severe swelling of my face, throat, tongue, hands and feet; raised, rope-like hives over my entire body; pain between my shoulder blades, in my throat, and under my right rib cage; vomiting after meals; diarrhea; and a weight gain of 50 pounds though I hardly eat. I have been to the emergency room 12 times since Christmas because my throat and tongue swell and I cannot breathe. I was fired due to illness and my life has become a nightmare. I never know how bad each day will be."

In addition to prednisone for her hives, Penelope had been given epinephrine (adrenaline), Prozac and doxepin (antidepressants), Hismanal® (antihistamine), and Zantac (an antacid needed after taking prednisone). At one point, she was taking nine different antihistamines to stop the hives and swelling of her throat, but nothing worked.

Although doctors told her that she had no allergy problems (based on blood tests), her urine test revealed serious allergies and Penelope reported being allergic to bee stings, molds, and cats. She had allergy symptoms of swollen glands, frontal headaches, nausea, and vomiting. In addition, Penelope's test showed severe fat and sugar intolerance, severe vitamin C deficiency, and excess acid reserves. A physical exam and palpation test revealed the need for 14 enzymes—something I have never encountered in all my years of practicing enzyme therapy. I put her on the following program, focusing first on her most urgent symptoms, the hives and vomiting:

- Thera-zymes Bil: for fat digestion
- Thera-zyme SvG: for sugar digestion
- Thera-zyme SmI: for candidiasis, parasites, and a toxic colon
- Thera-zyme Challenge Food Powder: to help cleanse her colon
- Thera-zyme MSCLR: for her hives
- Thera-zyme TRMA: for soft tissue trauma and her immune system
- Thera-zyme Kdy: an allergy formula

I also gave Penelope a thyroid glandular extract plus 10% natural progesterone in vitamin E oil for her lifelong hypothyroidism, which had probably led to her weight problems and hysterectomy to begin with.

During the first three months on this program, Penelope stopped taking all of her prescription drugs, with no adverse side effects. First, the hives went away, but it took both MSCLR (four capsules five times a day) and TRMA (four capsules three times a day) to accomplish this. Penelope noticed a difference within hours and, in less than 24 hours, the hives were gone. When they did return, they were no longer life-threatening and were controlled with enzyme therapy.

Next, she noticed less frequent vomiting and it stopped completely before the end of the third month. Finally, during the last six weeks of the three-month period, she dropped 25 pounds. In addition, she can now tolerate eating some raw fruits and vegetables, including green salads, whereas prior to the program, she could only eat meat, fish, potatoes, bread, and cooked vegetables.

Prevention and Elimination of Excess Weight

Before I tell you about my recommendations for a healthy weight-loss program, let me give you some common sense tips about weight loss.

■ Become more conscious of what you eat, why you eat, and when you eat. Do you eat to live or do you live to eat? Lots of people eat out of habit, not hunger. Some people eat late at night when the body won't utilize the calories, while others eat when they're under stress. As a child, did your mother stuff food into your mouth every time you cried to take your mind off your distress? Are you filling your cup with food because there is no love in it? Think about it.

■ Eat slowly. It takes time—about 30 minutes—for the body to know that it's satisfied. Have you ever noticed that if a friend phones you during dinner and you talk for awhile, when you hang up you are no longer hungry?

■ Do aerobic exercise. If you walk briskly 30 minutes a day (or do some other kind of aerobic exercise), you could lose 25 pounds in a year even without dieting (unless there is an organic condition underlying your excess weight).

Enzyme Therapy

As with all health conditions, the proper enzyme therapy depends on the cause of the condition, but the following formulas are ones I commonly use for weight problems.

■ Thera-zyme VSCLR: multiple digestive formula for people who have trouble losing weight, but other digestive problems must also be addressed, such as sugar and protein intolerance

■ Thera-zyme SmI: for people whose weight problem is due to candidiasis; contains a special form of cellulase that digests pathogenic yeast, plus probiotics to provide friendly bacteria to the colon

■ Thera-zyme TRMA: for a weak immune system, which is always present in a person with candidiasis; most effective when combined with SmI and a whole foods diet low in refined sugars

■ Thera-zyme IVD: can help decrease a big appetite

Thyroid Support

Most people who are over (or under) weight have a sluggish thyroid. If testing determines that your thyroid function is low, seek the advice of a health professional and take only natural thyroid glandular extract, not the popular synthetic synthroid. If you are a vegan and object to taking the animal-derived glandulars, you can take proloid, a synthetic drug which is a closer approximation to natural thyroid hormones than synthroid. (See Appendix A.)

Dietary Recommendations

■ Eat whole organic foods instead of counting calories. Processed foods don't eliminate hunger. Eating smaller portions happens naturally when you substitute whole foods for their processed counterparts.

■ Eat fiber: carrots are one of the best sources of fiber, which helps cleanse the colon and remove bowel toxins

■ Use coconut oil: a thyroid-stimulating oil which helps balance thyroid function and also has antiseptic and immune-stimulating properties

Nutritional Supplements

The following natural supplements, which can help you achieve your goal of losing weight, should not be treated as magic bullet solutions. They should only be used as part of a comprehensive approach that includes conscious effort, an exercise program, and awareness of foods and emotional triggers to eating.

■ Homeopathic appetite drops: used to control or balance appetite. They work to decrease or increase the appetite, whichever is needed. Don't wait to take this remedy until you are on your way to the refrigerator or are already pouring the hot fudge on your ice cream.

■ Spirulina, blue-green algae, and other "green foods": clinically associated with weight loss, perhaps because their high nutritional content satiates the appetite and reduces hunger.

■ Calorad: organic bovine-extracted collagen. It is not a diet drink nor a meal replacement, but a food beverage. The typical dosage is one tablespoon in a glass of water taken at least three hours after dinner and immediately before going to sleep, for those who desire to lose excess fat and build up muscle tissue. People who don't want to lose weight should take it in the morning. Its purported mechanism in weight loss is the exchange of fat for lean muscle.

There have been a number of studies of Calorad over the past ten years. Nutritionist Rina Davis, C.N., of Portland, Oregon, tested Calorad on over 300 people between the ages of 17 and 77, with various health histories, over a one-year period.[116] Although she advised her clients to eat a wholesome diet and to decrease sugar intake, she did not require them to exercise. She used hydrostatic weighing (an underwater weighing technique) to determine the percentage loss of fat tissue and the percentage gain of lean muscle tissue.

The average weight loss was four pounds per month and, for every pound lost, the body lost three inches of fat. In addition, 36% gained muscle mass whereas less than 1% lost any. In descriptive terms, the clients bodies got firmer, men lost their "love handles," and, in women, the flab underneath their arms and chins was decreased and their inner thighs got tighter.

For those who don't lose weight on Calorad, it may be because they have one or more of the following conditions: hypothyroidism; a bad diet of junk foods high in calories but low in nutrition, or a high-starch diet; or a genetically high LPL level. Since I address these issues in treatment, my patients have had good success with Calorad.

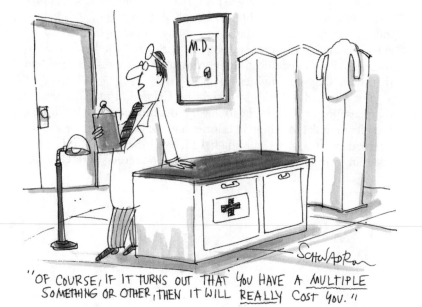

"OF COURSE, IF IT TURNS OUT THAT YOU HAVE A MULTIPLE SOMETHING OR OTHER, THEN IT WILL REALLY COST YOU."

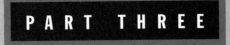

PART THREE

Appendices

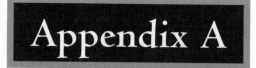

Appendix A

HORMONAL BALANCING

To give you more information on the importance of hormonal balancing in the restoration and maintenance of health, this appendix is devoted to discussion of hypothyroidism and the anti-aging steroidal hormones pregnenolone, progesterone, and DHEA.

Hypothyroidism

The thyroid gland is a small, butterfly-shaped gland located in the neck. It controls our metabolism, or the rate at which food is burned to create energy. Thyroid hormone is required to convert cholesterol into the vital anti-aging steroidal hormones pregnenolone, progesterone, and DHEA (dehydroepiandosterone). Pregnenolone converts to progesterone and DHEA in the body. Progesterone and DHEA are precursors for more specialized hormones, including estrogen, testosterone, and cortisol. The anti-aging steroids are responsible in part for the prevention of age-related diseases, such as cancer, heart disease, senility, and obesity.

There are two major forms of the thyroid hormone: the inactive form thyroxine or T4 (contains four iodine molecules) and the active form triiodothyronine or T3 (contains three iodine molecules). The healthy thyroid gland produces 93% T4 and 7% T3. The healthy liver converts T4 to T3 at just the rate needed. Excess estrogen and other thyroid toxins, along with faulty diet (inadequate protein, salt, and fruits) can inhibit this conversion. When thyroid function is low and/or when cholesterol is low, these hormones cannot be produced in adequate amounts. That is why low thyroid function (hypothyroidism) has so many varied and broad-spectrum symptoms.

It is easy to recognize severely low thyroid function in children who have edema with its characteristic appearance—round face, double chin, and fat, round belly plus abnormally bent knees and elbows. Subclinical hypothyroidism, however, is much more common and less easily recognized, because of the variety of its symptoms.

Causes of Hypothyroidism

The majority of people who come to see me have some form of thyroid

A Glossary of Hormones

DHEA (dehydroepiandrosterone) is naturally produced by the human adrenal glands and gonads with optimal levels occurring around age 20 for women and age 25 for men. After those ages, DHEA levels gradually decline. DHEA is an antioxidant, hormone regulator, and the building block from which estrogen and testosterone are produced. Low DHEA levels have been associated with cancer, diabetes, multiple sclerosis, hypertension, obesity, AIDS, heart disease, Alzheimer's, and immune dysfunction illnesses. Excess DHEA (more than 15 mg daily) in the body can convert to estrogen and thus contribute to hormonal imbalance. The safest way to raise DHEA levels is by supplementing with its precursor, the hormone pregnenolone.

Estrogen is a female sex hormone, produced mainly in the ovaries (some in the fat cells), which regulates the menstrual cycle. Estrogen is important for adolescent sexual development, prepares the uterus for receiving the fertilized egg by stimulating the uterine lining to grow, and affects all the body's cells; its levels decline after menopause. Estrogen slows bone loss, which leads to osteoporosis, and it can help reverse the incidence of heart attacks. It also improves skin tone, reduces vaginal dryness, and can act as an antiaging factor. For the first ten to 14 days in a woman's cycle, the uterus is mainly under the influence of estrogen. Estrogen levels begin to climb right before menstruation, from about days seven to 14, and peak at ovulation.

There are three natural types of estrogen: estradiol (produced directly in the ovary); estrone (produced from estradiol); and estriol (formed in smaller amounts in the ovary). Estradiol is the most potent of the three. It prepares the uterus for the implantation of a fertilized egg, and also helps mature and maintain the sex characteristics of the female organs.

Environmental estrogens are foreign compounds and/or chemical toxins that mimic the effects of estrogen. Environmental estrogens, also called xenoestrogens, are present primarily in man-made chemicals ("greenhouse gases," herbicides, and pesticides such as DDT) and industrial by-products (from manufacture of plastics and paper, as well as from the incineration of hazardous wastes). Environmental estrogens often cause an imbalance of estrogen relative to progesterone, another key hormone. The rise and fall of estrogen versus progesterone regulates the building up and, if no fertilization occurs, the eventual shedding of the uterine lining during the menstrual cycle. When a woman's body has too much estrogen (a condition called estrogen dominance), a variety of health problems can result, including breast cancer, fibroids, and endometriosis, among others. According to some researchers, environmental estrogens also affect men, and may contribute to testicular cancer, urinary tract disorders, and low sperm count.

continued on next page

A Glossary of Hormones (cont.)

Pregnenolone is a hormone which the brain and adrenal cortex synthesize from low-density lipoprotein (LDL) cholesterol in the presence of thyroid hormone and other nutrients, including vitamin A. Pregnenolone production slows down after age 45; by age 75, the body produces 60% less pregnenolone than it did during youth. Since pregnenolone converts to progesterone and DHEA, its effects will parallel these hormones. Pregnenolone repairs certain enzymes, helps restore hormones which decline during aging, protects from cortisone toxicity, relieves anxiety and panic attacks, and reduces exophthalmia (bulging eyes) in Graves' disease patients. As a brain power hormone, pregnenolone enhances memory, improves concentration, reduces mental fatigue, and generally keeps the brain functioning at peak capacity.

Progesterone is a female sex hormone (produced in the corpus luteum of the ovaries) which prepares the uterus for a fertilized egg and then stops the cell proliferation in the uterus if pregnancy does not occur. When estrogen is high, during days seven to 14 of a woman's cycle, the level of progesterone is at its lowest. Its levels climb to a peak from around days 14 to 24, and then dramatically drop off again just before the start of menstruation. When the cells stop producing progesterone, it's a signal to the uterus to let go of all the new cells produced during the month and to start afresh. In a sense, menstruation is progesterone withdrawal. Starting at age 35, a woman's progesterone production begins to decline.

Testosterone is the primary male sex hormone, made in the testes, important for the development of male sexual characteristics. Testosterone can help reverse male impotence, heighten virility, and increase muscle mass. After "male menopause" at midlife, testosterone levels decline. As one produces less testosterone, one of the safest ways to make the hormone more available to the body is through a skin-absorbed (percutaneous) gel. The gel is applied topically to the skin and absorbed slowly into the bloodstream.

dysfunction. Hypothyroidism is a condition of low or underactive thyroid gland function which can produce numerous symptoms. Among the 47 clinically recognized symptoms are: fatigue, depression, lethargy, weakness, weight gain, low body temperature, chills, cold extremities, general inappropriate sensation of cold, infertility, rheumatic pain, menstrual disorders (excessive flow, cramps), repeated infections, colds, upper respiratory infections, skin problems (itching, eczema, psoriasis, acne, dry, coarse, or scaly skin, skin pallor), memory disturbances, concentration difficulties, paranoia, migraines, oversleep, "laziness," muscle aches and weakness, hearing disturbances, burning/prickling sensations, anemia, slow reaction time and mental sluggishness, swelling of the eyelids, constipation, labored or difficult breathing, hoarseness, brittle nails, and poor vision. An underarm or oral temperature below 98° F in the morning and below the range of 98.6° F to 99.0° F during the day, along with a resting pulse of less than 85 beats per minute, may indicate hypothyroidism.

There are no accurate figures, but I believe that mild to severe hypothyroidism is a modern epidemic, not only among humans, but also among animals. Radiation is probably the greatest environmental cause of hypothyroidism and other thyroid problems, including tumors and thyroid cancer. Many radiogenic symptoms stem from damage to the thyroid that comes from radioactive iodine.

Other causes of hypothyroidism include:

■ Estrogen dominance (an excess of estrogen in relation to progesterone). Estrogen dominance inhibits thyroid function and can result from taking birth control pills, estrogen replacement therapy (ERT), or herbal estrogens such as black cohosh or sage, or exposure to environmental estrogens (see "A Glossary of Hormones"), such as pesticides, which mimic estrogen.

■ Synthetic and genetically engineered hormones (estrogen and others) in meat, dairy products, poultry, and eggs.

■ Excess intake of unsaturated fats (oils liquid at room temperature, excluding extra virgin olive oil), such as soybean, safflower, canola, corn, fish, flaxseed, borage, and evening primrose.[1]

■ Fluoride, common in water, foods, and toothpaste.[2]

■ Excess iodine. Most Americans get too much iodine, which in excess is a powerful thyroid inhibitor, because, besides being added to commercial salt, it is also used as a dough conditioner in baked goods, and is present in many supplements such as kelp.

■ Mercury, a toxic heavy metal, which comprises up to 50% of "silver" amalgam fillings. It poisons an enzyme critical in converting the inactive form of thyroid hormone (T4) into the active form (T3).[3]

■ Raw cruciferous vegetables (raw cabbage, broccoli, or cauliflower) which contain thyroid inhibitors; lightly steaming them kills these thyroid-suppressing substances.

■ Liver. While a nourishing food, it does contain thyroid inhibitors.

■ Soy products. There is some evidence that soy affects thyroid function.[4]

EDITOR'S NOTE

The position on unsaturated fats presented here is a controversial one. Many physicians advocate the dietary use and supplementation of essential fatty acids in the form of fish, primrose, borage, and flaxseed oils, among others, in the unsaturated category. There is research to support both positions.

■ Endurance exercise. Exercise accelerates the breakdown of thyroid hormones which results in a protective slowing of metabolism. This is why endurance athletes, such as long-distance runners, have a slow pulse rate and lower-than-average body temperature. The condition self-corrects when exercise is lessened.

Signs and Symptoms of Hypothyroidism
The following are indicators of low thyroid function:

Increased Cholesterol—Cholesterol rises because there is inadequate thyroid hormone to convert it to bile salts and the anti-aging hormones mentioned above. Many of the far-reaching effects of hypothyroidism result from a deficiency in these substances because of their importance in preventing cancer, heart disease, obesity, memory loss, and other conditions associated with aging.

Decreased Blood Sugar, Increased Adrenaline, and Cortisol—Glucose is required to convert T4 thyroid hormone into the active T3. This occurs mainly in the liver, if glucose is adequate, since glucose activates the enzymes that carry out the conversion. If T4 isn't converted, for whatever reason—stress, radiation, environmental toxins, estrogen dominance, a low-protein diet, or liver problems—T3 levels decrease and sugar is burned inefficiently, converting to lactic acid instead of easily eliminated carbon dioxide. So, the body gets less energy from the same amount of glucose. When the liver runs out of its stored sugar reserves, it stops converting T4 to T3.

The overall effect of this is low blood sugar, leading to increased adrenaline to compensate for the deficiency of energy, glucose, and oxygen. Low-thyroid patients excrete 10% to 40% more than the normal amounts of urinary adrenaline metabolites.[5]

At first, adrenaline attempts to mobilize glycogen (the form in which the body stores carbohydrates to be converted into glucose as needed) and stored fat. Then progesterone is converted to cortisol (adrenocortical hormone with similar physiological effects to cortisone) in the adrenal gland by a complex pathway involving a certain hormone which is released in response to adrenaline. Cortisol increases blood sugar via the breakdown of protein. Increased cortisol will decrease adrenaline and lead to a low pulse, common in hypothyroid people. But if the adrenal glands become exhausted and cannot produce enough cortisol, adrenaline will rise.

Sometimes people with hypothyroidism have a high pulse (greater than 100 and often 120 to 150) due to excess adrenaline. This is not as common as the low-pulse form. The production of cortisol is a life-saving response to stress, but in the hypothyroid person, it occurs abnormally in an attempt to keep the blood sugar up. Cortisol, like estrogen, inhibits the thyroid, creating a vicious cycle that can only be broken by proper hormonal balancing, such as thyroid therapy, and by opposing cortisone and/or estrogen with progesterone.

Heart Disease—Adrenaline (and its synthetic drug mimics, such as those used to treat asthma) is toxic when produced continuously in response to the stress of hypothyroidism or endurance exercise. Excess adrenaline is harmful to the heart because it damages heart mitochondria (the cell's energy factories) and causes chronic degeneration of the aorta (the main arterial trunk).

Cancer—According to Broda Barnes, M.D., a pioneering researcher in hypothyroidism, cancer risk increases in hypothyroid patients, both male and female.[6] This is directly related to increased production of estrogen and decreased production of the primary anti-aging steroids from cholesterol: pregnenolone, progesterone and DHEA. As noted previously, the anti-aging steroids cannot be made without adequate thyroid hormone and adequate cholesterol.

Blood Pressure Problems, Poor Circulation, Edema—The hypothyroid person can have high or low blood pressure, depending on the organ affected. If the adrenals are overly active, high blood pressure can result, but as the adrenals become exhausted, the blood pressure will drop below normal. Thyroid hormone will improve circulation, lower or raise blood pressure to normal, and increase blood glucose to normal. People with high adrenaline levels and high blood pressure should increase their thyroid dosage very slowly, because thyroid hormone makes the tissues sensitive to excess adrenaline and this can cause an increased pulse, an elevation in blood pressure, and sometimes a panic attack. Gradually, however, the adrenal glands stop overproducing adrenaline and blood pressure normalizes.

Another important factor in normalizing blood pressure and reversing edema (water retention and swelling) is adequate intake of noniodized sea salt. Intake of sea salt is inversely proportional to high blood pressure. Hypothyroid people cannot hold sodium, and inadequate sodium causes edema. Yet, many people believe that salt is bad, avoid it, become bloated, and then take diuretics.[7]

Hypothyroidism can lead to hypoxia (low tissue oxygen) and edema. People with hypothyroidism often complain of cold hands or feet, report

There are no accurate figures, but I believe that mild to severe hypothyroidism is a modern epidemic, not only among humans, but also among animals. Radiation is probably the greatest environmental cause of hypothyroidism and other thyroid problems, including tumors and thyroid cancer.

that their hands and feet "go to sleep" easily, and have poor circulation. Edema is involved in carpal tunnel syndrome (impingement on nerves in the wrist producing tingling or pain), in glaucoma, and in Grave's disease (in which the muscles behind the eyes swell). All of these problems can be relieved by the thyroid-dependent, anti-edema hormones, pregnenolone or progesterone, and proper thyroid therapy to correct the imbalance.

Colon Problems—Constipation is common among hypothyroid people, who have low intestinal tone. If not corrected, constipation leads to a toxic colon and serious conditions, such as chronic or acute appendicitis and, worse, colon cancer. Other colon conditions, such as colitis and irritable bowel syndrome, are also associated with hypothyroidism. Thyroid therapy will increase intestinal tone until the colon unloads the excess feces. Until this happens, some low thyroid people will wake up with a stuffy nose and sometimes a headache. A hypothyroid person can produce a similar response just by eating raw carrots, which stimulate the intestines.

Depression and Emotional Problems—Depression is a classic symptom of hypothyroidism. In women, this can lead to severe postpartum depression (following childbirth). Depression and other mental and emotional symptoms of hypothyroidism are sometimes present without any apparent physical symptoms.

Insomnia, Hyperactivity, and Fatigue—How can a hypothyroid person be tired, hyperactive, and have insomnia all at the same time? These symptoms do coexist in many hypothyroid people and may be remediated with thyroid therapy. In one study of 49 individuals diagnosed with hypothyroidism, 61% also were diagnosed with hyperactivity/attention deficit disorder (ADD).[8]

Thyroid hormone is essential for providing the necessary glucose to the brain and the body. When thyroid hormone is deficient, the nerves require abnormal stimulants to function or the body produces excess adrenaline to keep itself going. The result is that we get tired and tense at the same time—it's like drinking too much coffee. Instead of using Ritalin, caffeine, or other stimulants to raise the energy level of the brain, it makes more sense to correct the cause of the energy deficit—inadequate thyroid hormone.

When energy production is slowed due to lack of thyroid hormone, muscles tend to tire or cramp easily and to swell after exercise. Like the brain, all muscles need to restore their energy in order to relax. Whether it's leg cramps or brain fatigue, increasing the rate of energy production makes relaxation (and sleep) possible.

Many hypothyroid people report that they wake up exhausted, even after eight to ten hours of sleep. This is because a hypothyroid person can never go beyond stage II sleep; for adequate sleep, stage IV (deep sleep) must be reached. Thyroid therapy promotes deep sleep.

Weight Gain or Loss—Weight gain or inability to lose weight are common symptoms of hypothyroidism, but some hypothyroid people are underweight and even anorexic. In fact, most of the "weight" in the hypothyroid person is water, not fat.

Skin/Hair Problems—Many skin problems are associated with or aggravated by inadequate thyroid function. The most common symptom is dry skin. Many, but not all, people who suffer from acne, eczema, or psoriasis are relieved on thyroid therapy. Hair loss is also common among hypothyroid people, especially women after childbearing and women who diet frequently. In addition, low thyroid women tend to have abnormal facial hair (hirsutism) on the chin and above the upper lip. Abnormal facial hair in women is just one result of low thyroid, low progesterone, and excess adrenaline. These problems can be solved by hormonal balancing.

Headaches—Headaches, of course, have many causes; here we emphasize the thyroid/headache connection. There are two major causes of the hypothyroid headache. One is the "estrogen headache," common in estrogen-dominant hypothyroid women at ovulation or during menses. The second is the "colon headache," common in low thyroid people with a toxic colon. Most hypothyroid people are constipated, but hypothyroid people who are also severely sugar intolerant can have normal bowel function or even diarrhea, due to the sugar intolerance. Either of these types can get a "colon headache."

Immune Deficiency and Chronic Infections—Adequate thyroid hormone is required for proper immune system functioning. Hypothyroid people often have a low white blood cell count which is an indicator of a sup-

Thyroid hormone is essential for providing the necessary glucose to the brain and the body. When thyroid hormone is deficient, the nerves require abnormal stimulants to function or the body produces excess adrenaline to keep itself going. The result is that we get tired and tense at the same time—it's like drinking too much coffee.

pressed immune system.

Therefore, it is not surprising that hypothyroid people are subject to chronic infections, including frequent colds, respiratory infections, bronchitis, pneumonia, chronic sore throats, sinusitis, recurrent otitis media (middle-ear infection), tonsillitis, and recurrent bladder infections. Chronic fatigue syndrome, with its long list of viruses and other infections, may be an expression of low thyroid function.[9]

Multiple Sclerosis (MS)—The relationship between heavy metal poisoning and MS is probably more widely known than the relationship between MS and low thyroid function. Raymond Peat, Ph.D., explains the link as follows: certain cells, called oligodendrocytes, are responsible for creating the myelin sheath that covers nerve fibers and for producing pregnenolone. In MS, these cells appear to stop functioning. The clustering of these cells around deteriorating nerve cells may be an attempt to provide pregnenolone to the injured cells. Both pregnenolone and its end-product hormone, progesterone, protect against nerve damage by other substances, such as the excitotoxic amino acids glutamate (found in the condiment monosodium glutamate) and aspartate (found in NutraSweet™).

Hypothyroidism may go unrecognized in patients with MS symptoms who aren't overweight, lethargic, or severely disabled. Thyroid therapy can cause the MS symptoms to disappear in those patients who have no other obvious problems, such as heavy metal poisoning.[10]

Mitral Valve Prolapse—Common in chronic hypothyroidism, a mitral valve prolapse (also called floppy valve syndrome) is when the valve between the upper and lower chambers of the heart becomes floppy, disturbing normal blood flow. Thyroid-deficient women with PMS may have a premenstrual mitral valve heart murmur which is not present at other times of the month. Thyroid therapy can relieve both PMS and the mitral valve prolapse.[11]

Joint Pains– Joint pains, often diagnosed as arthritis, may be caused by a sluggish thyroid. In thyroid-deficient children, aching legs or calves, more noticeable after exercise, are often passed off as "growing pains." In fact, this can be a temporary exercise-induced hypothyroid edema of the leg muscles. In more severe cases, the cartilage in the joints swell, causing a knock-kneed appearance.

Women's Health Problems–Problems including infertility, miscarriage, fibrocystic breast disease, ovarian fibroids, cystic ovaries, endometriosis, PMS, and menopausal symptoms are usually caused or aggravated by hypothyroidism coupled with estrogen dominance. A relative excess of estrogen can occur with a normal estrogen level if progesterone is low, or with normal progesterone if the estrogen is high. Estrogen inhibits thyroid secretion; progesterone stimulates it.

Guidelines to Help Thyroid Function

Enzyme therapy, supplementation with thyroid glandular extracts (SEE QUICK DEFINITION), herbal remedies, hormonal balancing through the use of natural progesterone, and dietary changes can be integral parts of a treatment program for hypothyroidism.

Enzyme Therapy–Since the endocrine glands (SEE QUICK DEFINITION) are driven by digested food, my first effort in a treatment program is to correct digestive problems with food enzymes and to emphasize an organic, whole foods diet. When the organs are nourished with digested whole foods, many problems are ameliorated. Patients may find that they need lower doses of whatever drugs they are taking, including their thyroid medication. This is simply due to increased performance following organ nourishment.

Thyroid Support–For clients who do need additional thyroid therapy, whole food derivatives—whole bovine glandular extract—are preferable rather than synthetic thyroid hormones, because the glandulars contain the protein precursors to both thyroid hormones in a natural proportion of T4 to T3. Synthroid, a synthetic thyroid medication, is an ineffective form of thyroid therapy because it contains only thyroxine (T4).

For strict vegans who refuse bovine thyroid glandular, I

A **glandular extract** is a purified nutritional and therapeutic product derived from one of several animal glands including the adrenal, thymus, thyroid, ovaries, testes, pancreas, pineal, and pituitary. It is prescribed by a physician for a person whose corresponding gland is underfunctioning and not producing enough of its own hormone. The various glands are part of the endocrine system which, along with the nervous system, coordinates the functioning of all of the body's systems.

Endocrine glands, including the testicles, ovaries, pancreas, adrenals, thyroid, parathyroid, and pituitary, are central to the regulation and normalization of all the body's complex, interconnected systems, from metabolism and heat production to spermatogenesis and uterine preparations for pregnancy.

For information on **the oral temperature and resting pulse tests**, see Chapter 2: Diagnosing Enzyme Deficiencies, pp. 32-33.

recommend Proloid, a prescription drug which contains both T4 and T3. It is preferable to take the natural glandular extract, but Proloid will work and is much better than Synthroid.

In addition, patients need to consider the causes of hypothyroidism as enumerated above and work to eliminate or curtail as many of them as possible.

How to Use Thyroid Glandular Extract—Many people say that they have tried taking a thyroid glandular extract and it did not help them. They may have had an ineffective product or they may not have followed the instructions closely enough.

The following is general information (see Caution) that I typically provide to my clients on how to take thyroid glandular: Start with ¼ grain to one grain per day with food. Whatever dosage you take, divide it and take one portion with each meal. Monitor your oral temperature in the morning before arising; repeat at around noon and also take your resting pulse. Women should do the temperature test when they are sure they are not ovulating. Your oral temperature should be 98° F when rising and should go up to 98.6° F to 99° F between 11 a.m. and 3 p.m. Your resting pulse should be 85 beats per minute. The pulse and oral temperature should be at their optimum about 30 minutes after eating.

Slowly increase your dosage of glandular extract, by ¼ grain to one grain per day until you are feeling well and your oral temperatures and resting pulse are normal. Remember to divide your dosage of thyroid and take it with food throughout the day. The reason I give a varied dosage is that some people, especially those with a toxic colon, high blood pressure, or excess adrenaline, can have side effects if they increase their dosage too rapidly. This is not due to thyroid hormone but to the person's toxic condition or excess adrenaline.

The two major side effects of increasing your thyroid dose too fast are a transient racing pulse and headaches. The racing pulse is due to excess adrenaline. Thyroid hormone makes your tissues sensitive to adrenaline and, as this stabilizes, the adrenal glands will calm down and stop overproducing it. If you have a tendency for panic attacks, be careful, because increasing sensitivity to adrenaline can trigger a panic attack. If you feel your pulse racing or your heart beating, keep in mind that this is not a dangerous condition unless your pulse goes over 180 and you have high blood pressure. Most low thyroid people have simply never felt their heart beat.

If you do experience a racing pulse due to excess adrenaline, eat protein, salty snacks, and drink organic fruit juices, especially orange juice and tropical juices, to which ¼ tsp of organic noniodized sea salt has been added. This will raise your blood sugar and calm your adrenal glands in about 30 minutes. Adequate magnesium (found in fruit juice) is also important. In addition, an Epsom salt bath will increase body stores of magnesium. Use half a cup of Epsom salts in a tub of hot water and soak for 20 minutes. Finally, the herb stevia will help stabilize blood sugar and calm the adrenals.

As for headaches, thyroid affects circulation and the colon in a therapeutic way. A headache can be caused by either a transient change in blood pressure or a toxic colon. In either case, you may stop the thyroid therapy until the headache is gone. If you are getting colon headaches (more common than the blood pressure headaches), the best food to eat is raw carrots. Raw carrot fiber is one of the best colon cleansers available; it binds toxins and carcinogens, and helps relieve constipation. Some people are so toxic that even raw carrots will give them a morning headache. These people must just wait until the carrots have done their cleansing job.

The following is a good test to see if you're taking too much or too little thyroid extract: Take your oral temperature and pulse. If both are above normal, this indicates that you are taking too much thyroid glandular and have become hyperthyroid. If so, simply decrease your dosage and eat raw cabbage and cooked liver (both contain thyroid inhibitors and will slow down thyroid function). If both your oral temperatures in the morning and at noon and your resting pulse are low, you are not taking enough glandular extract. Also, if your oral temperatures are low, but your pulse is racing (above 90 beats per minute), the high pulse rate is due to adrenaline and you are still hypothyroid. Again, drink a glass of fruit juice with ¼ teaspoon of sea salt. The adrenaline rush is temporary and is a sign of healing.

In self-administration of thyroid glandular therapy, some people increase their dosage too fast or not fast enough, and they don't get well. Thyroid glandulars are not dangerous, but if not taken according to instructions, they can have unpleasant side effects such as a headache or a racing pulse. Thyroid therapy is therefore best undertaken with the guidance of a qualified health practitioner.

Herbal Remedies—There is almost always a plant equivalent to a human hormone. For example, the estrogen in yeast is chemically equivalent to the estrogen produced by the human body. I have been looking for plant analogs of thyroid glandular for my vegan clients. An herb which may meet this requirement is called *gugulipid*, an Ayurvedic herb that has been used in India for over 2,500 years. The second herb is *Coleus forskohlii*, which has been shown to increase thyroid hormone production as well as stimulate thyroid hormone release. However, I have never observed that these herbs, working alone, can correct a low thyroid function.

If you do experience a racing pulse due to excess adrenaline, eat protein, salty snacks, and drink organic fruit juices, especially orange juice and tropical juices, to which ¼ tsp of organic noniodized sea salt has been added. This will raise your blood sugar and calm your adrenal glands in about 30 minutes.

Hormonal Balancing—In addition to thyroid glandular therapy, natural progesterone therapy is also crucial for women, since it stimulates the thyroid to secrete hormones. Progesterone also opposes the toxic effects of estrogen and is a powerful immune system stimulant. I use progesterone in hypothyroid/estrogen-dominant women with PMS symptoms and other female problems, including breast pathology or uterine fibroids. In hypothyroid men, pregnenolone is preferred to progesterone because progesterone inhibits testosterone. Young men, in particular, may feel reduced libido and experience reduced facial hair growth if they take progesterone.

Dietary Recommendations—The following are important dietary elements to support your thyroid:

■ Adequate protein: organic beef or poultry; some kinds of fish, such as halibut and white fish; organic eggs; organic and especially raw milk or cultured milk products, such as kefir, yogurt, and cottage cheese. Vegans should eat lots of potatoes, which are a good source of protein.

■ Fruits or fruit juices: to help modulate blood sugar and calm the adrenal glands and to stimulate increased production of thyroid hormone. Also, fruit juice provides an important source of calcium and magnesium.

■ Salt: to mobilize glucose and calm the adrenal glands. A salty snack before bed will help induce sleep. Don't buy iodized salt—look for either organic sea salt or purified seawater with no added iodine. This is salt from the sea which contains, in addition to sodium chloride, all of the naturally occurring minerals plus 42 trace minerals.

■ Coconut oil: probably the most healthy saturated fat, other than raw butter. Coconut oil stimulates thyroid function and thus promotes weight loss in those who are overweight, and has all the anti-aging and anticancer effects of thyroid-stimulating foods.

■ Carrots: the fiber tones the bowel, binds toxins (including carcinogens), reduces the reabsorption of estrogen, and lowers cholesterol, if it is high.

The Anti-Aging Steroids

Following is a brief description of each of the anti-aging steroidal hormones, pregnenolone, progesterone, and DHEA, illustrating their importance to health and why it is dangerous to take drugs that artificially inhibit cholesterol formation (necessary for the production of these hormones) in the body.[12]

Pregnenolone

The need for supplemental pregnenolone increases as we age. In fact, the older and/or sicker you are, the more likely you are to feel an effect from taking pregnenolone. In a healthy person, the conversion of cholesterol to pregnenolone occurs inside the mitochondria, called "the lungs of the cell" because of their role in cell respiration. Once produced, pregnenolone leaves the mitochondria. Both natural progesterone and pregnenolone stimulate their own synthesis so that if you take them supplementally, the body's ability to synthesize them is not suppressed. Enzymes convert pregnenolone into either progesterone or DHEA, depending on the tissue and the need.

In addition to pregnenolone's ability to repair enzymes, the following are some of its anti-aging functions:

■ Impaired memory restoration: pregnenolone may help restore impaired memory, according to neurobiologist Eugene Roberts of the City of Hope Medical Center in Los Angeles, California, and his colleagues. In the March 1992 *Proceedings of the National Academy of Sciences*, these researchers reported that pregnenolone is several hundred times more potent than any memory enhancer that had been tested before. Their report stated that pregnenolone restores normal levels of memory hormones which decline during aging.

■ Protection from cortisone toxicity: the classic effects of toxic levels of cortisol include daytime euphoria, insomnia plus hot flashes at night, osteoporosis, brain aging, seizures, atrophy of the skin plus other signs of premature aging, and adrenal atrophy. Two injections of cortisone can destroy the beta cells of the pancreas in dogs, causing diabetes. A stress-induced elevation in cortisol or taking cortisone can cause diabetes in people as well. Pregnenolone can be used to withdraw from cortisone therapy over a period of a month or so without developing Addison's disease symptoms (from adrenal atrophy) because of its normalizing effects on the adrenal gland. In women, progesterone therapy may also be indicated.

■ Relief of anxiety and panic attacks: a deficiency of pregnenolone activates substances called endozepines which trigger anxiety and panic

There is some controversy about how progesterone is absorbed. Most authorities say that progesterone is best absorbed transdermally. However, progesterone, in my experience, is best absorbed orally, next vaginally, and third transdermally (anywhere on the skin).

attacks. Taking pregnenolone prevents the secretion of endozepine and is a safe and natural substitute for toxic drugs such as Xanax and Valium. The usual dose of pregnenolone is about 100 mg to 150 mg daily (about the size of a small pea, or a pinch on the end of a butter knife). However, severely anxious people may need ¼ teaspoon the first day.

■ Reduced exophthalmia (bulging eyes) in Graves' disease patients: in the 1950s, pregnenolone was tested on patients with exophthalmia from Graves' disease. It was reported that their eyes quickly receded to a more normal position in their sockets.

Progesterone

Women should have ten times more progesterone than estrogen, or a ten-to-one ratio. The lower the ratio of progesterone to estrogen, the more health problems a woman is likely to encounter. These include: PMS, cyclic seizures and/or estrogen headache (at ovulation and menses), breast, uterine, and ovarian pathology (fibrocystic breast disease, uterine fibroids, ovarian cysts), spontaneous abortion of the fetus at around the tenth week, osteoporosis, heart disease, gallbladder disease, and cancer of all kinds.

Progesterone opposes or balances estrogen, meaning that it opposes the unhealthy effects of estrogen. The major function of estrogen is cell division during a woman's fertile years, but cells also divide during the growth of cancer. That's why women need progesterone, to protect them from the carcinogenic effects of estrogen; these have been reported in the research literature since 1947.

When I speak of progesterone therapy, I am referring to natural progesterone. Synthetic progesterone (progestin) such as Depo-Provera has severe side effects, including increased risk of cancer and birth defects, and the inhibition of the ovaries' normal production of progesterone. Natural progesterone, on the other hand, stimulates the body's own production, inhibits or prevents cancer, and increases fetal intelligence. Sometimes only a few doses are sufficient to restore the body's ability to produce enough of its own progesterone.

Progesterone aids in controlling seizures, has antitumor properties,

Factors in Steroid Synthesis

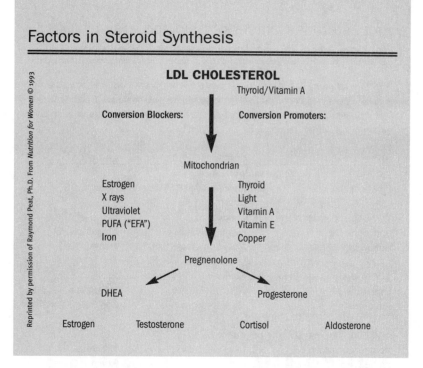

LDL CHOLESTEROL

Thyroid/Vitamin A

Conversion Blockers: Conversion Promoters:

Mitochondrian

Estrogen	Thyroid
X rays	Light
Ultraviolet	Vitamin A
PUFA ("EFA")	Vitamin E
Iron	Copper

Pregnenolone

DHEA   Progesterone

Estrogen   Testosterone   Cortisol   Aldosterone

and helps prevent and reverse osteoporosis, PMS, and menopausal symptoms, without toxic side effects. It also produces the anti-aging benefit of thickening and smoothing aged and atrophied skin by increasing pigment, cell size, and branching. It does not, however, cause healthy, young skin to thicken.[13]

How Progesterone is Absorbed

There is some controversy about how progesterone is absorbed. While many doctors view transdermal absorption as the most effective, I have concluded through research that progesterone is best absorbed orally, next vaginally, and third transdermally (anywhere on the skin).

Dissolved in natural vitamin E oil, progesterone enters the bloodstream almost immediately upon contact with any membrane such as the lips, tongue, or gums. If swallowed, it is absorbed during the digestive process. If eaten along with food, its absorption occurs at the same rate as the digestion and absorption of food. Due to this absorption route through the natural digestive process, progesterone is almost 100% absorbed and is distributed to all tissues.

Not just any fat will dissolve progesterone—only natural vitamin E oil will completely dissolve progesterone for maximum absorption, either

Progesterone Content of Selected Creams/Oils, As Reported By an Independent Laboratory

T he following list of natural progesterone products and their progesterone content was compiled by John Lee, M.D., of Sebastopol, California, based on laboratory tests conducted for him by Aeron LifeCycles in San Leandro, California (reprinted by permission of John R. Lee, M.D.).

PRODUCT	COMPANY	LOCATION
2,000-3,000 mg progesterone per ounce		
Progest-E Complex	Raymond Peat, Ph.D.	Eugene, OR
700-800 mg progesterone per ounce		
ProCreme Plus	Health Products	Manassas, VA
Renewed Balance	American Image Mktg.	Nampa, ID
500-700 mg progesterone per ounce		
Femarone-17	Wise Essentials	Hallendale, FL
Pro-Oste-All	Sarati International	Los Fresnos, TX
400-500 mg progesterone per ounce		
Adam's Equalizer	HM Enterprises	Norcross, GA
Angel Care	Angel Care	Atlanta, GA
Bio Balance	Elan Vitale	Scottsdale, AZ
Edenn Cream	SNM	Norcross, GA
E'Pro & Estrol Balance	Sarati International	Los Fresnos, TX
Equilibrium	Equilibrium Labs	Boca Raton, FL
Fair Lady	Village Market	Fond du Lac, WI
Femarone-17	Wise Essentials	Minneapolis, MN
Fem-Gest	Bio-Nutritional Formulas	Mineola, NY
Feminique	Country Life	Hauppauge, NY
Gentle Changes	Easy Way, Int'l.	Indianapolis, IN
Happy PMS	HM Enterprises	Norcross, GA
Heaven Sent	Answered Prayers, Inc.	Malibu, CA
Kokoro Balance	Kokoro, LLC	Laguna Niguel, CA
NatraGest	Broadmoore Labs	Ventura, CA
Natural Balance	South Market Service	Atlanta, GA
Natural Woman	Products of Nature	Ridgefield, CT
Natural Woman's Formula	Ultra Balance	Savannah, GA
New Woman	Pinnacle Nut, Inc.	Tulsa, OK
Nugest 900	Nutraceutics Corp.	Deerfield Beach, FL
Marpe Wild Yam	Green Pastures	Flat Rock, NC
Osterderm	Bezwecken	Beavertown, OR
PharmWest	PharmWest	Marina Del Ray, CA

PRODUCT	COMPANY	LOCATION
PhytoGest	Karuna	Novato, CA
Pro-Alo	Health Watchers	Scottsdale, AZ
ProBalance	Springboard	Monterey, CA
Progessence	Young Living	Payson, UT
Pro-G	TriMedica	Scottsdale, AZ
Pro-Gest	Transitions for Health	Portland, OR
Progest-DP	Life Enhancement	Petaluma, CA
Progonal	Bezwecken	Beaverton, OR
Serenity	Health & Science	Crawfordville, FL
Ultimate Total Woman	New Science Nutrition	N. Lauderdale, FL
Wild Yam Cream	Enrich, International	Orem, UT
10-20 mg progesterone per ounce		
Endocreme	Wuliton Labs	Palmyra, MO
EFX Wild Yam	Natural Efx, Inc.	Richardson, TX
Life Changes	MW Labs	Atlanta, GA
Novagest	Strata Dermatologics	Concord, CA
Nugestrone	Nutraceuticals	Boca Raton, FL
Phyto-Balance	Transitions for Health	Portland, OR
Progesterone Plus	Prof. Health Products	Sewickley, PA
Woman Wise	Jason Natural Cosmetics	Culver City, CA
Less than 5 mg progesterone per ounce		
Born Again	Alvin Last, Inc.	Yonkers, NY
Dioscorea Cream	Saroyal Int'l., Inc.	Toronto, Canada
Nutrigest	NutriSupplies, Inc.	West Palm Beach, FL
Progerone	Nature's Nutrition	Vero Beach, FL
Progestone 10	Dixie Health, Inc.	Atlanta, GA
Progestone-HP	Dixie Health, Inc.	Atlanta, GA
Yamcon	Phillips Nutrition	Laguna Hills, CA

orally or transdermally. Most formulas are suspensions of progesterone crystals in some kind of fat, such as corn oil or synthetic vitamin E. The undissolved progesterone is wasted. If the powdered form is taken, it cycles through the liver several times and then back through the blood and out the kidneys. This is a major reason why some women do not get the relief that they need from progesterone. They simply are not absorbing enough of it.

There are dozens of creams that claim to contain progesterone (see "Progesterone Content of Selected Creams/Oils," pp. 258-259). Most of them contain inadequate amounts of progesterone—not enough, in my experience, to effectively remediate female problems or relieve pain. Many contain wild yam (*Dioscorea villosa*) and claim that this is a source of

Comparison of Progesterone and Estrogen

Women who have an excess of estrogen relative to progesterone are estrogen dominant. Below are the symptoms and health effects associated with estrogen dominance, and the beneficial effects exerted by natural progesterone.[14] The benefits of progesterone do not apply to synthetic progesterone (progestin), which is carcinogenic, inhibits the natural production of progesterone, and causes birth defects.

Estrogen means all natural forms (estriol, estradiol, and estrone), synthetic forms (Premarin, oral contraceptives), phytoestrogens (black cohosh, sage, pennyroyal), and environmental estrogens (e.g., pesticides). Estrogen dominance can result from excess of any of these forms; some produce dominance faster than others.

Natural Progesterone	Estrogen Dominance
Prevents PMS, normalizes menses	Causes PMS, excessive bleeding, irregular or painful menses
Prevents/stops seizures regardless of cause	Causes seizures, especially at ovulation and menses
Antitumor, anticancer, anti-aging hormone	Carcinogenic
Prevents and cures fibrocystic breast disease	Causes fibrocystic breast disease
Increases fertility, protects fetus from abortion, when taken during pregnancy, it increases fetal intelligence	Causes spontaneous abortion of fetus around the 9th or 10th week of pregnancy (abortifacient)
Cardioprotective	Cardiotoxic
Improves brain structure and function, including memory	Inhibits memory, causes migraines
Decreases during menopause more than estrogen	Menopausal symptoms caused by estrogen damage to the pituitary gland
Prevents edema (fluid retention)	Causes edema
Increases body supply of oxygen, prevents hypoxia	Causes oxygen deprivation (hypoxia)
Decreases fat storage (oxidizes fat)	Increases fat storage
Anti-aging to skin. Makes aged, atrophied skin thicker, more regular. Increases pigment, cell size, and branching, but doesn't cause young healthy skin to thicken.	Causes aging of skin, makes skin thinner (skin atrophy) extending to pigment cells, decreases cell size, and eliminates dendritic branches.
Prevents age spots	Causes age spots
Prevents and reverses bone loss	Causes osteoporosis, rheumatoid arthritis, and other degenerative diseases
A factor in preventing gallbladder disease, especially in women	A causal factor in gallbladder disease, especially in women
Improves circulation	Causes blood clots and strokes
Shrinks fibroids, prevents/cures ovarian cysts	

progesterone. It is not—the body cannot convert wild yam to progesterone.[15]

How to Use Progesterone Oil or Cream

To use 10% progesterone oil, I typically recommend putting three drops on your finger and rubbing it on your gums. Three drops contain about 10 mg of progesterone. In severe cases (such as osteoporosis, severe cramps, heavy bleeding, breast or uterine pathology, hot flashes, and immune system problems), I typically recommend one drop every two hours, or five times a day for ten days or until well, and then reduce the dosage. The usual maintenance dose is three drops daily. The minimum dose for a healthy woman with no symptoms of female problems is three drops daily from mid-cycle to menses. Topical progesterone cream (3%) can be used to relieve pain anywhere as well as to lubricate the vaginal tissues, an important substance for women who experience painful intercourse. Along with the enzyme formula Chirozyme Rbs, it can also help repair sun damage.

DHEA

A number of studies have shown that DHEA has important effects on health, including possible roles in preventing breast cancer and obesity, while increasing youthful appearance.[16] One study of 242 men, 50 to 79 years old, reported that the DHEA levels in those who died were only one-third that of the survivors.[17]

DHEA can also have beneficial effects on libido. In men who have decreased testosterone production resulting in lowered libido, DHEA, which can convert to testosterone, can boost libido almost as well as testosterone. In addition, topical DHEA as well as topical progesterone can stop the pain of arthritis and other inflammatory conditions.

Dr. Peat advises a dosage of no more than 2 mg to 3 mg of DHEA for anyone other than an elderly, sick person, who can take 12 mg to 15 mg daily, but even then, not without pregnenolone, progesterone, and thyroid glandular. Since pregnenolone converts to both progesterone and DHEA, supplemental pregnenolone is a safer therapy.

CAUTION

In the wrong hormonal environment—low progesterone and/or low thyroid hormones—DHEA can convert to estrogen and testosterone. In women with cystic ovaries or cancer, DHEA can convert to estrogen. If you do take DHEA, you should know that at the peak of youth, between the ages of 20 and 30, the body produces 12 mg to 15 mg of DHEA daily. So, taking 25 mg to 200 mg daily is far greater than the physiological dosage and, in fact, can cause problems, such as liver enlargement. DHEA may also modify brain cells into the type associated with inflammation. Other research has shown that in some breast cancer cells in a low-estrogen environment, DHEA can convert to estrogen and stimulate tumor growth.

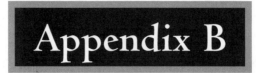

Appendix B

THERA-ZYME ENZYME FORMULAS

In the early 1980s, Howard Loomis, D.C., formulated his first line of enzymes called NESS (Nutritional Enzyme Support System), which was introduced in 1987. Over the past ten years, Loomis' research has led to Thera-zyme, his second generation line of enzymes. The following describes the Thera-zyme line, which is available to professional health practitioners from 21st Century Nutrition. These formulas have a counterpart in 21st Century's line of enzymes called Enzyme Solutions, which is available to the consumer.

In my experience, there are two unique qualities in the Loomis line of enzymes. First, these formulas nourish organs or tissues that are being negatively affected by subluxations (misalignments of vertebrae). Each formula corresponds to possible subluxations of several vertebrae. For example, there is a formula for stomach problems, Thera-zyme T5-T9 Stm, which is a multiple digestive enzyme formulated to nourish the mucosal tissues of the stomach disturbed by subluxations of the mid-thoracic spine (midback, between the fifth and the ninth thoracic vertebrae). If you have gastric problems (such as burning, an ulcer, hiatal hernia, or gastritis), you are likely to need a chiropractic adjustment of one of these thoracic vertebrae. Taking Thera-zyme T5-T9 Stm helps your body hold the adjustment. Formulas with no vertebrae listed are intended for the entire body, such as Thera-zyme TRMA for soft tissue trauma and Thera-zyme CLM for the nervous system.

The second unique quality in this line of enzymes is that all formulas have a pH (acid-alkaline) balancing system (designated pHBS on the label) which was designed to enhance the absorption and assimilation of the nutrients in the formula.

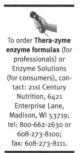

To order **Thera-zyme enzyme formulas** (for professionals) or Enzyme Solutions (for consumers), contact: 21st Century Nutrition, 6421 Enterprise Lane, Madison, WI 53719; tel: 800-662-2630 or 608-273-8100; fax: 608-273-8111.

You will note that there are several formulas which help relieve the same or similar conditions. This is because a condition or a symptom can have more than one cause and thus requires more than one remedy. For example, insomnia can be caused by restless legs due to calcium deficiency (Thera-zyme Para), muscle tension

(Thera-zyme MSCLR), sugar intolerance (Thera-zyme Adr), nervous or emotional problems (Thera-zyme CLM), or the inability to relax, become serene, and stop the mind from racing (Thera-zyme SvG).

If testing (see Chapter 2: Diagnosing Enzymes Deficiencies) reveals that you need one of the Thera-zyme formulas, you probably have at least one symptom on the list of those associated with the formula. However, from experience, I have learned that these formulas can relieve conditions not included on the list. Some of these discoveries are supplied by patients. For example, a client asked me for Thera-zyme SmI to help relieve a skin fungus. I told him that this formula was for candidiasis and would probably not help his skin. I was wrong. As soon as he took the formula, the skin fungus disappeared. When he discontinued it, the fungus returned.

The following list of Thera-zyme enzyme formulas and their applications was compiled from Loomis' research and my clinical experience. I have listed the contents of each Thera-zyme formula and symptoms that may be relieved simply by supplying the organ or tissue with the deficient enzymes or nutrients. The proportion of the primary enzymes (protease, lipase, amylase, and the disaccharidases sucrase, lactase, and maltase) in a given formula is directly related to the amount of protein, fat, carbohydrate, and sugars contained in the food or herb used in the formulation. In addition, some of these formulas contain catalase, an antioxidant enzyme that also reduces abnormal tissue fluids, such as edema following injury.

For those who prefer self-care, I have noted the comparable Enzyme and Herbal Formulas from the Enzyme Solutions line.

Please note: By symptom, I mean a condition felt by the client, such as headache, fatigue, or nausea, which cannot be measured by medical tests. By sign, I mean a condition which can be measured, such as high blood pressure, high blood sugar, and proteinuria (spilling protein into the urine). An undernourished or enzyme-deficient organ will develop symptoms long before the doctor can measure the condition by medical signs. When the organ becomes nourished, often the symptom goes away and never develops into pathology.

Multiple Digestive Formulas

Thera-zyme T4-T8 Bil (Biliary) or Enzyme & Herbal Formula #1

Contains the enzymes protease, amylase, lipase, and disaccharidases, plus fennel seeds, turmeric root, lecithin, cinnamon bark, and ginger root. Multiple digestive enzyme for people who are fat and protein intolerant.

Symptoms and signs: intolerant of fat and spicy foods; loss of appetite, especially for meat; burping or pain under the left rib cage, or nausea and/or vomiting after eating; frequent sour taste in mouth; gallstones or gallbladder surgery; frequent constipation with light colored stools.

Contraindication: gastric problems (ulcer, gastritis, hiatal hernia, frequent use of antacids or anti-inflammatory drugs).

Thera-zyme DGST (Digest)
or Enzyme & Herbal Formula #30

Contains the enzymes protease, amylase, lipase, and disaccharidases. A multiple digestive formula for mild digestive problems or colic in babies.

Symptoms and signs: mild digestive problems when unaware of the cause, flatulence, bloating, colicky abdominal pain, including colic in babies sometimes accompanied by projectile vomiting.

Thera-zyme HCL
or Enzyme & Herbal Formula #32

Contains protease, lipase, amylase, disaccharidases, invertase, pepsin, and betaine from beet root powder; contains no hydrochloric acid. A multiple digestive enzyme formula for both fat and sugar intolerance. For severe gluten intolerance, add Thera-zyme PAN; for severe lactose intolerance, add Thera-zyme LAC.

Thera-zyme LAC
or Enzyme & Herbal Formula #34

Contains lactase (as does PAN). May be needed in addition to PAN in severe cases of lactose intolerance.

Thera-zyme T5-T9 PAN (Pancreas)
or Enzyme & Herbal Formula #14

Contains enzymes only; protease, amylase, lipase, and disaccharidases. A multiple digestive enzyme formula for sugar and/or gluten intolerance. Sugar intolerance includes sucrose (white sugar), lactose (milk sugar), and maltose (grain sugar). Sugar-intolerant people may also need Thera-zyme T1-T2 SvG and/or Thera-zyme T9-T10 Adr.

Symptoms and signs: abdominal discomfort under left rib cage after eating; sensitive to air pollutants (perfumes, smoke, etc.); craving for cold liquids and foods; diarrhea worsened by eating sugar; history of asthma or bronchitis.

Thera-zyme T5-T9 Stm (Stomach) or Enzyme & Herbal Formula #12

Contains lipase, amylase, and cellulase, plus papaya leaf, marshmallow root, slippery elm bark, aloe vera, stomach intrinsic factor, vitamin B12, and folic acid. Formula for gastric problems; contains no protease.

Symptoms and signs: ulcers, gastritis, or hiatal hernia; frequent heartburn or indigestion with nausea and/or pain; acid rebound after eating (esophageal reflux); frequent use of antacids; stomach pain, nausea, or burning relieved by eating.

Thera-zyme VSCLR (Vascular) or Enzyme & Herbal Formula #2

Contains the enzymes protease, amylase, lipase (formula highest in lipase), plus the following herbs: bilberry extract, fenugreek seeds, *Ginkgo biloba* leaf, and dandelion root. For problems involving the cardiovascular system.

Symptoms and signs: diabetes; high cholesterol and/or triglycerides; high blood pressure and use of anti-hypertensive drugs; dizziness or light-headedness aggravated by movement; headaches on the side of the head and temples; obese or difficulty losing weight; history of varicose veins; fat-soluble vitamin deficiencies.

Formulas for Chronic or Acute Conditions

Thera-zyme T9-T10 Adr (Adrenal) or Enzyme & Herbal Formula #13

Contains the enzymes protease, amylase, lipase, and disaccharidases, brewer's yeast, Siberian ginseng root, gotu kola, rosehips, and *Ginkgo biloba*. For sugar intolerance.

Symptoms and signs: low blood sugar; dizziness or light-headedness, especially when bending over; low blood pressure; seizure disorders; trouble staying asleep or nightmares; hyperactivity/attention deficit disorder (ADD); depression, feel melancholic; mood swings, tendency toward violence; panic attacks; diagnosed with schizophrenic or bipolar disorders.

Thera-zyme Challenge Food Powder
or Enzyme & Herbal Formula #29

Contains fig, psyllium seed husk, fennel seed, flaxseed, pumpkin seed, and guar gum (no enzymes). Provides a balanced ratio of protein, carbohydrate, fat, and fiber. For parasites and a toxic colon.

Symptoms and signs: itching around rectum and groin; restless sleep, gnawing of teeth at night; loss of appetite, fatigue—unable to meet daily requirements; toxic colon with constipation or diarrhea.

Thera-zyme T1-T6 Circ (Circulation)
or Enzyme & Herbal Formula #9

Contains the enzymes protease, amylase, lipase, and disaccharidases, plus hawthorn berries, motherwort, collinsonia root, rosemary leaf, and white willow bark. This formula aids circulation and the cardiovascular system.

Symptoms and signs: poor circulation, irregular or skipped heart beats; pain under the breastbone upon exertion; poor circulation; anxiety with sighing or panting (hyperventilation); hemorrhoids, varicose veins, and sometimes bursitis.

Thera-zyme CLM (Calm)
or Enzyme & Herbal Formula #26

Contains the enzymes protease, amylase, lipase, and disaccharidases, plus valerian root, hops flowers, chamomile flowers, passionflower, and blue vervain. Nutritional support for the nervous system and a coccyx (tailbone) misaligned due to physical injury or emotional trauma such as sexual abuse.

Symptoms and signs: unresolved emotional problems; restlessness, nervousness; insomnia; inability to concentrate; frequent daydreaming or nightmares; unresolved physical problems such as migraine headaches, painful tailbone, lower back pain or hemorrhoids; history of severe emotional stress, mental, physical, or sexual abuse.

Thera-zyme ELXR (Elixir)
or Enzyme & Herbal Formula #31

Contains the enzymes protease, amylase, lipase, and disaccharidases, plus chlorella (source of vitamins, minerals, protein, and chlorophyll), yerba maté, astragalus, echinacea, American ginseng, hawthorn berries, licorice root, sarsaparilla, and ginger. An herbal maintenance formula.

Symptoms and signs: there are none here. This formula is for healthy people who don't like to take isolated vitamins or minerals.

Thera-zyme T10-L1 Fem (Female)
or Enzyme & Herbal Formula #23

Contains the enzymes protease, amylase, lipase, and disaccharidases, plus *dong quai*, yucca root, chasteberry fruit, and raspberry leaf.

Symptoms and signs: PMS, menstrual cramps and irritability; excessive, scanty, or no menstrual flow; irregular periods; vaginal discharge (not yeast); painful legs, especially down the sides or back of thighs; bone-aching flu (aches, fever); hidden viruses; arthritis.

Thera-zyme L1-L3 IrB (Irritable Bowel)
or Enzyme & Herbal Formula #21

Contains the enzymes protease, amylase, lipase, and disaccharidases, plus blackberry leaf and root bark, marshmallow root, mullein leaf, nettle leaf, plantain leaf, and psyllium seed husk.

Symptoms and signs: abdominal pain, especially in the lower left quadrant; diarrhea, frequent, loose, or painful bowel movements; blood or mucus in the stool; colitis or other disorders of the large intestine.

Thera-zyme C2-L5 IVD (Intervertebral Disc)
or Enzyme & Herbal Formula #5

Contains the enzymes protease, amylase, lipase, and disaccharidases, plus nettle leaf, prickly ash bark, marshmallow root, and rosehips. For musculoskeletal support.

Symptoms and signs: history of disc problems—herniated disc or back surgery; TMJ problems (clicking or painful jaw, sometimes leading to headaches); irritated or receding gums; inability to concentrate and slow reaction time; big appetite (may help decrease it).

Thera-zyme T10-T11 Kdy (Kidney)
or Enzyme & Herbal Formula #18

Contains the enzymes protease, amylase, lipase, and disaccharidases, plus alfalfa juice concentrate, rosehips, *Echinacea purpurea* root, mullein leaf, and ginger root. For lymphatic congestion leading to allergies.

Symptoms and signs: allergies; frontal headaches; dark circles under eyes; swollen glands; low blood sugar; nausea and sometimes vomiting (worse during menses and pregnancy in women); low-back (kidney) pain or pain under the left or right rib.

Thera-zyme L1-L3 Lgl (Large Intestine)
or Enzyme & Herbal Formula #20

Contains the enzymes protease, amylase, lipase, and disaccharidases, plus butternut bark, cascara sagrada bark, dandelion root and herb, gentian root, and ginger root. A liver formula to help relieve constipation due to liver problems.

Symptoms and signs: constipation or lack of daily bowel movements; lower abdominal pain, especially in the lower right abdominal quadrant; hard, painful stools; use of laxatives or enemas.

Thera-zyme T8-T10 Lvr (Liver)
or Enzyme & Herbal Formula #17

Contains the enzymes protease, amylase, lipase, and disaccharidases, plus safflower petals, barberry root, beet root, milk thistle extract, and gentian root. Specific for liver problems.

Symptoms and signs: hepatitis, jaundice, or other liver disorders; nausea after high-fat meals (see Thera-zyme Bil); coated tongue; inability to tolerate drugs, vitamins, and minerals or alcohol; frequent "hot," red, tender, or burning soles of feet.

Thera-zyme T10-T11 Mal (Male)
or Enzyme & Herbal Formula #22

Contains the enzymes protease, amylase, lipase, and disaccharidases, plus saw palmetto fruit, yucca root, alfalfa juice concentrate, safflower petals, and parsley leaf. For prostate problems and impotence (regardless of the cause).

Symptoms and signs: frequent night urination, dribbling, loss of libido or painful intercourse; feeling of incomplete bowel evacuation; pain in the groin or pain down the front of the leg; bone-aching flu (aches, fever); hidden viruses.

Thera-zyme MSCLR (Muscular)
or Enzyme & Herbal Formula #27

Highest in amylase of any formula. Also contains cellulase, burdock root, citrus bioflavonoids, and lecithin. Antihistamine. For skin, joint, and muscle problems.

Symptoms and signs: muscle soreness or pain after exercise; muscle and joint stiffness, especially after rest; abscesses (inflammation without infection, not relieved by antibiotics); allergies due to bee stings or insect bites; herpes (oral, genital, shingles) or other skin eruptions such as hives and rashes; insomnia due to restlessness. (Note: may also need Thera-zyme Lvr to help relieve skin problems;

Thera-zyme Rbs is another good formula for herpes.)

Thera-zyme T1-T3 Nsl (Nasal)
or Enzyme & Herbal Formula #4

Contains the enzymes protease, amylase, lipase, and disaccharidases, plus catalase, citrus bioflavonoids, carrot powder, fenugreek seed, odorless garlic, pau d'arco inner bark, rosehips, and grape seed extract. A potent antioxidant as well as a vitamin C formula.

Symptoms and signs: sinusitis; loss of sense of smell; obstructed nasal breathing (mouth breather); dry, stuffy or congested nose; nose bleeds; facial pain and/or paralysis (Bell's palsy); acute food allergies.

Thera-zyme T1-T2 Opt (Optical)
or Enzyme & Herbal Formula #3

Contains the enzymes protease, amylase, lipase, and disaccharidases, plus acerola cherries, rosehips, bilberry leaf, and calcium lactate. A vitamin C formula.

Symptoms and signs: bruising and slow wound healing; frequent head colds with wet, runny nose and watery eyes; eye pain or pain when moving the eyes; eyestrain headaches; conjunctivitis; poor vision and eye problems such as cataracts and glaucoma. (Note: may also need TRMA).

Thera-zyme OSTEO
or Enzyme & Herbal Formula #35

Contains the enzymes protease, amylase, and lipase, plus glucosamine sulfate, methylsulfonylmethane (MSM), vitamin D3, and the herbs FoTi, goldenseal, and chamomile. Relieves the pain of arthritis (degenerative joint disease), cartilage and ligament injury, or collagen tissue problems.

Symptoms and signs: pain or injury involving joints, bones, ligaments, or cartilage.

Thera-zyme S2-S4 Para (Sympathetic Support for Patients Who are Parasympathetic Dominant)
or Enzyme & Herbal Formula #1

Contains the enzymes protease, amylase, lipase, and disaccharidases, plus calcium lactate, fenugreek seed, horsetail rush, and Shitake mushroom (source of vitamin D). Calcium formula; parasympathetic dominant refers to people in whom

The **autonomic nervous system (ANS)** can be likened to your body's automatic pilot. It keeps you alive through breathing, heart rate, and digestion, without your being aware of it or participating in its activities. The ANS has two divisions: the sympathetic, which expends body energy; and the parasympathetic, which conserves body energy. The sympathetic nervous system is associated with arousal and stress; it prepares us physically when we perceive a threat or challenge by increasing our heart rate, blood pressure, and muscle tension. The parasympathetic nervous system slows heart rate and increases intestinal and most gland activity.

the parasympathetic branch of their autonomic nervous system (SEE QUICK DEFINITION) is more activated than the sympathetic branch.

Symptoms and signs: bone disorders, spurs, osteoporosis; sore or weak joints; loose teeth or poor-fitting dentures; hyperirritabilty, insomnia or restless legs during sleep; night cough; low-back pain due to sacral problems; bladder control problems; sore or weak joints or ligaments; fallen arches.

Thera-zyme T1-T12 Rbs (Ribs) or Enzyme & Herbal Formula #8

Contains the enzymes protease, amylase, lipase, and disaccharidases, plus wheat germ, lecithin, globe artichoke extract, chamomile flowers, and kelp. Specific for problems in the diaphragm and the ribs, such as pleurisy, as well as lung and skin problems.

Symptoms and signs: painful ribs, pleurisy, pain upon inhalation, worse with cough or sneeze; frequent canker sores on the lips, tongue, or inside the mouth; dry, flaky skin, hair falling out; sunburn or sun poisoning. (Note: for herpes, may also need Thera-zyme Lvr).

Thera-zyme T1-T7 Rsp (Respiratory) or Enzyme & Herbal Formula #10

Contains the enzymes protease, amylase, lipase, and disaccharidases, plus pleurisy root, mullein leaf, wild cherry bark, sarsaparilla root, and horehound herb. For the lungs.

Symptoms and signs: lung problems, including asthma, wheezing, chronic bronchitis; chronic cough, dry or producing mucus; emphysema; bursitis (more commonly needed than Thera-zyme Circ).

Thera-zyme T1-L3 Skn (Skin) or Enzyme & Herbal Formula #19

Contains amylase, fatty acids, and the following herbs: fumitory herb, burdock root, Oregon grape root, and figwort. A liver, kidney, and intestinal formula which is high in amylase and affects skin conditions.

Symptoms and signs: skin conditions including acne, psoriasis, eczema, and dermatitis; history of many warts and moles; skin eruptions or rashes; excess perspiration or a lack of perspiration.

Thera-zyme T9-L1 Sml (Small Intestine)

Contains cellulase, disaccharidases, and beneficial bacteria (*L. casei, L. acidophilus, Bacillus subtilis, Bifidobacterium longum,* and *L. salivarius*). For parasites and candidiasis.

Symptoms and signs: candidiasis; parasites; diarrhea or constipation.

Thera-zyme T6-T9 Spl (Spleen)
or Enzyme & Herbal Formula #15

Contains the enzymes protease, amylase, lipase, and disaccharidases, plus pau d'arco, yellow dock root, *Echinacea purpurea* root, astragalus, and mullein leaf. Improves oxygen-carrying ability. For the immune system.

Symptoms and signs: immune system problems, including mononucleosis, Epstein-Barr virus, and severe conditions such as cancer and AIDS; lung problems, including emphysema and pulmonary fibrosis; chronic fatigue syndrome; pale skin, lips, and nails due to iron deficiency; frequent mild, nagging headaches; low-grade fevers of unknown origin.

Thera-zyme SRB (Stabilized Rice Bran)
or Enzyme & Herbal Formula #33

This is a balanced whole food powder containing stabilized rice bran and germ, plus nutrients derived from garlic, tomatoes, barley, broccoli, alfalfa, cherries, pineapple, oranges, beets, spinach, parsley, and carrots. It contains a whole-food form of amino acids, fat- and water-soluble vitamins, minerals, and fiber. Adding one or two heaping tablespoons of this powder to juice, milk, or water and mixing in a blender provides a meal replacement for those who want to lose weight, or a between-meal snack for those who experience an afternoon slump or want to gain weight. In addition, this food product has been reported to enable both Type I and Type II diabetics to decrease their insulin dosage.

Symptoms and signs: there are none here, unless you want to consider weight problems, low blood sugar, afternoon slump, and diabetes as symptoms.

Thera-zyme T1-T2 SvG (Salivary Gland)
or Enzyme & Herbal Formula #6

Contains the enzymes protease, amylase, lipase, and disaccharidases, plus manioc root, citrus bioflavonoids, wheat germ, peppermint leaf, rosehips, and acerola extract. A source of vitamins A, E, and sugar-digesting enzymes. Manioc root is a source of tryptophan, precursor to the neurotransmitter (SEE QUICK DEFINITION) serotonin.

Symptoms and signs: sugar intolerance; frequent sore or irritated throat; sores on the tongue or in mouth; dry

QUICK DEFINITION

A **neurotransmitter** is a brain chemical with the specific function of enabling communications to happen between brain cells. Chief among the 100 identified to date are acetylcholine, gamma-aminobutyric acid (GABA), serotonin, dopamine, and norepinephrine. Acetylcholine is required for short-term memory and all muscle contractions. GABA works to stop excess nerve signals and thus keeps brain firings from getting out of control; serotonin does the same and helps produce sleep, regulate pain, and influence mood, although too much serotonin can produce depression. Norepinephrine is an excitatory neurotransmitter.

itchy eyes or dry mouth; history of speech impediment, stuttering, or stammering; loss of voice or laryngitis; inability to relax the mind, become serene, or meditate.

Thera-zyme C1-C3 Sym
or Enzyme & Herbal Formula #25

Contains the enzymes protease, amylase, lipase, and disaccharidases, plus chickweed herb, *Echinacea purpurea* root, chamomile flowers, and dandelion root and leaf. For the nourishment of body tissues affected by sympathetic irritation and subluxations of the upper cervical spine.

Symptoms and signs: neck (atlas) problems; history of head injury; history of headaches in back of head and neck or radiating to the forehead and behind the eyes; wandering pains; startled by sudden sounds; stiff joints, loss of mobility; sudden weak or sinking spells with complete loss of energy; high blood pressure; severe insomnia not relieved by natural remedies; seizures; digestive problems.

Thera-zyme C8-T1 Thy (Thyroid)
or Enzyme & Herbal Formula #7

Contains the enzymes protease, amylase, lipase, and disaccharidases, plus calcium citrate, fenugreek seed, kelp, magnesium amino acid chelate, and Irish moss. High in minerals including zinc, calcium, and magnesium.

Symptoms and signs: motion sickness; white spots on fingernails; neck, shoulder, arm, or hand pain; frequent leg cramps; poor circulation—cold hands and feet.

Thera-zyme TRMA (Trauma)
or Enzyme & Herbal Formula #28

Contains the enzymes protease, amylase, lipase, and disaccharidases, calcium lactate, and kelp, a source of minerals. Antioxidant inhibiting free-radical damage which is involved in all inflammatory conditions and pathologies.

Symptoms and signs: weak immune system; frequent infections of any kind (bacterial or viral); severe immune system problems including cancer and AIDS; ear problems (frequent infections or fluid in the ears); soft tissue trauma (accidental or surgical); anxiety—frequent sighing, taking tranquilizers; kidney disorders such as nephritis accompanied by edema (swelling of feet and ankles).

Thera-zyme T12-L2 UrT (Urinary Tract)
or Enzyme & Herbal Formula #24

Contains the enzymes protease, amylase, lipase, and disaccharidases, plus alfalfa juice concentrate, horsetail rush, buchu leaf, cranberry, hydrangea, meadowsweet, and uva ursi. Source of vitamins A and D.

Symptoms and signs: urinary tract problems, including frequent bladder infections, burning urination or cystitis; frequent urination, urgency or loss of bladder control, voiding small amounts; pain or discomfort during urination; hematuria (blood in the urine); kidney stones.

Appendix C

ENZYME THERAPY PRACTITIONERS

If there is not a listing in your area, contact: 21st Century Nutrition, 6421 Enterprise Lane, Madison, WI 53719; tel: 800-662-2630 or 608-273-8100; fax: 608-273-8111.

Below is a list of enzyme therapists who have been trained to use the Thera-zyme formulas, developed by Howard Loomis, D.C. As these practitioners use the 24-hour urinalysis, they can provide you with information on getting that test. (This list is not necessarily complete.)

Alaska
Marianne Miller, D.C.
3201 "C" Street,
Suite 107
Anchorage, AK 99503
tel: 907-562-1062

Arizona
Barry Kalinsky, D.C.
6122 East 22nd Street
Tucson, AZ 85711
tel: 520-790-2222

California
Mark Beigel, D.C.
Anaheim
Chiropractic Clinic
1440 South Anaheim Blvd.
Anaheim, CA 92805
tel: 714-956-1018

Eileen Kenny, D.C.
1911 North Lake Avenue
Altadena, CA 91001
tel: 626-398-0292

Colorado
Lou Depalma, D.C.
Depalma Chiropractic
2148 Broadway, Suite B2
Grand Junction, CO
81503
tel: 970-243-5164

Florida
David Frerking, D.C.
915 East Alfred Street
Tavares, FL 32778
tel: 352-343-9275

Larry Johnston, D.C.
905 East Martin Luther
King Jr. Drive, Suite 212
Tarpon Springs, FL
34689
tel: 813-938-9799

Joe Picone, D.C.
20488 West Dixie
Highway
North Miami Beach, FL
33180
tel: 305-935-9599

Georgia
Andrew Linial, Jr., D.C.
Chiropractic Arts
4501 Circle 75 Parkway
Atlanta, GA 30339
tel: 770-916- 9800

Hawaii
Armando Garza, D.C.
1744 Liliha Street,
Suite 201
Honolulu, HI 96817
tel: 808-533-2425

Illinois
Daniel Blue, D.C.
933 West 8th Street
Minonk, IL 61760
tel: 309-432-2922

Ross Hauser, M.D.
Marion Hauser, R.D.
Caring Medical
715 Lake Street,
Suite 600
Oak Park, IL 60301
tel: 708-848-7789

Doug Sandburg, D.C.
509 Old Northwest Hwy,
Suite 111
Barrington, IL 60010
tel: 847-382-0800

Indiana
Guy DiMartino, D.C.
180 South West Street
Crown Point, IN 46307
tel: 219-663-7750

Iowa
Dennis Hagemann, D.C.
2906 West Central Park
Avenue, Suite 3-A
Davenport, IA 52804
tel: 319-388-0842

Kansas
William Hafner, D.C.
Hafner Chiropractic
1309 Williams
Great Bend, KS 67530
tel: 316-792-3678

Tomm Hobbs, D.C.
215 Ames/56 Highway
Baldwin City, KS 66006
tel: 913-594-3144

Massachusetts
Jerry Brickley, D.C.
449 Route 6A
East Sandwich, MA
02537
tel: 508-888-1130

Michigan
Rich Easterling, N.D.
Rich Earth Clinic
P.O. Box 307
Grass Lake, MI 49240
tel: 800-253-1694

Winsen Zouzal, D.C.
15761 Mac Avenue
Detroit, MI 48224
tel: 313-885-3500

Minnesota
Rocco Bilazzo, D.C.
1020 Marie Avenue
St. Paul, MN 55075
tel: 612-455-5463

Mississippi
Louis Bookey, D.C.
17192 Highway 51
Hazlehurst, MS 39083
tel: 601-894-3314

Missouri
John Danz, D.C.
1205 Cedar Ridge Drive
St. Louis, MO 63146
tel: 314-275-2189

Doug Hays, D.C.
Kathy Gowans, R.N.
The Wellness Center
1350 South Glenstone,

Suite 10
Springfield, MO 65804
tel: 417-883-1936

New York
Deborah Cutler, D.C.
101 Perry Street, Suite 1K
New York, NY 10014
tel: 212-741-6285

Paul Inselman, D.C.
Mineola Chiropractic
476 Jericho Turnpike
Mineola, NY 11501
tel: 516-747-1122

Anthony Leroy, D.C.
55 Old Nyack Turnpike,
Suite 601
Nanuet, NY 10954
tel: 914-624-1634

Ohio
Leon Neiman, M.D.
Carol Martin, R.N.
120 West Bowery Street
Akron, OH 44308
tel: 330-535-3101

Oklahoma
Jim Suiter, D.C.
913 North 11th
Duncan, OK 73533
tel: 405-252-6210

Oregon
Ivan Kelley, D.C.
530 NW 3rd Street,
Suite A
Newport, OR 97365
tel: 541-265-5132

Sylvia Zook, Ph.D.
12293 Summit Loop SE
Turner, OR 97392
tel: 503-743-2631

Texas
Dayton Boyd, D.C.
205-B North University
Lubbock, TX 79415
tel: 806-762-4507

Larry Breedlove, D.C.
3839 Bee Cave Ed.,
Suite 202
Austin, TX 78746
tel: 512-327-2921

Washington
Jennifer Huntoon, N.D.
1329 North 45th Street
Seattle, WA 98103
tel: 206-632-8804

Wisconsin
Su Aberle, N.D.
Promise Outreach
Route 2, Box 61
Cashton, WI 54619
tel: 608-634-2440

Colleen Keen, R.D.
Pam Wollin, N.D.
The Wellness Center
128 West 8th Street
Monroe, WI 53566
tel: 608-328-3438

Katherine Walker, D.C.
235 North Seymour
Street
Fond Du Lac, WI 54935
tel: 920-929-9599

Appendix D

PRODUCT CONTACT INFORMATION

For **soil-based organisms:**
GanEden Ltd.
15355 72nd Drive North
Palm Beach Gardens, FL 33418
tel: 800-622-8986 or 561-748-2478
fax: 561-575-5488

Life Sciences
321 North Mall Drive, Building F-201
St. George, UT 84790
tel: 801-628-4111
fax: 801-628-6114

For **Citricidal** (health practitioners only):
Nutribiotic
P.O. Box 238
Lakeport, CA 95453
tel: 800-255-435 or 707-263-0411
fax: 707-263-7844
The consumer's equivalent is
Nutribiotic's Standardized Extract
of Grapefruit, available in health
food stores.

For **RC, Raven, Immupower, Thieves,
Forgiveness, Joy, Ravensara,** and
other **Young Living Essential Oils:**
Baker Health Foundation
204 East North El Camino Real,
Suite 402
Encinitas, CA 92024
tel: 760-737-5000
fax: 760-737-5090

Another source of essential oils is:
Phyto Medicine Company
6701 Sunset Drive, Suite 100
Miami, FL 33143
tel: 305-662-6396
fax: 305-667-5619

Progest-E Complex (10%
progesterone oil) and **EV** (3% topical
progesterone cream) are available in
some health food stores. Health
practitioners only:
Raymond Peat, Ph.D.
P.O. Box 5764
Eugene, OR 97405
fax: 503-683-4279
For a list of other natural
progesterone products, see Appendix
A: Hormonal Balancing, pp. 258-259.

For **Stress Release:**
Bioenergetics
P.O. Box 127
Sandy, OR 97055
tel: 800-334-4043 or 503-668-7478

For fumaric acid products **Psorex**
and **Psoractin:**
Cardiovascular Research
1061-B Shary Circle
Concord, CA 94518
tel: 800-888-4585 or 510-827-2636
fax: 510-676-9231

For **Alticort** (cream containing
licorice root):
Phyto-Pharmica
P.O. Box 1745
Green Bay, WI 54305
tel: 800-376-7889 or 920-469-9099
fax: 920-469-4418

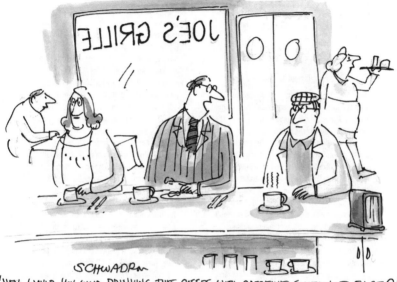

"HEY, WOULD YOU MIND DRINKING THAT COFFEE WITH CAFFEINE SOMEPLACE ELSE?"

Endnotes

Chapter I
Why Enzymes?

1 Stephen E. Langer, M.D., with James F. Scheer. *Solved: The Riddle of Illness* (New Canaan, CT: Keats Publishing, 1995), 25.

Chapter 2
Diagnosing Enzyme Deficiencies

1 Tom Valentine. "What Happens When Americans Consume Tons of Microwaved Foods?" *Search for Health* 1:1 (September/October 1992), 2-13. G. Lubec et al. "Amino Acid Isomerization and Microwave Exposure." *The Lancet* (December 9, 1989), 1392. Paul Brodeur. "Radiation in Daily Life." *Health Watch* (December 1, 1986), 45-48.

2 Howard Loomis, D.C. "Clinical Nutrition and the Chiropractic Practice." *American Chiropractor* (September 1990). Howard Loomis, D.C. *The Nutritional Value and Clinical Appreciation of Food Enzymes* (Madison, WI: 21st Century Nutrition, 1986).

3 Howard Loomis, D.C. "Muscle Contraction and Body Distortions, How to Recognize Disease." (Madison, WI: 21st Century Nutrition) Seminar Presentation, San Francisco, California (April 4, 1998).

Chapter 3
What Causes Enzyme Deficiencies?

1 "Changing Profile of Pesticide Poisonings." *New England Journal of Medicine* 316:13 (1987), 807-809.

2 Russell Jaffee, M.D. "Sixteen Million Americans Sensitive to Pesticides." *Townsend Letter For Doctors* 89(1990), 869-872.

3 "Pesticides: The Hidden Threat of 'Inerts'." *Safe Food News* (Fall 1994), 14. (Now called *Food and Water Journal*. Available from: Food & Water, Inc., RR1, Box 68D, West Danville, VT 05873.)

4 Norma Grier. "Taking the Secrets Out of Pesticide Products: How to Use 'Inerts' to Promote Alternatives." *Journal of Pesticide Reform* 12:3 (Fall 1992), 6-9.

5 Betty Kamen, Ph.D. Kamut: the Ancient Grain (Available from: Green Kamut Corporation, 1965 Freeman Avenue, Long Beach, CA 90804.)

6 Brian Tokar. "Exchange." *Safe Food News* (Fall 1993),

6. (Now called *Food and Water Journal*. Available from: Food & Water, Inc., RR1, Box 68D, West Danville, VT 05873.)

7 William Campbell Douglass, M.S. *The Milk Book: How Science Is Destroying Nature's Nearly Perfect Food* (Atlanta, GA: Second Opinion Publishing, 1994).

8 C. Bhaskaram and G. Sadasivan. "Effects of Feeding Irradiated Wheat to Malnourished Children." *American Journal of Clinical Nutrition* 28:2 (February 1975), 130-135. Morton Walker, D.P.M. "Raw Capitalism at Its Worst: Food Irradiation, Part 1." *Townsend Letter for Doctors* (August/September 1992), 774-777. Morton Walker, D.P.M. "Raw Capitalism at Its Worst: Food Irradiation, Part 2." *Townsend Letter for Doctors* (December 1992), 1094-1098. Tony Webb et al. *Food Irradiation: Who Wants It?* (Marshfield, VT: Food & Water, 1993). Available from: Food & Water, Inc., R.R. 1, Box 30, Marshfield, VT 05658.

9 "Bill Would Require Red Meat Irradiation." *Register Guard* (September 17, 1997), 4A.

10 C.J. Meade et al. *Advanced Lipid Research* 127(1978), 165.

11 A.J. Honour et al. "The Effect of Changes in Diet on Lipid Levels and Platelet Thrombosis Formation." *British Journal of Experimental Pathology* 59:4 (1978), 390-394. C.F. Lim et al. "Influence of Nonesterified Fatty Acid and Lysolecithins on Thyroxine Binding to Thyroxine-Binding Globulin and Transthyretin." *Thyroid* 5:4 (1995), 319-324. Stephen E. Langer, M.D., with James F. Scheer. *Solved: The Riddle of Illness* (New Canaan, CT: Keats Publishing, 1995), 25.

12 S. Ikemoto et al. "High-Fat Diet-Induced Hyperglycemia." *Proceedings of the National Academy of Sciences* 92 (1995), 3096-3099.

13 C.F. Lim et al. "Influence of Nonesterified Fatty Acid and Lysolecithins on Thyroxine Binding to Thyroxine-Binding Globulin and Transthyretin." *Thyroid* 5:4 (1995), 319-324. Stephen E. Langer, M.D., with James F. Scheer. *Solved: The Riddle of Illness* (New Canaan, CT: Keats Publishing, 1995), 25.

14 E.A. Mascioli et al. "Medium Chain Triglycerides and Structured Lipids as Unique Nonglucose Energy Sources in Hyperalimentation." *Lipids* 22:6 (1987), 421-423.

15 H. Selye. "Sensitization by Corn Oil for the Production of Cardiac Necrosis," *American Journal of of Cardiology* 23: (1969), 719-22. G. Byster and R.

Vles. "Nutritional Effects Of Rapeseed Oils In Pigs," Proceedings of the Fifth International Rapeseed Conference (1978). F.Z. Meerson. *Adaptive Protection of the Heart: Protecting Against Stress and Ischemic Damage* (Boca Raton, FL: CRC Press, 1991). S. Parthasarathy and S.M. Rankin. "Role of Oxidized Low-Density Lipoprotein in Atherogenesis." *Progress in Lipid Research* 31:2 (1992), 127-143.

16 C. Ip et al. "Requirement of Essential Fatty Acids for Mammary Tumor," *Cancer Research* 45 (1985), 997-2001.

17 S. Kitada, E.F. Hays, and J.F. Mead. "A Lipid-Mobilizing Factor in Serum of Tumor-Bearing Mice." *Lipids* 15 (1989), 168-174.

18 H.S. Black et al. "Relation of Antioxidants and Level of Dietary Lipids to Epidermal Lipid Peroxidation and Ultraviolet Carcinogenesis." *Cancer Research* 45 (1985), 6254-6259.

19 J.M. Bell and P.K. Lundberg. "Effects of a Commercial Soy Lecithin Preparation on Development of Sensorimotor Behavior and Brain Biochemicals in the Rat." *Developmental Psychobiology* 8 (1985), 59-66. D. Harman et al. "Free Radical Theory of Aging: Effect of Dietary Fat on Central Nervous System Function." *Journal of the American Geriatric Society* 24 (1976), 292-298. F.Z. Meerson et al. "Effect of the Antioxidant Ionol on Formation and Persistence of a Defensive Conditioned Reflex During Peak Exercise." *Bulletin of Experimental Biology and Medicine* 96 (1983), 70-71.

20 Raymond Peat, Ph.D. *From PMS to Menopause: Female Hormones in Context* (self-published), 175. Available from: Raymond Peat, P.O. Box 5764, Eugene, OR 97405; website: www.efn.org/~raypeat.

21 L.L. Wang and E.A. Johnson. "Inhibition of Listeria Monocytogenes by Fatty Acids and Monoglycerides." *Applied and Environmental Microbiology* 58:2 (1992), 624-629.

22 "Coco Q10™." Available from: Carotec, P.O. Box 9919, Naples, FL 34101; tel: 800-522-4279 or 941-353-2348; fax: 941-353-2365.

23 Mary Enig, Ph.D., F.A., C.N. "Lauric Acid-Rich Coconut Oil 'Saturated' Yet Outstanding." *Search for Health* (March/April 1996), 11-18.

24 F. Berschauer et al. "Nutritional-Physiological Effects of Dietary Fats in Rations for Growing Pigs. 4. Effects of Sunflower Oil and Coconut Oil on Protein and Fat Retention, Fatty Acid Pattern of Back Fat and Blood Parameters in Piglets." *Archiv fur Tierernahrung* 34:1 (1984), 19-33. J. Yazbech et al. "Effects of Essential Fatty Acid Deficiency on Brown Adipose Tissue Activity in Rats Maintained at Thermal Neutrality." *Comparative Biochemistry and Physiology A: Comparative Physiology* 94:2 (1989), 273-276.

25 I. Liscum and N.K. Dahl. "Intracellular Cholesterol Transport." *Journal of Lipid Research* 33 (1992), 1239-1254.

26 F. Berschauer et al. "Nutritional-Physiological Effects of Dietary Fats in Rations for Growing Pigs. 4. Effects of Sunflower Oil and Coconut Oil on Protein and Fat Retention, Fatty Acid Pattern of Back Fat and Blood Parameters in Piglets." *Archiv fur Tierernahrung* 34:1 (1984), 19-33. J. Yazbech et al. "Effects of Essential Fatty Acid Deficiency on Brown Adipose Tissue Activity in Rats Maintained at Thermal Neutrality." *Comparative Biochemistry and Physiology A: Comparative Physiology* 94:2 (1989), 273-276.

27 Raymond Peat, Ph.D. "Coconut Oil." *Ray Peat's Newsletter* (July 1994). Available from: Raymond Peat, P.O. Box 5764, Eugene, OR 97405; fax: 503-683-4279; website: www.efn.org/~raypeat. Weston Price, D.D.S. *Nutrition and Physical Degeneration: A Comparison of Primitive and Modern Diets and Their Effects* (La Mesa, CA: Price-Pottenger Nutrition Foundation, 1970).

28 C. Ip and D.K. Sinha. "Enhancement of Mammary Tumorigenesis by Dietary Selenium Deficiency in Rats With a High Polyunsaturated Fat Intake." *Cancer Research* 41:1 (1981), 31-34.

29 Stephen E. Langer, M.D., with James F. Scheer. *Solved: The Riddle of Illness* (New Canaan, CT: Keats Publishing, 1995), 25.

30 Tom Valentine. "What Happens When Americans Consume Tons of Microwaved Foods?" *Search for Health* 1:1 (September/October 1992), 2-13. G. Lubec et al. "Amino Acid Isomerization and Microwave Exposure." *The Lancet* (December 9, 1989), 1392. Paul Brodeur. "Radiation in Daily Life." *Health Watch* (December 1, 1986), 45-48.

31 Lita Lee, Ph.D. *Radiation Protection Manual* (self-published, 3rd edition, 1990). Available from: Lita Lee, P.O. Box 516, Lowell, OR 97452. Paul Brodeur. *Currents of Death* (New York: Simon and Schuster, 1989).

32 "Deadly Zones, Degeneration from Geopathic Interference." Available from: The Royal Rife Research Society, 7040 Avenida Encinas #104-291, Carlsbad, CA 92009.

33 Ibid.

34 John Yiamouyiannis, Ph.D. *Fluoride: The Aging Factor* (Delaware, OH: Health Action Press, 1983).

35 Richard G. Foulkes, M.D. "Celebration or Shame? Fifty Years of Fluoridation (1945-1995)." *Townsend Letter for Doctors & Patients* (November 1995), 52-63. John Yiamouyiannis, Ph.D. *Fluoride: The Aging Factor* (Delaware, OH: Health Action Press, 1983). John Yiamouyiannis, Ph.D. "Fluoride." *Mothering* (Winter 1989).

36 L.J. Hahn et al. "Dental 'Silver' Tooth Fillings: A Source of Mercury Exposure Revealed by Whole-Body Image Scan and Tissue Analysis." *FASEB Journal* 3:2644 (1989).

37 M. Vimy. "Toxic Teeth: The Chronic Mercury Poisoning of Modern Man." *Dental Amalgam Mercury Syndrome* 2 (1995), 1-6.

A-Z of Health
Conditions

----

1 Broda Barnes, M.D., and L. Galton. *Hypothyroidism: The Unsuspected Illness* (New York: Harper & Row, 1976). Stephen E. Langer, M.D., with James F. Scheer. *Solved: The Riddle of Illness* (New Canaan, CT: Keats Publishing, 1995). U. Kabadi et al. "Familial Hypothyroidism Manifested by Painful, Swollen Joints." *New York State Journal of Medicine* 77:9 (1977), 1489-1491. P. Wahlberg et al. "25 Year Follow-Up of the Aland Thyroid Study of 1956: Thyroid Status and Incidence of Rheumatoid Arthritis." *Acta Endocrinologica Supplementum* 251 (1983), 47-52.

2 John R. Lee, M.D. *What Your Doctor May Not Tell You About Menopause* (New York: Warner Books, 1996). John R. Lee, M.D. "Osteoporosis Reversal." *International Clinical Nutrition Review* 10:3 (July 1990).

3 William Campbell Douglass, M.S. *The Milk Book: How Science Is Destroying Nature's Nearly Perfect Food* (Atlanta, GA: Second Opinion Publishing, 1994).

4 P.F. Adams and V. Benson. "Current Estimates from the National Health Interview Survey, National Center for Health Statistics." *Vital Health Statistics* 10:181 (1991). Centers for Disease Control and Prevention. *Vital and Health Statistics, Current Estimates from the National Health Interview Survey*, 1994 DHHS Publication No. PHS 96-1521 (Washington, DC: U.S. Department of Health and Human Services, Public Health Service, National Center for Health Statistics, 1995).

5 Centers for Disease Control and Prevention. *Vital and Health Statistics, Current Estimates from the National Health Interview Survey*, 1994 DHHS Publication No. PHS 96-1521 (Washington, DC: U.S. Department of Health and Human Services, Public Health Service, National Center for Health Statistics, 1995).

6 E. Rubenstein and D.D. Felderman, eds. *Scientific American Medicine* (New York: Scientific American Medicine, 1982).

7 Centers for Disease Control and Prevention. *Vital and Health Statistics, National Hospital Discharge Survey: Annual Summary*, 1993 DHHS Publication No. PHS 95-1782 (Washington, DC: U.S. Department of Health and Human Services, Public Health Service, National Center for Health Statistics, 1995).

8 American Lung Association statistics cited in: Joe Rojas-Burke. "Study Seeks Improved Asthma Care." (Eugene, OR) *Register-Guard* (January 24, 1997), 1A.

9 "Study Links Asthma Drug to Death." *San Jose Mercury News* (February 20, 1992), 5A.

10 "Deadly Zones: Degeneration from Geopathic Interference." Available from: The Royal Rife Research Society, 7040 Avenida Encinas #104-291, Carlsbad, CA 92009.

11 P. Ebeling and V.A. Koivisto. "Physiological Importance of Dehydroepiandrosterone (DHEA)." *The Lancet* 343:8911 (June 11, 1994), 1479-1481.

12 William Campbell Douglass, M.S. *The Milk Book: How Science Is Destroying Nature's Nearly Perfect Food* (Atlanta, GA: Second Opinion Publishing, 1994), 132, 253.

13 Stephen E. Langer, M.D., with James F. Scheer. *Solved: The Riddle of Illness* (New Canaan, CT: Keats Publishing, 1995), 25.

14 Connie and Alan Higley. *Reference Guide for Essential Oils* (Olathe, KS: Abundant Health, 1998).

15 Arthur C. Guyton, M.D. *Textbook of Medical Physiology* 7th Ed. (Philadelphia: W.B. Saunders, 1986), 825.

16 C.F. Lim et al. "Influence of Nonesterified Fatty Acid and Lysolecithins on Thyroxine Binding to Thyroxine-Binding Globulin and Transthyretin." *Thyroid* 5:4 (1995), 319-324. Tom Valentine. "If You Eat Soy, Watch Your Thyroid Function: New Study." *True Health* (Autumn 1997), 1-3. R.L. Divi et al. "Anti-Thyroid Isoflavones from Soybean: Isolation, Characterization, and Mechanisms of Action." *Biochemical Pharmacology* 54:10 (November 15, 1997), 1087-1096. Stephen E. Langer, M.D., with James F. Scheer. *Solved: The Riddle of Illness* (New Canaan, CT: Keats Publishing, 1995), 25. Richard G. Foulkes, M.D. "Celebration or Shame? Fifty Years of Fluoridation (1945-1995)." *Townsend Letter for Doctors & Patients* (November 1995), 52-63. John Yiamouyiannis. *Fluoride: The Aging Factor* (Delaware, OH: Health Action Press, 1983), 8, 87.

17 C.F. Lim et al. "Influence of Nonesterified Fatty Acid and Lysolecithins on Thyroxine Binding to Thyroxine-Binding Globulin and Transthyretin." *Thyroid* 5:4 (1995), 319-324. F.Z. Meerson. *Adaptive Protection of the Heart: Protecting Against Stress and Ischemic Damage* (Boca Raton, FL: CRC Press, 1991). S. Parthasarathy and S.M. Rankin. "Role of Oxidized Low-Density Lipoprotein in Atherogenesis." *Progress in Lipid Research* 31:2 (1992), 127-143.

18 W.C. Young. *Sex and Internal Secretions* (Baltimore, MD: Williams & Wilkins, 1961). Raymond Peat, Ph.D. *From PMS to Menopause: Female Hormones in Context* (self-published), 7. Available from: Raymond Peat, P.O. Box 5764, Eugene, OR 97405; website: www.efn.org/~raypeat.

19 M.S. Seelig and H.A. Heggtveit. "Magnesium Interrelationships in Ischemic Heart Disease: A Review." *American Journal of Clinical Nutrition* 27:1 (January 1974), 59-79. V. Beral. "Cardiovascular Disease Mortality Trends and Oral Contraceptive Use in Young Women." *The Lancet* 2 (1976), 1047-1051. B.V. Stadel. "Oral Contraceptives and Cardiovascular Disease." *New England Journal of Medicine* 305 (1981), 612. F. von Kaulla et al. "Conjugated Oestrogens and Hypercoagulability." *American Journal of Obstetrics and Gynecology* 122 (1975), 688. Collaborative Group for the Study of Stroke in Young Women. "Oral Contraceptives and Stroke in Young Women." *Journal of the American Medical Association* 231 (1975), 718-722.

20 Kilmer S. McCully, M.D. "Atherosclerosis, Serum Cholesterol and the Homocysteine Theory: A Study of 194 Consecutive Autopsies." *American Journal of Medical Science* 229 (1990), 217-221.

21 Kilmer S. McCully, M.D. "Homocysteine Theory: Development and Current Status." *Atherosclerosis Review* 11 (1983), 157-246. Kilmer S. McCully, M.D. *The Homocysteine Revolution: Medicine for the New Millennium* (New Canaan, CT: Keats Publishing, 1997).

22 Joseph C. Hattersley. "Vitamin B6: The Overlooked Key to Preventing Heart Attacks." *Journal of Applied Nutrition* 47:1-2 (1995), 2431. Reprints may be ordered from: Joseph C. Hattersley, 7031 Glen Terra Court S.E., Olympia, WA 98503.

23 J. Regnstrom et al. "Susceptibility to Low Density Lipoprotein Oxidation & Coronary Atherosclerosis in Man." *The Lancet* 339 (1992), 1183-1186.

24 Melvin Page, D.D.S. *Degeneration Regeneration* (St. Petersburg, FL: Nutritional Development, 1977). Available from: Nutritional Development, 5235 Gulf Blvd., St. Petersburg, FL 33706. Or from: PPNF, P.O. Box 2614, La Mesa, CA 92041.

25 J.T. Salonen et al. "High Stored Iron Levels Are Associated with Excess Risk of Myocardial Infarction in Eastern Finnish Men." *Circulation* 86 (1992), 803-811.

26 William Campbell Douglass, M.D. "Iron, Chickens and Hyperferremia." *Health Freedom News* 5:8 (September 1986), 10-12.

27 T.E. Strandberg et al. "Long-Term Mortality after Five-Year Multifactorial Primary Prevention of Cardiovascular Diseases in Middle-Aged Men."
Journal of the American Medical Association 226 (1991), 1225-1229.

28 Raymond Peat, Ph.D. "The Edema of Stress." *Blake College Newsletter* 1:3.

29 Raymond Peat, Ph.D. "Optimizing Respiration." *Ray Peat's Newsletter* (October 1997. Raymond Peat, Ph.D. "Recharging the System." *Ray Peat's Newsletter* (1998). Available from: Raymond Peat, P.O. Box 5764, Eugene, OR 97405; fax: 503-683-4279; website: www.efn.org/~raypeat. M.V. Riley et al. "The Roles of Bicarbonate and CO2 in Transendothelial Fluid Movement and Control of Corneal Thickness." *Investigative Ophthalmology and Visual Science* 36:1 (1995), 103-112.

30 Alexander G. Schauss, Ph.D. *Minerals, Trace Elements and Human Health* (Tacoma, WA: Life Sciences Press, 1996), 8.

31 "The Unique Pharmacology of Coleus forskohlii." *American Journal of Natural Medicine* 1:3 (November 1994), 10-13.

32 Personal communication with Raymond Peat, Ph.D., of Portland, Oregon.

33 Personal communication with Howard Loomis, D.C., of Madison, Wisconsin.

34 David Hoffman. *The New Holistic Herbal* (Rockport, MA: Element Books, 1991). Richard Mabey, ed. The New Age Herbalist (New York: Collier Books, 1988).

35 William Campbell Douglass, M.S. *The Milk Book: How Science Is Destroying Nature's Nearly Perfect Food* (Atlanta, GA: Second Opinion Publishing, 1994).

36 Melvyn R. Werbach. *Nutritional Influences On Illness* (Tarzana, CA: Third Line Press, 1987), 197-201,

37 C.F. Lim et al. "Influence of Nonesterified Fatty Acid and Lysolecithins on Thyroxine Binding to Thyroxine-Binding Globulin and Transthyretin." *Thyroid* 5:4 (1995), 319-324. Stephen E. Langer, M.D., with James F. Scheer. *Solved: The Riddle of Illness* (New Canaan, CT: Keats Publishing, 1995), 25.

38 Broda Barnes, M.D., and L. Galton. *Hypothyroidism: The Unsuspected Illness* (New York: Harper & Row, 1976).

39 B.K. Chakravarthy et al. "Pancreatic Beta-Cell Regeneration in Rats by Epicatechin." *The Lancet* 2 (1981), 759-760.

40 X.M. Xu and M.L. Thomas. "Estrogen Receptor-Mediated Direct Stimulation of Colon Cancer Cell Growth in Vitro." *Molecular and Cellular Endocrinology* 105:2 (1994), 197-201. B.T. Zhu et al. "Conversion of Estrone to 2- and 4-Hydroxyestrone by Hamster Kidney and Liver Microsomes: Implications for the Mechanism of Estrogen-Induced Carcinogenesis." *Endocrinology* 135:5 (1994), 1772-1779. H.V. Thomas et al. "A Prospective Study of Endogenous Serum Hormone Concentrations and Breast Cancer Risk in

Premenopausal Women on the Island of Guernsey." *Journal of Steroid Biochemistry and Molecular Biology* 63:4-6 (1997), 175-188.

41 H.J. Roberts. *Aspartame (NutraSweet): Is It Safe?* (Philadelphia: Charles Press Publishers, 1990), 191-192.

42 H.J. Roberts. *Aspartame (NutraSweet): Is It Safe?* (Philadelphia: Charles Press Publishers, 1990). H.J. Roberts. *Sweet'ner Dearest: Bittersweet Vignettes About Aspartame (NutraSweet)* (West Palm Beach, FL: Sunshine Sentinel Press, 1992).

43 Michael T. Murray, N.D. "Are Botanical Medicines Useful in Diabetes?" *American Journal of Natural Medicine* 1:3 (November 1994), 5-7.

44 Ibid.

45 Connie and Alan Higley. *Reference Guide for Essential Oils* (Olathe, KS: Abundant Health, 1998).

46 Maureen K. Salaman. "President's Message: It May Be Better Business But We're Not Buying." *Health Freedom News* (October 1988), 6.

47 R.L. Smith and E.R. Pinckney. *The Cholesterol Conspiracy* (Sherman Oaks, CA: Vector Enterprises, 1992).

48 Melvyn R. Werbach, M.D. *Nutritional Influences on Illness: A Sourcebook of Clinical Research* (Tarzana, CA: Third Line Press, 1988), 197. "How Sugar Can Get You Stoned." *Scientist* 14 (March 21, 1985).

49 C.F. Lim et al. "Influence of Nonesterified Fatty Acid and Lysolecithins on Thyroxine Binding to Thyroxine-Binding Globulin and Transthyretin." *Thyroid* 5:4 (1995), 319-324. Stephen E. Langer, M.D., with James F. Scheer. *Solved: The Riddle of Illness* (New Canaan, CT: Keats Publishing, 1995), 25.

50 Melvyn R. Werbach, M.D. *Nutritional Influences on Illness: A Sourcebook of Clinical Research* (Tarzana, CA: Third Line Press, 1988), 199.

51 S.A. Jenkins. "Vitamin C and Gallstone Formation: A Preliminary Report." *Experientia* 33 (1977), 1616-1617.

52 J.C. Breneman. "Elimination Diet as the Most Effective Gallbladder Diet." *Annals of Allergy* 26 (1968), 83.

53 M.R. Werbach. *Nutritional Influences on Illness* (Tarzana, CA: Third Line Press, 1987), 197-201.

54 Ibid.

55 D. Golledge. "Getting Rid of Gallstones." *Alive* 115 (1992), 30-32.

56 Allan Sachs, D.C., C.C.N. *The Authoritative Guide to Grapefruit Seed Extract* (Mendocino, CA: LifeRhythm, 1997), 97-99. Available from: LifeRhythm, P.O. Box 806, Mendocino, CA 95460; tel: 707-937-1825.

57 Howard F. Loomis, Jr., D.C. "Indigestion: Why HCl, Antacids, and Pancreatin Are Not the Answer." *American Chiropractor* (April 1988), 82-87. Howard F. Loomis, Jr., D.C. *The Nutritional Value and Clinical Application of Food Enzymes* (Madison, WI: Howard Loomis, EFI–Enzyme Formulations, 1986).

58 *Physicians' Desk Reference* (Montvale, NJ: Medical Economics, 1994), 2404. William Campbell Douglass, M.D. "Cortisone Use Can Be Fatal." *Second Opinion* 6:1 (January 1996), 1.

59 *Physicians' Desk Reference* (Montvale, NJ: Medical Economics, 1994), 1866.

60 Morton Walker, DPM. "Soil-Based Organisms Support Immune System Functions from the Ground Up." *Townsend Letter for Doctors & Patients* 169 (August/September 1997), 85-92.

61 Leslie N. Johnston, D.V.M. *Iron Overload = Hemochromatosis = Too Much Iron* (self-published monograph, 1993). Available from: Leslie N. Johnston, 4632 N. Peoria, Tulsa, OK 74055-6917; tel: 918-425-6209 or 918-272-3745.

62 Joe Rojas-Burke. "Common Genetic Defect Cause of Excess Iron." *The Register Guard* (September 1, 1997), C1.

63 Leslie N. Johnston, D.V.M. *Iron Overload = Hemochromatosis = Too Much Iron* (self-published monograph, 1993). Available from: Leslie N. Johnston, 4632 N. Peoria, Tulsa, OK 74055-6917; tel: 918-425-6209 or 918-272-3745.

64 Stephen E. Langer, M.D., with James F. Scheer. *Solved: The Riddle of Illness* (New Canaan, CT: Keats Publishing, 1995), 25.

65 Connie and Alan Higley. *Reference Guide for Essential Oils* (Olathe, KS: Abundant Health, 1998).

66 J.C. Breneman. "Elimination Diet as the Most Effective Gallbladder Diet." *Annals of Allergy* 26 (1968), 83.

67 R.N. Rao et al. "Dietary Management of Urinary Risk Factors in Renal Stone Formers." *British Journal of Urology* 54 (1982), 578-583.

68 R. Scott et al. "The Importance of Cadmium as a Factor in Calcified Upper Urinary Tract Stone Disease: A Prospective 7-Year Study." *British Journal of Urology* 54 (1982), 584.

69 C.F. Lim et al. "Influence of Nonesterified Fatty Acid and Lysolecithins on Thyroxine Binding to Thyroxine-Binding Globulin and Transthyretin." *Thyroid* 5:4 (1995), 319-324. Stephen E. Langer, M.D., with James F. Scheer. *Solved: The Riddle of Illness* (New Canaan, CT: Keats Publishing, 1995), 25. Richard G. Foulkes, M.D. "Celebration or Shame? Fifty Years of Fluoridation (1945-1995)." *Townsend Letter for Doctors & Patients* (November 1995), 52-63. John Yiamouyiannis. *Fluoride: The Aging Factor* (Delaware, OH: Health Action Press, 1983), 8, 87.

70 Tom Valentine. "If You Eat Soy, Watch Your Thyroid Function: New Study." *True Health* (Autumn 1997), 1-3. R.L. Divi et al. "Anti-Thyroid Isoflavones From Soybean: Isolation, Characterization, and

Mechanisms of Action." *Biochemical Pharmacology* 54:10 (1997), 1087-1096.

71 J.C. Prior. "Progesterone as a Bone-Trophic Hormone." *Endocrinology Review* 11:2 (1990), 386. J.C. Prior et al. "Osteoporosis: Prevention and Control." *New England Journal of Medicine* 327:9 (August 27, 1992), 620. J.C. Prior et al. "Reproduction for the Athletic Woman." *Sports Medicine* 14:3 (September 1992), 190. J.C. Prior et al. "The Prevention and Treatment of Osteoporosis." *New England Journal of Medicine* 328:1 (January 7, 1993), 65.

72 P. Ball et al. "Interactions Between Estrogens and Catechol Amines: Purification and Properties of a Catechol-O-methyl-transferase From Human Liver." *Research on Steroids* 5 (1973), 377-383.

73 P.W.F. Wilson et al. "Postmenopausal Estrogen Use, Cigarette Smoking, and Cardiovascular Morbidity in Women Over Fifty." *New England Journal of Medicine* 313 (1985), 1038.

74 D. Goldgaber et al. "Molecular Analysis of Alzheimer Disease Cloning of the Mouse Amyloid Beta Protein Gene." Paper presented at the 38th Annual Meeting of the American Society of Human Genetics, San Diego, California (October 7-10, 1987).

75 John R. Lee, M.D. *What Your Doctor May Not Tell You About Menopause* (New York: Warner Books, 1996). Raymond Peat, Ph.D. *From PMS to Menopause* (self-published). Available from: Raymond Peat, P.O. Box 5764, Eugene, OR 97405; website: www.efn.org/~raypeat. V.C. Musey et al. "Age-Related Changes in the Female Hormonal Environment During Reproductive Life." *American Journal of Obstetrics and Gynecology* 157:2 (1987), 312-317. J.C. Prior et al. "Osteoporosis—Prevention and Control." *New England Journal of Medicine* 327:9 (August 27, 1992), 620. J.C. Prior et al. "The Prevention and Treatment of Osteoporosis." *New England Journal of Medicine* 328:1 (January 7, 1993), 65.

76 Raymond Peat, Ph.D. "Recharging the System." *Ray Peat's Newsletter* (1998). Available from: Raymond Peat, P.O. Box 5764, Eugene, OR 97405; fax: 503-683-4279; website: www.efn.org/~raypeat. M.V. Riley et al. "The Roles of Bicarbonate and CO2 in Transendothelial Fluid Movement and Control of Corneal Thickness." *Investigative Ophthalmology and Visual Science* 36:1 (1995), 103-112.

77 Susan E. Brown, Ph.D. *Better Bones, Better Body* (New Canaan, CT: Keats Publishing, 1996), 125.

78 Howard F. Loomis, Jr., D.C. *The Nutritional Value and Clinical Application of Food Enzymes* (Madison, WI: Howard Loomis, EFI-Enzyme Formulations, 1986).

79 John R. Lee, M.D. *What Your Doctor May Not Tell You About Menopause* (New York: Warner Books, 1996).

80 C.F. Lim et al. "Influence of Nonesterified Fatty Acid

and Lysolecithins on Thyroxine Binding to Thyroxine-Binding Globulin and Transthyretin." *Thyroid* 5:4 (1995), 319-324. Stephen E. Langer, M.D., with James F. Scheer. *Solved: The Riddle of Illness* (New Canaan, CT: Keats Publishing, 1995).

81 Michael B. Schachter, M.D. *The Natural Way To a Healthy Prostate* (New Canaan, CT: Keats Publishing, 1995).

82 David Steinman. "Treating Prostate Troubles." *Natural Health* (November/December 1993), 56.

83 M. Yu and S. Ho. "Selective Increase in Type II Estrogen Binding Sites in the Prostates of Nobel Rats." *Cancer Research* 53 (1993), 523.

84 J.C. Carraro et al. "Comparison of Phytotherapy (Permixon) with Finasteride in the Treatment of Benign Prostatic Hyperplasia: A Randomized International Study of 1098 Patients." *Prostate* 29 (1996), 231-240. Donald Brown, N.D. "Saw Palmetto Extract—Efficacy Shown in Long-Term Study." *Quarterly Review of Natural Medicine* (Winter 1996), 253-255. Donald Brown, N.D. "Comparing Saw Palmetto Extract and Finasteride for BPH." *Quarterly Review of Natural Medicine* (Spring 1997), 13-14.

85 Michael B. Schachter, M.D. *The Natural Way to a Healthy Prostate* (New Canaan, CT: Keats Publishing, 1995).

86 K. Savolainen et al. "Phosphoinositide Second Messengers in Cholinergic Excitotoxicity." *Neurotoxicology* 15:3 (1994), 493-502.

87 W.C. Young. *Sex and Internal Secretions* (Baltimore, MD: Williams & Wilkins, 1961). Raymond Peat, Ph.D. *From PMS to Menopause: Female Hormones in Context* (self-published), 7. Available from: Raymond Peat, P.O. Box 5764, Eugene, OR 97405; website: www.efn.org/~raypeat.

88 H.V. Thomas et al. " A Prospective Study of Endogenous Serum Hormone Concentrations and Breast Cancer Risk in Premenopausal Women on the Island of Guernsey." *Journal of Steroid Biochemistry and Molecular Biology* 63:4-6 (November 1997), 175-188. B.V. Stadel. "Oral Contraceptives and Cardiovascular Disease." *New England Journal of Medicine* 305 (1981), 612. V. Beral. "Cardiovascular Disease Mortality Trends and Contraceptive Use in Young Women." *The Lancet* 2 (1976), 1047-1051. X.M. Xu and M.L. Thomas. "Estrogen Receptor-Mediated Direct Stimulation of Colon Cancer Cell Growth in Vitro." *Molecular and Cellular Endocrinology* 105:2 (1994), 197-201. B.T. Zhu et al. "Conversion of Estrone to 2- and 4-Hydroxyestrone by Hamster Kidney and Liver Microsomes: Implications for the Mechanism of Estrogen-Induced Carcinogenesis." *Endocrinology* 135:5 (1994), 1772-1779.

89 Raymond Peat, Ph.D. *From PMS to Menopause: Female Hormones in Context* (self-published), 155. Available from: Raymond Peat, P.O. Box 5764, Eugene, OR 97405; website: www.efn.org/~raypeat.

90 Raymond Peat, Ph.D. "Oils in Context." *Townsend Letter for Doctors* (December 1989), 5. H.H. Draper et al. "Metabolism of MDA." *Lipids* 21:4 (1986), 305-307. L.P. Belcheva et al. "Influence of Some Anticonvulsants on the Brain Lipid Peroxidation in Generalized Seizures." *Dokaldi Bolgarskoi Akademii Nauk, Comptes Rendus de l'Academia Bulgare des Sciences* 38:1 (1985), 141-143. L.P. Belcheva et al. "Influence of Some Convulsants and Anticonvulsants on the Brain Lipid Peroxidation in vitro." *Dokaldi Bolgarskoi Akademii Nauk, Comptes Rendus de l'Academia Bulgare des Sciences* 38:2 (1985), 255-257.

91 H.J. Roberts. *Aspartame (NutraSweet): Is It Safe?* (Philadelphia: Charles Press Publishers, 1990), 82.

92 J.W. Olney and O.L. Ho. "Brain Damage in Infant Mice Following Oral Intake of Glutamate, Aspartame or Cysteine." *Nature* 227 (1970), 609-611.

93 H.J. Roberts. *Aspartame (NutraSweet): Is It Safe?* (Philadelphia: Charles Press Publishers, 1990). H.J. Roberts. *Sweet'ner Dearest: Bittersweet Vignettes About Aspartame (NutraSweet)* (West Palm Beach, FL: Sunshine Sentinel Press, 1992).

94 H.J. Roberts. *Aspartame (NutraSweet): Is It Safe?* (Philadelphia: Charles Press Publishers, 1990).

95 H.J. Roberts. *Sweet'ner Dearest: Bittersweet Vignettes About Aspartame (NutraSweet)* (West Palm Beach, FL: Sunshine Sentinel Press, 1992).

96 John Yiamouyiannis. *Fluoride: The Aging Factor* (Delaware, OH: Health Action Press, 1983), 9. John Yiamouyiannis. "Fluoride." *Mothering* (Winter 1989).

97 John Yiamouyiannis. *Fluoride: The Aging Factor* (Delaware, OH: Health Action Press, 1983), 3-4, 7, 26.

98 J.M. Faccini. "Fluoride-Induced Hyperplasia of the Parathyroid Glands." *Proceedings of the Royal Society of Medicine* 62 (1969), 241. L. Spira. "Fluorosis and the Parathyroid Glands." *Journal of Hygiene* 42 (1942), 500-504. S.P.S. Teotia and M. Teotia. "Hyperactivity of the Parathyroid Glands in Endemic Osteofluorosis." *Fluoride* 5 (1972), 115-125.

99 Robert S. Mendelsohn, M.D. *How to Raise a Healthy Child...In Spite of Your Doctor* (Chicago: Contemporary Books, 1984), 76.

100 Alexander G. Schauss, Ph.D. *Minerals, Trace Elements and Human Health* (Tacoma, WA: Life Sciences Press, 1996), 8.

101 E.C. Ditkoff et al. "The Impact of Estrogen on Adrenal Androgen Sensitivity and Secretion in Polycystic Ovary Syndrome." *Journal of Clinical Endocrinology and Metabolism* 80:2 (1995), 603-607. A. Dunaif et al., eds. *The Polycystic Ovary Syndrome* (Cambridge, MA: Blackwell Scientific, 1992).

102 C.F. Lim et al. "Influence of Nonesterified Fatty Acid and Lysolecithins on Thyroxine Binding to Thyroxine-Binding Globulin and Transthyretin." *Thyroid* 5:4 (1995), 319-324. Stephen E. Langer, M.D., with James F. Scheer. *Solved: The Riddle of Illness* (New Canaan, CT: Keats Publishing, 1995), 25. Richard G. Foulkes, M.D. "Celebration or Shame? Fifty Years of Fluoridation (1945-1995)." *Townsend Letter for Doctors & Patients* (November 1995), 52-63. John Yiamouyiannis. *Fluoride: The Aging Factor* (Delaware, OH: Health Action Press, 1983), 8, 87.

103 Tom Valentine. "If You Eat Soy, Watch Your Thyroid Function: New Study." *True Health* (Autumn 1997), 1-3. R.L. Divi et al. "Anti-Thyroid Isoflavones from Soybean: Isolation, Characterization, and Mechanisms of Action." *Biochemical Pharmacology* 54:10 (November 15, 1997), 1087-1096.

104 Raymond Peat, Ph.D. *Nutrition for Women* (self-published, 1993). Available from: Raymond Peat, P.O. Box 5764, Eugene, OR 97405; website: www.efn.org/~raypeat.

105 Richard G. Foulkes, M.D. "Celebration or Shame? Fifty Years of Fluoridation (1945-1995)." *Townsend Letter for Doctors & Patients* (November 1995), 52-63. John Yiamouyiannis. *Fluoride: The Aging Factor* (Delaware, OH: Health Action Press, 1983), 8, 87. Burton Goldberg and the Editors of Alternative Medicine Digest. *Chronic Fatigue, Fibromyalgia, and Environmental Illness* (Tiburon, CA: Future Medicine Publishing, 1998), 198-199.

106 Anthony di Fabio. "A Surprising Psoriasis Treatment." *Townsend Letter for Doctors* 6 (June 1990), 351-358.

107 Ibid.

108 Robert B. Francis, ed. *Atherosclerotic Cardiovascular Disease, Hemostasis and Endothelian Function* (New York: Marcel Dekker, 1992), 183. K.S. McCully. "Atherosclerosis, Serum Cholesterol and the Homocysteine Theory: A Study of 194 Consecutive Autopsies." *American Journal of Medical Science* 299 (1990), 217-221. K.S. McCully. "Homocysteine Theory: Development & Current Status." *Atherosclerosis Reviews* 11 (1983), 157-245.

109 A. di Fabio. "A Surprising Psoriasis Treatment." *Townsend Letter for Doctors* 6 (June, 1990), 351-358.

110 John Pagano. *Healing Psoriasis* (Englewood Cliffs, NJ: Pagano Organization, 1991).

111 Ibid.

112 David Hoffmann. *The New Holistic Herbal* (Rockport, MA: Element, 1993).

113 A. di Fabio. "A Surprising Psoriasis Treatment." *Townsend Letter for Doctors* 6 (June, 1990), 351-358.

114 W. Wayt Gibbs. "Gaining on Fat." *Scientific American* (August 1996), 88.

115 Howard Loomis, D.C. *Enzyme Replacement Therapy* (Madison, WI: 21st Century Nutrition).

116 From the records of Rina Davis, C.N., of Portland, Oregon. Her work has been reported in: Pete Billac. *Lose Fat While You Sleep: No Dieting, No Drug, No Exercise* (Alvin, TX: Swan Publishing, 1998); and Robert E. DeMaria, D.C. *Clinical Observations in the Utilization of CALORAD* (Amherst, OH: Creativity Unlimited, 1997).

Appendix A
Hormonal Balancing

1 C.F. Lim et al. "Influence of Nonesterified Fatty Acid and Lysolecithins on Thyroxine Binding to Thyroxine-Binding Globulin and Transthyretin." *Thyroid* 5:4 (1995), 319-324. Stephen E. Langer, M.D., with James F. Scheer. *Solved: The Riddle of Illness* (New Canaan, CT: Keats Publishing, 1995).

2 Richard G. Foulkes, M.D. "Celebration or Shame? *Fifty Years of Fluoridation* (1945-1995)." *Townsend Letter for Doctors & Patients* (November 1995), 52-63. John Yiamouyiannis. *Fluoride: The Aging Factor* (Delaware, OH: Health Action Press, 1983), 8, 87.

3 Burton Goldberg and the Editors of Alternative Medicine Digest. *Chronic Fatigue, Fibromyalgia, and Environmental Illness* (Tiburon, CA: Future Medicine Publishing, 1998), 198-199.

4 Tom Valentine. "If You Eat Soy, Watch Your Thyroid Function: New Study." *True Health* (Autumn 1997), 1-3. R.L. Divi et al. "Anti-Thyroid Isoflavones From Soybean: Isolation, Characterization, and Mechanisms of Action." *Biochemical Pharmacology* 54:10 (November 15, 1997), 1087-1096. Stephen E. Langer, M.D., with James F. Scheer. *Solved: The Riddle of Illness* (New Canaan, CT: Keats Publishing, 1995).

5 P. Coulombe et al. "Catecholamine Metabolism in Thyroid Disease. II. Norepinephrine Secretion Rate in Hyperthyroidism and Hypothyroidism." *Journal of Clinical Endocrinology and Metabolism* 44:6 (June 1977), 1185-1189. J. Vavrejnova. "Increased Levels of Noradrenaline in Hypothyroidism and Its Association with Cardiovascular System Function." *J Endokrinologicky Ustav, Praha* 38:12 (December 1938), 1195-1200.

6 Broda Barnes, M.D., and L. Galton. *Hypothyroidism: The Unsuspected Illness* (New York: Harper & Row, 1976).

7 Raymond Peat, Ph.D. "The Edema of Stress." *Blake College Newsletter* 1:3.

8 Alan R. Gaby, M.D. "Thyroid Hormone and Attention Deficit-Hyperactivity Disorder." *Townsend Newsletter for Doctors* (April 1994), 280.

9 Broda, Barnes, M.D., and L. Galton. *Hypothyroidism: The Unsuspected Illness* (New York: Harper & Row, 1976). Stephen E. Langer, M.D., with James F. Scheer. *Solved: The Riddle of Illness* (New Canaan, CT: Keats Publishing, 1995).

10 Raymond Peat, Ph.D. *Nutrition for Women* (self-published, 1993), 51-52. Available from: Raymond Peat, P.O. Box 5764, Eugene, OR 97405; fax: 503-683-4279; website: www.efn.org/~raypeat.

11 Raymond Peat, Ph.D. *Generative Energy* (self-published), 110. Available from: Raymond Peat, P.O. Box 5764, Eugene, OR 97405; fax: 503-683-4279; website: www.efn.org/~raypeat.

12 M. Kalimi and W. Regelson. *The Biological Role of Dehydroepiandrosterone* (Berlin, NY: Walter de Gruyter, 1990). T.H. McGavack, M.D., et al. "The Use of Pregnenolone in Various Clinical Disorders." *Journal of Clinical Endocrinology* 11:6 (June 1951), 559. Raymond Peat, Ph.D. "Steroids." *Blake College Newsletter* 1:4. Raymond Peat, Ph.D. "Solving Some of the Problems of Aging." *Townsend Letter for Doctors* (January 1991), 60. Raymond Peat, Ph.D. "The Progesterone Deception." *Townsend Letter for Doctors* (November 1987), 416. Raymond Peat, Ph.D. *From PMS to Menopause: Hormones in Context* (self-published). Available from: Raymond Peat, P.O. Box 5764, Eugene, OR 97405; fax: 503-683-4279; website: www.efn.org/~raypeat.

13 Cathy Perlmutter, with Maureen Sangiorgio. "Beyond Estrogen, the Miracle Pill for Women Over 35." *Prevention* (February 1993), 76.

14 Compiled from Dr. Raymond Peat's books, articles, and newsletters. Available from: Raymond Peat, P.O. Box 5764, Eugene, OR 97405; fax: 503-683-4279; website: www.efn.org/~raypeat.

15 John Lee, M.D. *What Your Doctor May Not Tell You About Menopause* (New York: Warner Books, 1996). Tori Hudson, N.D. "Wild Yam, Natural Progesterone, Unraveling the Confusion." *Townsend Letter for Doctors and Patients* (July 1996), 125-127.

16 Warren Froelich. "Miracle Drug From Mexican Yam?" *San Diego Union* (February 12, 1989).

17 E. Barrett-Connor et al. "A Prospective Study of Dehydroepiandrosterone Sulfate, Mortality, and Cardiovascular Disease." *New England Journal of Medicine* 315:24 (December 11, 1986), 1519-1524.

Index

Abcesses, 23
Abscisic acid, 92
Accutane, 224
Acidity. *See* pH
Acne, 217–24
ADD. *See* attention deficit disorder
Addison's disease, 255
Adrenal glands
  in hypothyroidism, 243, 247, 252–53, 254
  normalizing, 255–56
Adrenaline
  cardiovascular disease and, 101
  in hyperactivity, 115
  in hypothyroidism, 105, 246, 247, 248, 252
  surges, 176, 181
Adrenaline mimics, 80, 104
Aeron LifeCycles, 258
Aflatoxin, 51
Age pigment, 101
Aging, 75
Agribusiness, 46, 48, 49, 123
AIDS, 22, 89
Alkalinity. See pH
Allergens, 41
Allergies, 65–70
  acne from, 218
  enzyme depletion by, 49, 65–66
  food, 17, 25, 224
  headaches and, 152–53
  incontinence and, 112
  overweight and, 234–35
Alternative medicine, 9, 12, 13
Alzheimer's disease, 181
Amaranth, 48
American Dental Association, 60, 152
Amino acids, 20, 21, 81, 162
  excitatory, 208, 209–10
  imbalance, 233
Amylase, 17, 19, 20, 22–23, 164
Anaphylactic shock, 65
Anemia, 112
Angina pectoris, 97
ANS. *See* autonomic nervous system
Antacids, 137
Anti-aging hormones, 54, 101, 242, 247, 255–61

Antibiotics, 25
  for acne, 219
  allergies to, 66, 67
  repeated use, 94
  resistance to, 60
Antifungals, 94
Antigens, 218
Antihistamines, 22, 68, 70
Antimicrobials, 73, 74, 148. *See also*
  Citricidal
Antioxidants, 16, 110, 164, 226
Antiseptics, 53, 148
Anxiety, 21, 159, 256
  insomnia and, 166
  metabolic dysfunctions and, 183
Appendicitis, 71–74, 139, 140
Appendix, 71, 72
Arachidonic acid, 226–27
Arginine, 162
Aromatherapy
  for asthma, 86
  for cancer, 93
  for diabetes, 126
  for injuries, 165
  for intestinal disorders, 148
Arrhythmia, 97
Arteries, thickening of, 98
Arteriosclerosis, 97
Arthritis, 75–79, 165, 225
Ascorbic acid, 42
Aspartame, 165, 208, 209–10, 215, 250
Aspartate, 250
Asthma, 22, 80–86
  allergies and, 65
  drugs, 80, 104
Atherosclerosis, 97, 98, 102, 103
Atlas headache, 149
Attention deficit disorder (ADD), 25, 115–17, 248
Autoimmune disorders, 75
Autonomic nervous system (ANS), 111, 269
Ayurveda, 83

Bacteria
  bowel, 147
  friendly. *See* probiotics; *see also* soil-

diet and, 25-27
  inhibition of, 52
Digestive leukocytosis, 55
Disaccharidase deficiency, 24, 156, 182
Disaccharidases, 17, 19, 23-25
Disaccharides, 17, 19, 22
Disc problems, 165
Disease mimics, 60. *See also* illness
Diverticulitis, 139
DNA (deoxyribonucleic acid), 47, 57
Drugs, 66
  antiepileptic, 210, 211, 214-15
  asthma, 80, 104
  cholesterol-lowering, 104, 130-31
  damage from, 12
  effect on body temperature, 32
  prescription, 39, 130
  psychiatric, 183, 185
  for sleep, 166
  steroids, 94
  synthetic, 12, 103
Dunphy, Daniel, 125
Duodenum, 17, 129

Eating, 234, 237, 238. *See also* diet; foods
Eczema, 227
Edema, 21, 206, 242, 247-48
Eggs, 27
Electrolytes, 39, 41
Electromagnetic fields (EMFs), 56-57, 102
EMFs. *See* electromagnetic fields
Emotional problems, 24-25, 150, 152, 157.
  See also anxiety; mental disorders; stress
Emotional stress, 82, 83, 112, 132
Emotions, 218, 248
  asthma and, 82, 83
Endocrine glands, 78, 251
Endometriosis, 251
Endozepines, 256
Environmental estrogens, 87, 180, 191, 243,
  245, 260
Environmental illness, 25
Environmental Protection Agency (EPA), 48
Environmental toxins, 41, 59, 66
Enzyme deficiencies, 25, 28, 55
  allergies and, 65
  cholesterol and, 99
  development of, 69
  diagnosing, 28-44, 64, 69
  PMS and, 200
  symptoms, 28
Enzyme depletion, 46, 47

Enzyme inhibitors, 26, 27, 55. *See also* thyroid inhibitors
Enzyme profile (questionnaire), 30, 38
Enzyme supplementation, 30, 64. *See also* enzyme therapy
Enzyme therapists, 28, 43, 64, 274-75
Enzyme therapy, 12, 68-69. *See also* enzyme supplementation; nutritional supplementation
  for acne, 222-23
  for allergies, 69-70
  for appendicitis, 73
  for arthritis, 78
  for asthma, 84-85
  for cancer, 89-90
  for candidiasis, 95
  for cardiovascular disease, 108-9
  choosing, 44
  for diabetes, 122
  for gallbladder disorders, 133-34
  for headaches, 156-57
  for herpes, 161-62
  for hypothyroidism, 251
  for incontinence, 113
  for injuries, 164-65
  for insomnia, 167, 168-69
  for intestinal problems, 145
  for kidney stones, 174
  for menopausal symptoms, 179
  for mental disorders, 188
  for osteoporosis, 195-96
  for overweight, 237-38
  for parasitic infections, 199
  with plant enzymes, 19, 27
  for PMS, 203
  practitioners, 274-75
  products for, 64, 276
  for prostate enlargement, 207
  for psoriasis, 229
  for seizures, 215-16
  Thera-zyme formulas, 43, 64, 262-73
Enzymes, 16, 64. *See also* digestive enzymes; metabolic enzymes; pancreatic enzymes; plant (food) enzymes
  categories, 16-17
  deactivating, 17
  destroying, 17, 47, 50, 66. *See also* cooking
  ratios, 27
EPA. *See* Environmental Protection Agency
Epstein-Barr virus (EBV), 158
ERT. *See* estrogen replacement therapy
Essential fatty acids, 51, 123, 131, 209, 245

arthritis and, 76-77
on asthma, 81
on gallbladder flushes, 133
on neck problems, 212
palpation test, 44
on stomach acid, 137
on structural problems, 149, 150,
153-54, 212
Low-density lipoprotein (LDL) cholesterol,
244, 257
LPL. See lipoprotein lipase
Lupron, 127
Lymphatic system, 41, 42, 49, 65
Lysine, 162

Magnesium, 99, 171, 174, 211, 253, 254
Magnetism, 56-57, 102
Mallouh, Camille, 204
Maltase, 182
Maltose, 18, 24, 28, 81
Manganese, 124, 211
McCully, Kilmer S., 102
Meat, 27, 56, 124. See also diet; foods
Medications. See drugs
Memory enhancers, 244, 255
Men
environmental estrogens and, 243
progesterone use by, 223
Mendelsohn, Robert, 211
Menopausal symptoms, 75, 127, 175-81
Menopause, 175, 251
Menstrual cycle, 201, 243
Mental disorders, 24-25, 182-89. See also
emotional problems
Mercury, 60, 245
Metabolic enzymes, 16, 47, 52, 66
Metabolism, 129
calcium, 159, 170, 179, 191-93
psoriasis and, 225-26
thyroid and, 242, 246
Metals, heavy, 58-59, 171, 181, 250
Microorganisms, 46. See also bacteria;
parasites; soil-based organisms
Microwaving, 30, 46, 55, 56. See also cook-
ing; radiation
Migraines, 153-54
Milk. See dairy products
Minerals, 30, 99, 254
deficiencies, 68-69
sources, 110, 216
Miscarriage, 251
Miso, 91-92

Mitochondria, 104, 255
Mitral valve prolapse, 250
Mononucleosis, 158
Monosaccharides, 22
Monounsaturated fatty acids, 52
Mouth, 16, 17, 20, 159
MS. See multiple sclerosis
Mucous membranes, 137, 138-39
Multiple sclerosis (MS), 250
Murray, Michael T., 125
Myocardial infarction, 97

Nasal specifics, 157
Naturopathic remedies (for gallstones), 135
Nausea, 140
Neck problems, 212
Nerves, 250
Nervous system, 42
Neuralgia, 25
Neurotoxins, 25
Neurotransmitters, 188, 271
Nitrite, 41
NutraSweet. See aspartame, see also sugars;
sweeteners
Nutrients, 19
absorption, 18, 68
destruction, 46, 47, 51
dietary sources, 124, 223
fat-soluble, 23
in urine, 39-43
Nutritional deficiencies, 131-32
cholesterol and, 99
herpes and, 159
kidney stones and, 171
seizures and, 211
symptoms questionnaire, 30, 36-37
urinalysis for, 31, 39-43
Nutritional supplementation, 193
absorption/assimilation of, 18-19, 262
anti-gallstones, 135
for cardiovascular support, 110
diet and, 99-100, 133, 171
enzyme support of, 18-19, 68
enzymes, 27. See also enzyme therapy
for parasitic infections, 199-200
for seizures, 216
for weight loss, 238-39
Nuts, 26, 27, 55

Oils, 23, 51-52. See also fats
gallbladder contraction and, 133
hydrogenated, 52, 99

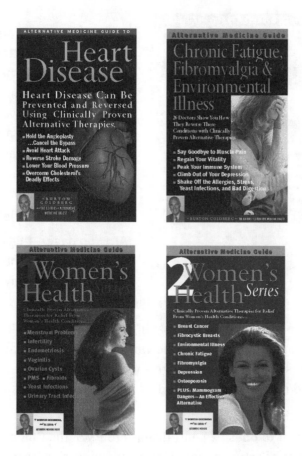

These titles are part of our *Alternative Medicine Guide* paperback series—healing-edge advice that may mean the difference between sickness and robust health. We distill the advice of hundreds of leading alternative physicians from all disciplines and put it into a consumer-helpful format—medical knowledge without the jargon. Essential reading before—or instead of—your next doctor's visit. Because you need to know your medical alternatives.

TO ORDER, CALL 800-333-HEAL

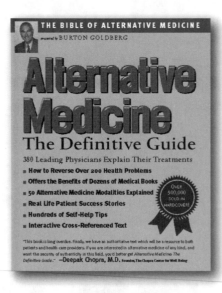

Millions of people are searching for a better way to health—this is the book they're reaching for. *Alternative Medicine: The Definitive Guide* is an absolute must for anyone interested in the latest information on how to get healthy and stay that way.

At 1,100 pages, this encyclopedia puts all the schools of alternative medicine—50 different therapies—under one roof.

The *Guide* is packed with lifesaving information and alternative treatments from 380 of the world's leading alternative physicians. Our contributors give you the safest, most affordable, and most effective remedies for over 200 serious health conditions.

From cancer to obesity, heart disease to PMS. the Guide gives you dozens of actual patient stories and physician treatments to show you how this medicine really works.

The Guide does something no other health book has ever done. It combines the best clinical information from doctors with the most practical self-help remedies all in a format that is easy-to-read, practical, and completely user-friendly.

The Guide gives you the knowledge you need today so you can make intelligent choices about the future of your health.

TO ORDER, CALL 800-333-HEAL

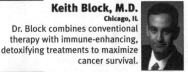

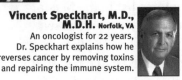
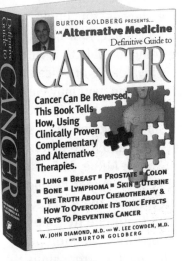

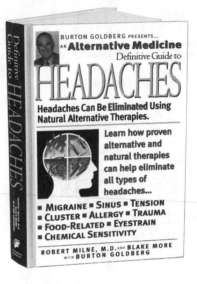

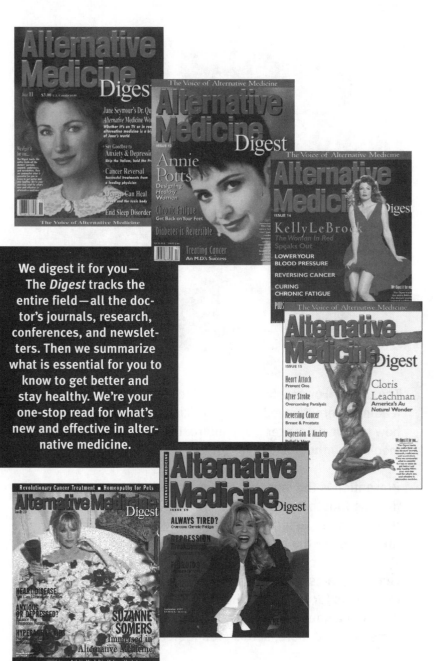

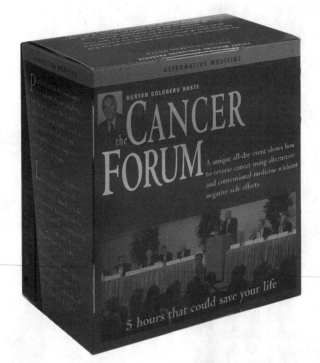

The Cancer Forum—five hours of lifesaving information from leading alternative medicine physicians who show you how to reverse cancer using alternative and conventional medicine without negative side effects.

Prevention is the most important and reliable cancer-fighting tool that exists today. The fact that cancer can be treated and reversed and that it can be detected early and prevented are the most significant messages of this forum.

Learn the latest proven, safe, nontoxic, and successful treatments for reversing cancer, including herbs, nutrition and diet, supplements, enzymes, glandular extracts, homeopathic remedies, and more, in this groundbreaking video.

TO ORDER, CALL 800-333-HEAL